THE POLITICS OF HEALTH IN INDIA

COMPARATIVE STUDIES OF HEALTH SYSTEMS
AND MEDICAL CARE

General Editor
John M. Janzen

Founding Editor
Charles Leslie

Editorial Board

For a list of titles in the series
Comparative Studies of Health Systems and
Medical Care, see back of book.

THE POLITICS OF HEALTH IN INDIA

ROGER JEFFERY

University of California Press

BERKELEY • LOS ANGELES • LONDON

University of California Press
Berkeley and Los Angeles, California

University of California Press, Ltd.
London, England

Copyright © 1988 by The Regents of the University of California

Library of Congress Cataloging-in-Publication Data

Jeffery, Roger.
The politics of health in India.

(Comparative studies of health systems and medical care)
Bibliography: p.
1. Medical care—India—History.   2. Public
health—India—History.   3. Medical policy—
India—History.   I. Title.   II. Series.
RA395.I5J44   1988   362.1'0954   87–10869
ISBN 0–520–05938–7 (alk. paper)

Printed in the United States of America

1 2 3 4 5 6 7 8 9

Contents

Acknowledgments

I have been very dependent on the help of many people, including many librarians, for whose assistance I am very grateful. In particular I would mention Margaret Dowling and the Inter-Library Loan staff in Edinburgh University for their help in searching for books and articles from almost inaccessible sources. I am also grateful to the Social Science (now the Economic and Social) Research Council in London which funded my research in India in 1975–1976 and in 1982–1983; to the Overseas Development Agency for allowing me to use some material collected while I was a consultant; to the British Council, whose scholarship took me to India in 1973–1974; and to my colleagues in Edinburgh University for travel funds on several occasions and for permission to take leaves of absence for my research trips to India. None of these bears any responsibility for the views expressed here. My debt to Patricia Jeffery is enormous; without her stimulus I would probably never have completed this work.

R. J.

University of Edinburgh

Chronology

DATE	General History	Public Health History
1802–1804	Defeats of Marathas and of Scindia	Famine in Bombay, Madras & North India
1807		Madras famine
1812–1814	Charter of East India Company renewed.	Madras and Bombay famine
1822		Founding of Native Medical Institution, Calcutta.
1823		Madras famine
1824–1826	First Burmese War	
1832–1833	Abolition of Thuggee and Sati	Famine in Guntur area, Madras
1835		Closure of Native Medical Institution
		Founding of Calcutta Medical College
1837–1838	Afghan campaign begins	Famine in Northern India
1849	Annexation of Punjab	
1856	Annexation of Oudh	
1857	Mutiny/Sepoy Revolt	Creation of Indian Universities
1858	End of Company Rule	
1860		Famine in North-West, Punjab
1862–1863		Royal Commission on Sanitary Conditions of the Army in India
1866		Orissa famine
1873–1874		Bihar and Bengal famine
1876–1878		Madras famine
1882	Local Self-Government Act	
1896		Plague returns to Bombay
1896–1898		Northern India famine
1899–1900		Central India famine
1906	Partition of Bengal	
1907–1909	Morley-Minto Reforms	
1919	Montagu-Chelmsford Reforms and Government of India Act	

1919–1920		Influenza epidemic
1935		Government of India Act
1938		National Planning Committee
1942	Quit India Movement	
1943		Bengal famine
1943–1946		Bhore Committee
1947	Independence	Partition and mass migrations
1950		Planning Commission established
1951–1956		First-Plan Period
1953–1958		National Malaria Control Program
1956–1961		Second-Plan Period
1958–1970		National Malaria Eradication Program
1961–1966		Third-Plan Period
1962	War with China	
1965	War with Pakistan	
1966–1969		Annual Plans Period
1969–1974		Fourth-Plan Period
1974–1979		Fifth-Plan Period
1975–1977	''Emergency''	
1977	Janata wins elections	Community Health Workers scheme introduced
1980	Mrs. Gandhi wins elections	
1979–1980		Annual Plan only
1980–1985		Sixth-Plan Period

Abbreviations

AAS	Association for Asian Studies
ADB	Asian Development Bank
ANM	Auxiliary nurse-midwife; since 1977, health worker (female)
BAR	Bengal Administration Report
BHU	Benares Hindu University
BMA	British Medical Association
BMPS	Bombay Medical and Physical Society
CAHP	Coordinating Agency for Health Planning
CBHI	Central Bureau of Health Intelligence
CCH	Central Council of Health
CDR	Crude death rate
CHS	Central Health Services
CHV	Community health volunteer; previously, community health worker; since 1981, often referred to as village health guide
CFPC	Central Family Planning Council
CHEB	Central Health Education Bureau
CMH	Central Ministry of Health
CPHB	Central Provincial Health Board
CSIR	Council for Scientific and Industrial Research
DGHS	Director-general of health services
EPI	Expanded Program on Immunization
ESIC	Employees State Insurance Corporation; also, ESI, ESIS (scheme)
FWD	Family Welfare Department
GMC	General Medical Council
GOI	Government of India
GOO	Government of Orissa
IAMR	Institute of Medical Research
IAMS	Indian Academy of Medical Sciences
ICDS	Integrated Child Development Scheme

ICSSR   Indian Council of Social Science Research
IIM   Indian Institute of Management
IMA   Indian Medical Association
IMC   Indian Medical Council
IMR   Infant mortality rate
IMS   Indian Medical Service
IOL   India Office Library and Records, London
ISC   Indian Statutory Council
JIMA   Journal of the Indian Medical Association
LHV   Lady health visitor; since 1977, health assistant
          (female)
MCI   Medical Council of India
MP   Madhya Pradesh; also, member of parliament
NAI   National Archives of India
NIHFW   National Institute of Health and Family Welfare;
          earlier, National Institute of Health Administration
          and Education (NIHAE) and National Institute of
          Family Planning, combined.
NMI   National Medical Institution
NPC   National Planning Committee
NSS   National Sample Survey
ODA   Overseas Development Administration
ODM   Overseas Development Ministry
OUP   Oxford University Press
PHC   Primary Health Center
PL   Public law
PMPAI   Private Medical Practitioners Association of India
RAMC   Royal Army Medical Corps
Rs, Re   Rupees, Rupee
RUHSA   Rural Unit for Health and Social Affairs
SPM   Social and Preventive Medicine
SRS   Sample Registration Scheme
UNCTC   United Nations Center for Transnational Corporations
UNIDO   United Nations Industrial Development Organization
UP   Uttar Pradesh; United Provinces (United Provinces
          formerly included North-West Provinces and Oudh)
USAID   United States Agency for International Development
WMA   World Medical Association

Introduction

The health services of India affect the lives of some 700 million people in one of the world's poorest countries. This alone would make it a worthy subject for study, but surprisingly there are no good accounts of the Indian health system in the literature on comparative health systems or on health systems of individual countries or regions. A comparison with China is instructive. Far less is known about health-care provision and development in China than in India. This has stimulated almost every visitor to write at least an article describing what they saw, if not a book surveying what is known and placing it into perspective for a wider audience (e.g., Bowers [ed.] 1973; Quinn [ed.] 1972; Sidel 1972). There are also several more analytic accounts, of which those by Lampton (1977, 1978) are the most detailed (see also Hillier and Jewell 1983; Lucas 1982). Of course, China is seen as a success story potentially relevant for the rest of the world, whereas India is regarded as a failure. Thus, in the appendixes to the WHO (World Health Organization) and UNICEF (United Nations Children's Fund) books outlining alternative approaches to meeting health-care needs, the Chinese system as a whole merits a case study, whereas the Indian examples are of a small voluntary-sector project in Maharashtra (Jamkhed) and of Ayurvedic medicine (Newell [ed.] 1975; Djukanovic and Mach 1975). Similarly, a recent collection on comparative health systems includes China as its one example from outside the developed capitalist world (Raffel 1984).

Furthermore several of the existing accounts of India are severely flawed: Jaggi's multivolume history of medicine in India is little more than a compilation of reports (1979–1980). On the other hand, Elling's short discussion of India (1979) is so concerned with the context that very little emerges about the health services themselves.

Most accounts of health and health services in India fall into one of two categories; either descriptive/uncritical accounts, essentially

1

within the modernization tradition, seeing health services moving toward a western model through technological transfer and culture contact (e.g. Dutt et al. 1963); or radical/Marxist critiques, in which health services are regarded as warped and rendered irrelevant (if not positively harmful) by the imperialistic dependency relationships within which technologies are transferred and indigenous elites retain power (e.g. Banerji 1984; Zurbrigg 1984).

The former approach when applied to India is insufficiently critical, while the latter approach too sweepingly ignores variations among countries, is too deterministic in simple economic ways, and is incapable of theorizing change. In these pages, then, my first concern is to provide evidence about changes in health services in India, and my second, to analyze the significance and causes of these patterns. My goal is to avoid the two extremes described above—that is, neither to exclude a political economy of health-care services nor to make it the sole element in the account. Of course, evidence is not free from theoretical presuppositions. Several decisions have guided the material I have searched out and how I have presented it. In the rest of this introduction I shall spell out some of these theoretical concerns.

My first priority was to understand the patterns of health provision and their developments since 1947, but this requires a picture of their position when the British left. Several critics have blamed the imperial legacy for postindependence weaknesses. Health services in India today are conditioned in important ways by the legacy of health services established under British rule. "Incrementalism" is a major feature of change even in "revolutionary" contexts, as the accounts of medical policy in postliberation China make clear (Lampton 1977; Lucas 1982). Even workers near the bottom of a hierarchy have interests in restricting changes which might cost them their jobs or cause their jobs to be radically redefined or require their own retraining and create uncertainty. Those workers near the top are likely to have scarce skills (socially defined), enabling them to limit proposals that might reduce or change their positions. In order to set the background and context for health policy in independent India, Part I sketches, all too briefly, the development of health policy under the British—explored in much greater detail by others (Arnold 1985; Ramasubban 1982; Hume 1985). The starting point for the historical discussion is set largely by my interest in health-policy making; few sources and little evidence of such policy concerns exist prior to 1800. However, this starting point could be too generous to imperialism, effectively ignoring the period of conquest and rapacious plunder. I will return to this point in Chapter 4.

I have used recent discussions on the nature of the state in developing societies to provide a framework for the material I am considering and have usually bracketed off the issue of whether or not health services lead to better health. Thus I assume that health changes as a result of wider social changes and not only through systematic attempts to heal or cure or protect people from illness and disease. Indeed, those attempts may make matters worse. But health policy is worth investigating in itself, without trying too hard to decide what effects it has on health. Other decisions will become clearer as the material unfolds, but these two require some discussion here.

Discussions of the nature of the state in India fall into two general categories. In the pluralist view power is exercised through alliances forged by groups on the basis of a number of common and competing characteristics—caste, language, religion, and education, for example, all providing bases for common action as well as (and often overriding) narrow economic interests. But in addition, state bureaucracies are often seen as central to an understanding of the chances of any policy being implemented—as in the accounts which came from Ralph Braibanti and his associates in the early 1960s (Braibanti 1961). These two strands are often poorly integrated. For those who focus on the state the issues are the quality of recruitment policies, structure of control, or the quality of bureaucratic procedures, as if the bureaucracy were divorced from the everyday political world and just "holds the ring." Failure to maintain this divorce is then castigated by calling the result corruption without posing questions about the interests of the bureaucrats or the social groups favored by these "corrupt" practices.

The major alternative view of the state in modern India is derived from debates within Marxism on the character of capitalist states. Problems are posed for Marxism by the different kinds of capitalist states and the uncertain tendencies of these states toward fascism or not, or toward the conditions necessary for socialist transformations. As Urry (1980) has recently argued, much of the discussion of the state by Marxists tends to deal with the state solely in terms of the class dominance of the bourgeoisie—in Marx's own phrase, the state as the executive committee for managing its common affairs. The difficulties with this reductionist position are enormous: politics and ideology are not determined in a close way by the demands of capital, social institutions (such as health services) vary quite dramatically among different capitalist states, and the "needs of capital" are rarely unambiguous, self-evident, or followed with relentless logic.

Althusser and others responded to this kind of problem by suggesting that political and ideological "instances" (levels) have varying degrees of autonomy from the economic base; an alternative response, such as that of E. P. Thompson (1979), is to return to class struggle and the conscious aims of historical actors as the central elements in an account. However, developments in social policy cannot be explained solely by referring to the twin concepts of capital's needs and labor's demands (Harris 1980). These formulations may seem plausible, but they do not indicate well why welfare provisions developed when they did, at different times and in different ways in different countries, and in the state rather than in the private sector in some countries but not in others (ibid.).

Marxists and others now are pointing also to the similarities between these discussions and those within orthodox sociology, concerned with relationships between structure and action. Some authors have even described two sociologies, one of functions and systems and one of processes (Dawe 1970). Urry argues that Marxist accounts are similarly polarized. Marxist functionalists are concerned with the state in terms of its functions for capitalism, while Marxist humanists focus on class struggles, without looking at the effects of these struggles (Urry 1980:5; Harris 1980:245).

Earlier Marxist discussions of the state in India drew on these traditions, presuming that the state reflects or is an instrument of dominant classes. Debate (as, for example, between the various Marxist parties in India) focused on which classes are aligned together and whether to collaborate with the so-called national bourgeoisie, seen as particularly powerful in the Congress party (Kurien [ed.] 1975; Hawthorn 1983). However, more recent Marxist discussion of the Third World state looks to the work of Alavi (1972), who argues that the state in postcolonial societies is overdeveloped because it inherited bureaucratic and military institutions resulting from the colonialists' concern to maintain order and control. Alavi suggests that these institutions are strong enough to be relatively autonomous of the propertied classes in postcolonial societies and of their metropolitan allies abroad: what distinguished the colonial state from the postcolonial one was the alien character of the former, not its institutions or primary concerns.

Alavi's formulation has been attacked from several quarters. The following points are most crucial here. Firstly, Alavi exaggerates the colonial state's capacity to control civil society. Saul (1974), for example, argued that in the African context it is difficult to sustain the case, certainly without more clear-cut indicators of what might count as an "overdeveloped" state. In India, following Frykenberg (1965), some authors stress the limits to state control over local politics (Bayly 1979; Washbrook 1978), local economies (Whitcombe 1972), and local social structures (Kumar 1965). Washbrook, for example, argues that the British state in India exercised a less "developed" range of modes of control over civil society than did the states that preceded it in South India—to such an extent that land-revenue collection became almost the only connection between the state and the local population (Washbrook 1977; see also Moore 1980). Furthermore, Indians were incorporated into positions of influence and, eventually, power from the 1880s onwards, probably because the British recognized the limits of the control their state apparatus could wield. Of course, this argument cannot be taken too far; in terms of the control of legitimate force and the ability to coerce agreement in the last resort, the Indian army (with the British army in India), the Indian police, and the Indian civil service, together could still forge an instrument of domination more efficient and flexible than any previously seen on the subcontinent. However, since Alavi's case seems to be based on the ability to manage everyday politics and bureaucratic matters without reliance on landed classes, his critics have considerable validity.

The second weakness in Alavi's account is his assumption that the imperial state was straightforwardly a tool of the "metropolitan bourgeoisie." The imperial state *was* alien and answerable to its masters in Britain, but that control was restricted by distance and lack of knowledge. The interests of the "metropolitan bourgeoisie" were rarely clear, unambiguous or unchanging. Even the extreme case—"ensuring a stable environment for trade, commodity production, and revenue collection" (Wood 1978)—gave few guidelines by the 1920s to Indian bureaucrats attempting to cope with world recession and Japanese competition (Charlesworth 1982). Further, Alavi's formulation not only cannot help us understand the pressure on the state to provide for the needs of capital; it also cannot help us understand social policy, such as British suppression of *sati* and female infanticide, and the introduction of programs of general education (particularly female education) and in the field of health. Here, imperial ideology (and the variations in form this took among individuals in the imperial system at different times and in different places) has to be considered seriously.

The third difficulty with Alavi's formulation is the meaning to be attached to the transfer of power at the time of independence. The Indian Congress party was a party of "step-in-your-shoes" nationalists—wanting power but without a clear idea of what to do when they had it—as opposed to the Chinese Communist party, for example (Maddison 1971). By taking over the existing bureaucracy, the Chinese Communists and the Congress party alike could cope with immediate problems of administration in desperate times, but they were also constrained in the kinds of policy innovations they were then able to make. Whereas the Chinese Communists appreciated their limitations however, and tried to overcome bureaucratic inertia through a policy of increasing political control at all levels, the Congress party was largely content with what it had. Alavi argued that this was not because of an identity of interests with the British, but because the social classes represented by the political parties in India were ineffectual. The bureaucracy had developed ways of by-passing political leaders. Wood (1978) suggests that increasing the complexity of bureaucratic routine was the main technique for blunting political pressures.

Alavi was, of course, talking specifically about Pakistan and Bangladesh where the very shortness of the periods of civilian rule make his case more plausible. The bureaucracy and the military certainly can work well together in situations where political interference is minimized. But Wood's extension of Alavi's argument to India is more difficult to defend. In particular, ministerial office in the Indian states permits the exercise of several controls which the bureaucracy is almost powerless to prevent—for example, the transfer and promotion of state (rather than all-Indian) civil servants. The departments with the largest employment (such as education and health) are often prized ministerships because they offer such scope for patronage and corruption (Wade 1984). Yet they are also ministries where policies change. In trying to understand this we do not get very far by referring to bureaucratic methods of coping with politicians, nor to the competing classes whose interests are (or are not) articulated by the postcolonial state.

Alavi (1982) provides some answers to these issues by distinguishing four levels of analysis of the state. The first draws on the so-called "capital-logic" school and focuses on the state's role in creating and reproducing a social order that permits the economy to function. In Alavi's terms, India is a "peripheral capitalist" economy, so minimally the state must make it possible for capitalists to make a profit, to benefit personally, and to continue to invest. The second level relates to the questions Alavi raised in 1972 about the classes and groups that can be said to control the state; at this level the actions of the state in specific spheres have to be considered. The third level entails analyzing the bureaucracy, its social origins and interests, and the extent of its autonomy; while the fourth level is the state as an arena for competing interests—party and pressure-group politics.

Alavi argues that state action at the second level is set by a context in which a "structural imperative" exists in which the basic notions of profitability, calculation, and capital accumulation affect the consequences of state action, but do not determine those actions in advance. Rather, the other two levels (the bureaucracy and the political) play a role, making for deviations from the strict logical requirements of capitalist enterprises and capital in general. It may still be very difficult to define what that strict logic might require in any particular historical situation. In this model of political and social life strict logic never applies, but politics and society tend in this direction in the long run.

Alavi's recent position, then, allows that "mistakes" can be made and that not everything done by the state can be understood as meeting the needs of dominant classes. In addition, it provides a space for sociological analysis of the ideas and interests of bureaucratic and other groups without making them seem either hypocrites or idiots—either consciously dissembling about the real reasons for policy or unaware of the benefits to particular classes— which is all classical Marxist analyses tend to permit. Alavi's position can also clarify some of the differences between the two kinds of accounts of health policy in India which I outlined at the beginning. In general, the uncritical accounts focus on Alavi's third and fourth levels, taking what doctors and bureaucrats say they are doing, and why, very much at face value and taking a similar approach to the pressure groups which try to influence policy. The critical writers, on the other hand, generally concentrate on Alavi's first and second levels, the structural imperatives of capitalism and the class interests of powerful groups.

Plausibly, a fuller account encompassing all four levels would be more satisfactory. State interests cannot be assumed once a particular country has been identified as "peripheral capitalist." The forms taken by health services have varied from country to country, and they have changed through time. The obvious problem lies in how to analyze the relationships among levels without creating a picture of either total autonomy or total determination. This is the framework I shall use to look at health policy in India. Roemer presents a superficially similar account in a systems approach distinguishing historical determinants, economic levels, political policies, and other cultural influences as the "determinants of health-care systems" (1977:1). However, he classes all non-Socialist, underdeveloped, health-care systems together solely on the basis of economic levels, but then places India in a "transitional" category (ibid.:198). By contrast, I want to discuss the extent to which India is unlike the patterns described for other countries in the "capitalist periphery," and this needs a more sophisticated discussion of the state than the "political policies" and "ideology" described by Roemer.

Some demands impinge more directly on health services than others—men's complaints rather than women's or children's, town-dwellers' complaints rather than villagers', ruling races', classes', and parties' rather than complaints of the ruled. Experiences of diseases and interpretations of their meaning vary. Therefore, even if health services were to respond in a direct manner to the effective demands made on them, they would not necessarily reflect any real disease pattern. Other interests also affect health services; the interests of the state may be paramount, or health services may be mediated by the interests of the occupation that dominates among members of the medical division of labor. Their views of appropriate patterns of health services would be conditioned by their theories of the causes and treatments of diseases as well as by their views of their own proper position in society. In a colonial situation, indigenous and colonial views may differ widely. Many would argue that this mismatch continues in the postindependence world as a result of neocolonialism. This raises the problem of whose perceptions should be used for the analysis.

Diseases are experienced and interpreted as social events (illnesses), and the demands people make of healers are based on these cultural processes. The classic (and over-generalized) example from India is that some people explain smallpox as a curse from a particular goddess and they respond to a smallpox sufferer very differently from the way they treat someone with plague or cholera, for example (Arnold 1985). Some writers have argued that the cultural specificity of disease categories makes it impossible to use Western categories in the discussion of other populations. However desirable it might be in principle to use Indian disease categories in what follows, there are considerable problems. Firstly, there is no uniform set of Indian disease categories, but variations regionally and culturally. Secondly, the sources I am consulting all use a version of Western categories, even if these change through time. Finally, I (and most of my readers) implicitly order their view of the world of health and illness using Western categories, and any attempt to use an alternative set would be partial and not genuine. But it should always be remembered that for most Indians a 'humoral' view of health and illness, sometimes extended by the use of concepts derived from the classical Indian traditions, gives a closer approximation to how they see the world.

These alternative views of the disease reality pose a problem in explaining improvements in health. In general, I do not presume that health services are the major determinants of health. The debates in Western Europe and North America concerning the causes of mortality decline in the nineteenth century, and the current relationships between health services and levels of life expectancy, are well known (McKeown, 1966; Powles, 1972; Illich, 1976; Lalonde, 1975). Except for a few interventions directly under medical stimulus (such as clean water supplies, or a few mass preventive campaigns) the major killers of the nineteenth century declined in significance well before specific remedies or protections were provided by medical science. The relevance of this debate for twentieth century changes in the rest of the world is more uncertain (see, e.g. Ruzicka, 1984). I shall discuss this issue in more detail, when I consider the impact of changes in living standards, the control of famine, and the role of good nutrition in reducing mortality. Usually, I maintain an agnostic position: I do not go as far as Illich and his followers, who maintain that health services are a major cause of ill-health and no benefit at all, but equally, I find there is often little evidence that hospital attendance, vaccination campaigns, and town water supplies have made a marked difference to people's health. However, I will discuss the arguments where the evidence seems more powerful or where the issue of the likely causes of mortality decline is more central. Nonetheless, my main concern is with how services were provided, at what cost, when, and in what form, even if, in strictly medical terms, they had little effect on people's health.

In these pages I hope to tease out some of these relationships in the Indian context, and in particular to throw light on why current patterns of health services in India took the forms they have. These patterns are generally agreed to be inadequate, either for dealing with the needs of the Indian population today or as a foundation for the goal of "Health for All by the Year 2000." Understanding better the historical roots of these patterns and their significance for present-day policy-making may help those trying to overcome these inadequacies.

The material is presented in two sections. Part I deals with the historical background, the story up to 1947. Here I am concerned to describe the likely effects of British rule on health and on the development of health services in India. In Part II I deal with post-Independence policy in its social, political and economic context, taking health expenditure, policy with respect to health personnel, foreign assistance, medical migration and pharmaceutical policy as case studies for more detailed attention. In general, I have restricted myself to analyses of what happened, rather than with alternative desirable patterns, though the policy implications of this material will become clear, and are brought out most directly in chapter 11.

Sources and Methods

The material reported here comes from a variety of sources, and has been collected over the last fifteen years or so. My interest in the topic was stimulated during a stay in Pakistan in 1970–1971, when I carried out fieldwork in Lahore hospital casualty departments and also collected data on health policy and planning in Pakistan (Jeffery 1973; 1974). I visited Punjab (India) in 1974, and made some preliminary analyses of Punjab government materials available in Chandigarh, but a more substantial collection of data took place in 1975–1976, when I was based in New Delhi.

I collected material from the reports of the Central Council of Health, newspapers in the Nehru Memorial Library, other documents from the National Medical Library in the All-India Institute of Medical Sciences, and archival material from the National Archives of India in New Delhi. I also used sources provided by the Indian Medical Association at its national headquarters as well as by the Delhi branch, and interviewed their office-holders and one former minister of health and a former director-general of health services. I then created a listing of doctors in Delhi, and interviewed a 2 percent sample.

After returning to the United Kingdom I consulted materials held by the India Office Library in London and by the Edinburgh University Library, and undertook as well several other shorter trips to India to investigate conditions on tea estates in Assam and to advise on a United Kingdom health-aid program in Orissa. These visits widened my understanding of government processes. Finally, in 1982–1983 I spent a year carrying out a joint research project (with Patricia Jeffery and Andrew Lyon) on childbearing in rural Uttar Pradesh, providing a new perspective on health services as seen by a villager, however privileged and temporary. Material on various aspects of this research has already been published; the bibliography includes a complete listing. In particular, the data on foreign aid, used in Chapter 8, has appeared in the *International Journal of Health Services* (Jeffery 1986a); some of the material in Chapters 2 and 4 has appeared in *Social Science and Medicine* (Jeffery 1983) and in *Modern Asian Studies* (Jeffery 1979); and an early version of chapter 6 formed the basis of an article in *Health Policy and Planning* (Jeffery 1986b).

In what follows I transgress a number of disciplinary boundaries, most notably of sociology, history, and health economics, and I shall not satisfy specialists in any of these fields. In developing the material for this case study I have been restricted by the availability of sources. The material drawn from Orissa was available only because of my regular visits to that state in a semiofficial capacity, and I did not select the state on any theoretical grounds. Some of the gaps in the arguments reflect similar problems and some of my arguments may reflect the existence of sources I have been able to use, rather than the most important arguments one might want to have made. Nonetheless, I hope these pages will shed light on an area much discussed, but not much studied.

A Note on Terminology

I have generally referred to doctors trained in the medical colleges and schools established by the British as Western doctors, and the kind of medicine in which they were educated as Western medicine. This is controversial; Leslie, for example, has urged the use of the term *cosmopolitan medicine* to denote the fact that this kind of treatment no longer has its roots solely in Europe and North America (Leslie 1976). Referring to Western medicine is also problematic in India, since both *Unani* (''Greek'') and homoeopathic medicine also came from the West. However, it reflects usage in India, especially in the period before 1947 when this system of medicine was identified with the British and when ''cosmopolitan'' strikes an anachronistic note. The alternative terminology in India is *allopathic*, a term derived from homoeopathy and contested by Western doctors as being too narrow. I do not feel that there is an ideal solution, but I feel happiest with Western medicine and Western doctors and have used the terms in this way.

PART I:

Health and Health Policy Under the British

Introduction to Part I

Many writers have wrestled with the attempt to disentangle and evaluate what Marx called England's double mission in India—one destructive and one regenerative—which others have regarded as a characteristic of industrial capitalism in general (Marx 1973:320). The inclusion of India in a world economy was certainly helped by British direct rule over much of what we now call India. The British Raj oversaw the construction and operation of the new economic order, but it was finally responsible to political control outside India; this undoubtedly had specific consequences. In the field of tariff control and land revenue British rule may have been decisive. But in many other areas it becomes a hopeless task to try to assess how things might have been different had political control remained in India. Even some Marxists have returned to themes which Weberian writers have stressed, namely, that changes in social and political institutions and cultural patterns would have been necessary before economic changes could have taken hold (Worsley 1980; Warren 1980). The absence of colonial rule in India would not, by itself, have led to faster, more thoroughgoing, or more equitable processes of social and economic change.

Similarly, historians are increasingly stressing the degree of integration in pre-British India, the level of monetization of the economy, and the extent of agrarian landlessness (Kumar, ed. 1982). Colonial rule was neither as all-encompassing nor as destructive as many early writers claimed and the social and cultural impact was perhaps as important in the long run as the "drain" of booty to England in the eighteenth century or the lack of protection for the

hand-loom cotton industry in the eighteenth and early nineteenth
century (Charlesworth 1982). Some Marxists have contributed to
these reinterpretations of nineteenth-century Indian history. For example, Warren (1980) attempted to refocus Marxist thought on the
generative side of imperialism and modern capitalism and stressed
the improvements in health brought about by the colonizers. He
cited rapid population growth and declines in mortality rates within a few decades of colonial rule. Warren's view is at odds with
most Marxist analyses in which colonialism's contribution to an expansion of misery and a decline in the quality of life are more
usually stressed.

But Frank (1967) was wrong to treat the whole imperial period
as though it were static. Three main periods in the history of the
imperial state can be identified. Prior to 1860, the state was a cu-
rious amalgam of commercial, administrative, and military
machines; from 1860 to 1920 we can see the "High Noon" of the
British state in India; from 1920 onward the process of Indianization began in earnest. Independence in 1947 ushered in a further
set of changes. These dates are of course only approximations; not
only are the stages reached at different times in different parts of
the subcontinent (Punjab often seeming to lead the way) but the
turning points are often spread out over several years. Thus the
new order established by the 1919 Government of India Act can be
traced back to Curzon's attempt to partition Bengal, in 1906, and
to the Morley-Minto reforms of 1907.

The history of the British annexation of India does not need
much rehearsal; the main signposts of the political history are
familiar enough. From the founding in 1601 of the trading company, the East India Company, until the military campaigns of 1757
which included the Battle of Plassey and Clive's victorious march
on Calcutta, British power was largely confined to control over
different aspects of foreign trade. Their European competitors—the
Dutch and the French—were comparable in military strength and
trading ability. (The ebb and flow of competition among the European powers was overshadowed by the growth and decline of the
Moguls who reached their furthest geographical spread in the reign
of the Emperor Aurangzeb who died in 1707.) But the events of
1757 established the superiority of the British over the other European powers and demonstrated Britain's ability to intervene effectively in Indian politics. An almost irresistible chain of conquests
and advances was set in train, culminating in the overthrow of the

Sikh kingdom in the Punjab in 1847 and the takeover of Oudh in 1856. The East India Company developed into a ruling body partly to defend and extend its commercial interests, but one result of conquering territory and taking on the collection of land revenue was to reduce steadily the relative significance of its trading activities. The problems and rewards offered by rulership and land revenues led the British Parliament, in Acts of 1833 and 1853, to exercise increasing supervision of events in India.

In 1800 the processes of territorial spread and institutional transformation were still under way. In the last half of the eighteenth century the British in India had acted rapaciously, looting and laying waste the lands of defeated enemies, using force to insist on unequal contracts or the payment of penal fines, and extorting very high land revenues. As the aggressive conquests of new territory in the core of the Indian subcontinent came to an end, the British government in India was steadily bureaucratized (in almost the classical Weberian sense). By 1860 the process was almost complete. Private functions and finances were steadily separated from public ones, efforts were made to establish recruitment procedures which were free from elements of purchase and sale of office, and clear lines of control were set up between London and Calcutta and on down into the countryside.

The events of 1857 (the Mutiny or Sepoy Rebellion) hastened the changes. The 1858 Government of India Act required regular reporting of Indian financial affairs and efforts to promote "moral and material progress" in the country. These reinforced moves to regularize and systematize the organizational structure within India. The forms of government established at this time dominated developments for the next sixty years. Most of the reforms, such as the increasing involvement of Indians at the higher levels of the government, were brought in without changing the basic structure; others, such as the establishment of local self-government after 1882, only began to have a serious impact toward the end of the period. This sixty-year spell saw British rule at its most self-confident and typifies the image usually held of racial pride, a concern for official superiority and efficiency, and mountains of paperwork.

In this period policy in India was most clearly stimulated by the changing context of ideas in England, with Liberal and Conservative viceroys and secretaries of state attempting to influence developments in the light of their ideas of the imperial role (Moore

1966; Stokes 1959). In subjects such as public education and public-health provision the state took a much more prominent role in India than in Britain, because vested interests and alternative institutions in civil society were absent. But these innovations were always limited by the main demands on the state—the maintenance of law and order, protection of the external boundaries, and financial rectitude.

The reforms associated with Montagu (as secretary of state) and Chelmsford (as viceroy), in 1918–1919, mark a decisive shift. They were heralded by the Morley-Minto reforms of 1907–1909 which Moore (1966) characterized as "the shadow of reform and the substance of repression." Both reform packages extended the principles of representation and ministerial government responsible to an elected legislature, but the Montagu-Chelmsford reforms were of much greater long-term significance. The 1919 reforms drew on two royal-commission reports and other proposals to extend "Indianization" and to transfer several spheres of government to provincial ministers, responsible to elected assemblies. The division of powers between the center and the provinces, established in 1919, was left virtually unchanged by the reforms of 1935 and is the basis of the Indian constitution after independence.

Although the Congress party never fully committed itself to working the 1919 constitution, the interwar period saw real power exercised for the first time by Indian ministers and a dramatic growth in the Indian share of all the elite bureaucratic services. The India Office's ability to control events in India steadily declined, so that independence became increasingly predictable and well within established patterns despite the apparently chaotic conditions of 1946 and 1947. Post-1947 policies in many areas followed the lines already laid down.

Critical arguments about imperial impact, with specific reference to health and health services in India, were produced both by nationalists and Marxists (e.g., Naoroji 1901; Digby 1901; Baran 1958; Banerji 1975). Put simply, the critical case against imperial rule is that it had a number of negative consequences for Indian society. Living standards were reduced (particularly through excessive land revenue demands, trading patterns in which the surplus was creamed off by European traders, and the drain to London). As a result, development potentials were thwarted, limiting technical and social change in India and lowering the technical level in certain key areas. These changes adversely affected health conditions in India.

But a conundrum remains. What caused the rise in population (especially after 1920) if not an improvement in general living standards? But what was the result of that population increase if it was not a decline in general living standards? Banerji (1974) follows the nationalist tradition dating from Naoroji (1901) and Digby (1901). They argue that imperialism destroyed existing balances between people and their environments (including coping mechanisms like indigenous healing traditions) and led to a decline in standards of living (indicated by such variables as income per head and reports of the rise of urban slums and rural distress). In addition, Indian healers were "deskilled," because they were deprived of elite patronage, and local village-based society was destroyed by commercialization and the syphoning of surplus by the state. Furthermore, many developments had "unhealthy" consequences; for example, the conditions that were permitted in towns, the spread of malaria (accompanying canal and road and rail developments) and the plague (introduced into Bombay along colonial trade paths). The critics continue by arguing that the measures adopted by the government in India were totally inadequate to deal with these problems, partly because of the racist basis of rule: interests of the European minority received undue concern, while the Indian majority received little more than crumbs from the white table (Ramasubban 1982).

Thus the Indian Medical Service (IMS) was designed to service the Indian Civil Service and the army; only incidentally were services provided for the mass of the population. Hospitals and dispensaries were urban and designed with the interests of European civil servants as their highest priority; and the training of medical practitioners provided subordinates for Europeans in the medical service. Little was made available to provide private medical services to the mass of the population, services whose potential was limited not merely by inadequate training, but also by denial of the relevance of the local culture and systematic derision of local medical traditions. The provision of health services was excessively medical in character with preventive and sanitary measures given low priority; most concern was for European troops and European quarters of towns. Sanitary measures were often restricted to attempts at social control, most obvious in the antiplague measures.

Thus, what little was spent on health could have had virtually no benefit for the mass of the local population. Any improvements in the health of Indians was no more than accidental and the unintended consequences of quite other policies.

Critics, however, are too willing to generalize on the basis of very little material. In fact, there are few good discussions of the impact of British rule on health in India. The critics also tend to apply anachronistic standards—to blame colonial health services for their inadequacy when, prior to the 1920s, medical services were inadequate everywhere and even public-health services had an uncertain impact on health, particularly on infant and child health (Powles 1973; Oakley 1985).

Apologists for empire, especially from the colonial period, focus on the benefits of British imperialism (Griffiths 1952; Anstey 1926; Davis 1951). From their perspective, British rule brought peace to a subcontinent racked by local wars and declining public order as the Mogul Empire collapsed. It also provided railways, roads, canals, trade, improved living standards, and economic security. Health services based on "scientific" medicine replaced "medieval" medicine or superstition. Famine policy—the provision of jobs and relief in times of scarcity—was a major benefit of imperial rule, leading to major savings of lives. The limits of imperial achievements were set by the poverty of India and the ignorance and resistance of its population, not by the inadequacies of imperial policy.

Many apologists assume the significance of health services because they were provided at all, rather than assessing their real contribution. The apologists too quickly conclude that health services are an unmitigated good, and that "the natives" were living in benighted squalor before they received the benefit of such "civilizing" influences as education and medicine. After the 1820s few British avoided the temptation to ignore both the positive aspects of existing institutions and the contribution to the squalor made by foreign rule. Influential Orientalists made efforts to learn Sanskrit and to find valuable aspects of Hindu culture to preserve and pass on. Their influence over British ruling ideology seems to have been almost totally lost and only isolated commentators (e.g., Leitner 1886; Digby 1901) stand out against the complacent assessments of British superiority.

The two major viewpoints may be addressed by three interrelated questions: What happened to the health of the Indian population in this period? How did British rule affect the indigenous ways of coping with illness, with local medical systems and their practitioners? How successful were British attempts to provide medical care and public health services?

CHAPTER ONE

Health Status in India Before 1947

> Another by-product of British rule which served to worsen
> the position of the peasantry was the increase in popula-
> tion. . . . In the years since (1880) the population has in-
> creased considerably. The amount of land available to the
> average peasant family has become less. Because of the com-
> petition for land, the landowners and moneylenders have
> been able to make the peasants agree to more and more oner-
> ous terms for the use of the soil and of credit. (Thorner and
> Thorner 1962:109–110)

The first substantial and reliable censuses in India
were held around the middle of the nineteenth century with the
first attempt at an all-India census held between 1869 and 1872. Decennial national censuses date from 1881. While they provide out-
standingly good information compared to many other countries,
their main weakness is underenumeration, usually not random but
larger for some age groups than for others, for some areas than for
others, and of women more than of men; estimating the extent of
this is a tricky and inexact art (Visaria, 1971).

The other demographic sources are much less valuable; the registration of births and deaths which started in the main cities at about
the same time has yet to reach an acceptable level of coverage. The
Sample Registration Scheme was instituted by the government of
India in the mid-1960s when the inadequacy of the National Sample Survey became obvious. This provides fairly reliable estimates
of mortality and fertility. The Model Registration Scheme provides
seriously inadequate estimates on causes of death, and national
morbidity figures are even now nonexistent. For the period of British rule evidence about causes of death have to be inferred from
small surveys or from special enumerations during epidemics, as
of plague or cholera.

To estimate population totals and mortality and fertility levels prior to 1871, sketchy information must be interpreted (Morris 1974). For my purposes (to assess population changes in the nineteenth and twentieth centuries) I need an estimate of the total population as well as mortality and fertility rates in 1800. Two basic methods have been used: extrapolating forward from 1600, or backwards from 1871. The sources for 1600 are Akbar's revenue collection documents (the *'Ain-i-Akbari*), first used for this purpose by Moreland (1920:22). Habib (1982) has recently argued plausibly that Moreland's original figure for all-India (100 million) was an underestimate, probably by as much as 50 percent. Habib's revised estimate of about 140 million to 150 million seems a reasonable figure. But what happened to the population between 1600 and 1800? Das Gupta and his colleagues (1972) argued that the growth in population was largely during the relatively stable years of Mogul power between 1600 and 1675, with little growth from 1675 to 1800 when that power declined under internal strains and external pressures. Using Habib's revised 1600 figure, an estimate for 1800 of 190 million to 220 million would be generated.

Others have preferred to work back from 1871 and ensure that the implications for the period between 1600 and 1871 seem reasonable. Writers doing this have produced a variety of estimates for 1800. Davis (1951) assumed a population in 1800 of around 125 million by trebling a contemporary estimate for British territories of 41 million. But as he notes himself, in order to make this compatible with his corrected 1871 census figure of 255 million, he had to assume quite dramatic increases in population from about 1845. The estimates produced by Das Gupta (1972) and Morris (1974) assume less substantial population growth in the nineteenth century, of around 0.4 percent per year. Das Gupta used the same regional growth rates for the area of present-day India as for those that occurred between 1871 and 1921; Morris used the average annual rate of growth between 1871 and 1921 for the whole subcontinent. His estimate of the population of all-India in 1800 was 197 million.

But little evidence supports this line of argument, or any particular set of assumptions. As Cassen (1978:3) notes, neither kind of estimate can be regarded as precise and all should be treated skeptically. Visaria and Visaria (1983:464) also note that more recent estimates of the population in 1800 are much higher than the earlier ones. But the current view, for what it is worth, is that the population of all-India in 1800 was between 190 million and 210 million. In the preceding 200 years the population grew only slowly and unevenly, by as much as one-third overall. After 1800, population growth remained uneven but was at a higher average rate, rising by between 25 percent and 33 percent in only seventy years, and at a similar rate until 1921.

Fertility fluctuates in the short term, because famines and epidemics affect fecundity and the numbers of married couples in the reproductive age groups. Although fertility may have risen in the nineteenth century as Dyson and Murphy (1985) argue is plausible for Madras and Bombay during the first half of the twentieth century, a substantial rise in fertility is unlikely, because almost all women were probably married at a young age. Thus the key determinant of population increase was probably a fall in the mortality rate. However, estimates of mortality and fertility between 1800 and 1870 have to be based on data derived from the censuses after 1871 and more insubstantial material from 1851 (see table 1). The life expectancy figures are heavily dependent on demographic models which may be made unrealistic if ages are wrongly recorded or if people in some age groups are under-recorded. As Alice Clark (1985) has demonstrated, newer techniques less vulnerable to these problems, would produce much lower estimates of life expectancy at birth, especially for females, and correspondingly higher death rates.

The general view, then, is that from 1800 to 1921 India had high birthrates (fluctuating to a small extent, but over 40 per 1,000 population in most years) and high death rates (fluctuating much more, sometimes above and sometimes below 40 per 1,000 population). The peaks in mortality are particularly associated with droughts and famines; in "normal" years, mortality was affected more by endemic diseases and poor living standards. Famines were often followed by epidemics whose effects were magnified by malnutrition suffered by vulnerable groups in the preceding year. Mitra (1978:II, 764–818) lists droughts and famines reported between 1729 and 1973. They rarely affected the whole of the country. From the 1830s on, when reporting improved, a famine, scarcity, or drought was reported from somewhere in the country every three years or so. Bhatia (1967) argued that there was a much higher frequency of famines in the nineteenth century than in the preceding period, especially in Bengal, with the worst occurring during the fifty years

TABLE 1
POPULATION FIGURES FOR ALL-INDIA: 1871–1941

Year	Population (millions) Gujral	Davis	Crude birth rate	Crude death rate	Life Expectancy at birth males	females
1851	224					
1861	241					
1871	253	255	n.a.	n.a.	24	26
1881	258	257	49	41	25	26
1891	282	282	46	44	24	24
1901	285	285	48	43	23	23
1911		303	49	49	19	21
1921		306	46	36	27	27
1931		338	45	31	32	31
1941		389				

SOURCE: Gujral 1973; Davis 1951:36, 62, 69.
NOTE: These figures are for what is now India, Pakistan, and Bangladesh.
KEY: n.a. = not available

after 1860. Widespread and severe famines and droughts occurred in 1877 and 1878; in 1897 and 1898 (accompanied by an epidemic of plague); and in 1919 and 1920 (preceded by the influenza epidemic). After 1921 only the Bengal famine of 1943 compares with these earlier disasters.

Sen's recent detailed reanalysis of excess mortality after the Bengal famine clarifies the processes involved (Sen 1980). The famine and the deaths directly and obviously from starvation were over by November 1943, but mortality from malaria, smallpox, and to a lesser extent cholera continued at above-normal levels for the next three years or so. Of the excess mortality registered between 1943 and 1946, 37 percent were attributed to malaria. Sen argues that official estimates ignored almost half the famine-related deaths, because people in the later stages of malnutrition contract diseases from which they then are recorded as dying. The concept of "excess mortality" is hard to define, but famines seem to increase mortality partly by helping to turn endemic diseases into epidemic ones. (It is puzzling that in India, unlike Europe, tuberculosis deaths do not normally rise during and after famines.) Famines also affect sanitary arrangements and water supplies, and diseases spread more easily as desperate populations (usually men) search the countryside for work and public-health services break down. These patterns account partly for the peaks of mortality. However, the generally high level had more to do with malaria which possibly accounted for one death in five at the end of the nineteenth century and after (Klein 1973). Respiratory diseases—pulmonary tuberculosis, pneumonia, bronchitis—may have been the next largest contributor to mortality, and then the digestive-tract diseases, of diarrhea, dysentery, cholera. Probably as many as 10 million people died from plague in the twenty years after 1896 when it spread from Bombay.

As with other poor populations, infants contributed most to the mortality levels and were particularly vulnerable to most of these diseases mentioned. Estimates of infant mortality are over 250 per 1,000 live births in the nineteenth century, falling to around 160 to 200 per 1,000 by 1941 (Visaria and Visaria 1982). It is surprising that most estimates of infant and early childhood mortality rates for females are lower than for males even in North India, where female infanticide was practiced among some groups until the 1870s and where neglect of female children remains more common than in south India. But of those who survived childhood, women at each age were more likely to die than men (Visaria and Visaria 1983:498–500). During peaks of mortality, the reverse was often the case for reasons not yet clear (Mitra 1978; Sen 1980).

Mortality rates tend to be higher among the poor, but records were kept by caste or community that straddle economic categories. In the 1880s and 1890s mortality figures were kept in Bombay and Calcutta with some degree of accuracy. In normal periods the registered crude death rates of the low castes were about 50 percent above those of clean caste Hindus and twice European rates. In periods of famine and epidemic the lower castes suffered catastrophically. As late as 1920 low-caste Hindus in Bombay had a registered crude death rate of 120 per 1,000, in contrast to figures for other categories ranging from 25 per 1,000 (for Europeans) to 41 per 1,000 for non-Brahman clean-caste Hindus (Klein 1973). It is not surprising that famine relief services were most sought by agricultural laborers, often Harijan in caste, and some of the village artisans, especially weavers (Bhatia 1967:10–11).

In the Indian subcontinent as a whole, mortality levels were probably lower during the first century or so of British dominance than previously. However, any tendency for mortality to decline was halted during the 1890s and the 1910s (because of the plague and famines of 1896–1900 and the influenza epidemic of 1919–1920). In addition, the potency of some epidemic diseases, especially malaria, probably rose in this period. After 1921, by contrast, population grew quite dramatically.

This apparently straightforward national pattern, however, is made up of quite varied local ones. In some areas the picture is complicated by the results of administrative decisions—the siting of cantonments or the choice of a railway route—which might dramatically affect the population of one district as compared with another. Migration always has a greater potential significance for total population the smaller the unit studied. Considerable short-distance or short-term mobility occurred from the eighteenth century onward. After 1860 substantially longer distance and longer term mobility, to tea plantations or as indentured labor abroad, affected regions such as Chota Nagpur, Punjab, Gujarat, and south India more than others (Tinker 1979).

Census commissioners dealing with provincial variations in population histories often failed to discern any clear pattern. Sometimes the districts that grew in population were the most densely populated to begin with, while elsewhere there was an expansion of cropped land to account for population growth. Distinguishing mortality changes from other demographic changes in smaller areas is very difficult. Some long-term studies of individual districts or villages try to show the causes of local population changes. Kumar (1968:302) shows that the population of Indapur taluka, near Poona, rose by 65 percent between settlements of land revenue in 1835–1836 and 1895–1896. Yet, this area was particularly badly hit by the influenza epidemic and the population, which had risen by almost a further 20 percent by 1911, was recorded at the same level in 1931. Kessinger (1974:85–93) shows that Vilyatpur, in Punjab, was relatively densely populated even in the nineteenth century and that the population rose steadily from 1855 to 1891 before falling until 1931 and rising again thereafter. He suggests that the population decline was largely accounted for by emigration, though epidemics of cholera in 1892, plague in 1897–1898, 1903, and 1915, and influenza in 1918 also played a part.

Local variations were not restricted to the area of British India. In the princely states, those parts of India left under indirect rule, population changes were roughly comparable to those of the surrounding British areas. Major exceptions are the states of Travancore and Cochin (roughly the modern state of Kerala), particularly interesting exceptions since mortality and fertility rates are currently much below the levels in the rest of India. After making allowances for underenumeration, Rayappa and Prabhakara (1981:2018–2031) estimated that the population of Travancore rose by over 10 percent in every decade after 1881, and by nearly 25 percent in the decade 1921–1931. They attributed only a small part of this rise to net immigration. The Cochin rises are only slightly less dramatic. As table 2 shows, the two other sizable south Indian princely states, Mysore, and one part of Hyderabad (the eastern Telengana) show similar patterns. The steady overall increase in Mysore is held down by population decline in some areas in the forested hills in the west of the state—the "malnad"—where malaria and continuing poverty made recovery from famines a slow affair. Over the sixty years from 1891 to 1951 total population growth in this area was only about 2 percent, compared with over 50 percent in the rest of the state (UN 1961:13–14). In the other part of Hyderabad (southern Mahratwara), population change was closer to that of India as a whole, with declines in population between 1891 and 1901 and again between 1911 and 1921.

Thus the transition to declining mortality patterns took place much earlier in parts of south India than in the rest of the country and the idea of a national pattern to population change is suspect. Ecological variation, such as climate, accounts for some of this; in other cases geographical factors interact with social ones, as in the impact of the route by which a disease was introduced into India, or the trading routes along which it spread. But there are also sources of variation which are more clearly social in character, and I shall now consider some of these.

TABLE 2

POPULATION GROWTH IN PRINCELY SOUTH INDIA: 1871 TO 1941

State	*Population in millions*							
	1871	1881	1891	1901	1911	1921	1931	1941
Cochin	0.60[a]	0.60	0.72	0.81	0.92	0.98	1.21	1.42
Travancore	2.3[a]	2.4	2.6	2.9	3.4	4.0	5.1	6.1
Hyderabad								
Telengana		4.3	5.2	5.4	6.7	6.4	7.5	n.a.
Mahratwara		5.5	6.3	5.7	6.6	6.1	6.9	n.a.
Mysore	5.1	4.2	4.9	5.5	5.8	6.0	6.6	7.3

SOURCE: Decennial Census reports.
[a] The Cochin and Travancore census was held in 1875, not in 1871.

Effects of British Rule

ON INCOME LEVELS

This is one of the most contested topics in modern Indian economic and social history. A major debate on the issue in
the 1960s left the question unresolved (Morris et al. 1972) and has
given rise to a further substantial debate (Heston 1982). Several
necessary elements in the analysis are difficult to assess and all
show considerable regional variation. First, total output over the
period was affected by growth or decline of industry, by changes
in agricultural productivity, cropping patterns, cropped area, and
so on. Second, the distribution of the income generated by this output between the state, which transmitted some of its share to Britain, and various sectors of the local population was affected by
changing patterns of rights and obligations with respect to the land.
As the form of the output changed (for example, rising cash crops,
changing exports and imports) it affected the distribution of income
too. In Marxist shorthand, we need to comprehend the changes in
the forces and relations of production over this period of 150 years
to assess their likely impact on the health of the Indian population.
Thus, per capita income is a very crude indicator of changes in
levels of living, but it remains the best we have for comparing the
nineteenth and the early twentieth century.

The classical view (as Morris terms it) is that per capita income in the period from 1800 to 1947 was stagnant or declined (Morris 1970). For example, Mukherji (1965:700–702) concluded that real incomes rose between about 1860 and about 1885, declined slightly until around 1900, rose again until about 1925, then stagnated before declining again from about 1940 to 1950. Blyn (1961) analyzed crop statistics and derived a series for the gross availability of food grains which rose during the 1890s but was stable from then until Indian independence—thus implying a steady decline in per capita availability from 1921 onwards (see table 3). However, Blyn's analysis relies on crop statistics provided by officials who had little interest in the subject, little support, and no training. It is unclear whether these estimates vary randomly or whether there might be consistent tendencies for which allowances could be made (Dewey 1978:304; P. Chaudhuri 1979). Dewey, perhaps the harshest critic of these figures, nevertheless suggests that the picture of regional variations they portray is useful. The deteriorating conditions in Bihar and the steady expansion in Punjab, for example, are reflected in the figures (Dewey 1978:314; see also Charlesworth 1982). Some have argued that the criticism is unwarranted, at least in certain regions for certain purposes. Islam (1978) uses these sources for his study of Bengal and Mishra (1983) argues that the statistics for Bombay are more reliable than Dewey and others have suggested (see also Hill 1984; Farmer 1986).

Once again even this regional picture needs to be looked at carefully. Thus for Bengal, Islam (1978:201) agrees with Blyn that most of the decline in per capita output was attributable to declines in Bihar and Orissa. Within Bengal, per capita crop output seems to differentiate the area around Calcutta and the Rajshahi region—where official figures indicated there was an increase from 1920/1924 to 1940/1944 of over 20 percent—from Burdwan and Chittagong regions—where there were declines of about 20 percent (ibid:52). Islam revises these figures and reduces them by about 20 percent in each case, giving a picture of stability in the Calcutta and Rajshahi regions and around a 40 percent decline in Burdwan and Chittagong (ibid.).

These changes in average incomes need to be complemented by an account of changes in their distribution. As Tomlinson (1986) notes, four schools can be described. The "stratifiers" see polarization occurring during the nineteenth century; for "pessimistic stratifiers" small landholders were impoverished and the rural

TABLE 3

AVERAGE CHANGE IN PER CAPITA ALL-CROP OUTPUT FROM
1896/97–1906/07 TO 1936/37–1946/47 IN
BRITISH INDIA AND REGIONS

Region	*Average*		% change
	1896/97–1906/07 Rs	*1936/37–1946/47* Rs	
Greater Bengal	41.6	32.5	− 22.0
United Provinces	37.1	36.7	− 1.0
Madras	37.0	37.6	+ 1.5
Greater Punjab	34.4	42.3	+ 23.0
Bombay-Sind	38.7	40.7	+ 10.5
Central Provinces	58.0	42.9	− 26.0
BRITISH INDIA	41.5	32.5	− 21.7

SOURCE: Blyn 1961:309.
NOTE: Greater Bengal includes Bihar, Orissa and Assam; Greater Punjab includes Northwest Frontier Province, and Delhi.

proletariat expanded, a process assisted by the destruction of handicraft manufacturing in competition with Lancashire textiles and Birmingham metalworks and because the state took an increasing share of the output of the land. The share remaining with actual cultivators was further reduced since larger shares went to those with a variety of higher claims to rights in the land. Landlord classes were protected by a legal and state system that buttressed their position. On the one hand this led to a great growth in intermediate holders of rights in the land with the position of cultivator stagnating and the numbers of landless laborers growing where there had been few before (Thorner and Thorner 1962:109). On the other hand, "optimistic stratifiers" have argued that "elite wealth-creation had signifiant trickle-down and multiplier effects" (Tomlinson, 1986:11).

The alternative "populist" schools draw on Morris (1963). He stressed regional variations; he pointed to the evidence of considerable numbers of landless laborers in the pre-British periods and little sign of a proportional increase in the nineteenth century; and he argued that during that period the rise in total output and the increasing commercialization of the economy suggest a rise in real per capita income which was not restricted to the landholding classes. In the early twentieth century a different picture is presented: real levels of output stagnated, so the rising population after 1921 caused a fall in real incomes, especially marked for the lower groups (Heston 1982). Some "populists" have been optimistic, seeing growth from below, while others have been pessimistic, seeing a deepening poverty for all.

Some of these variations can be explained by the regional focus of an author. Thus Islam suggests for Bengal that the population dependent on subsistence crops saw its living standards stagnate or decline and only landlords able to take advantage of land pressure and uncertain urban markets were likely to have experienced a rise in real incomes (1978:201–203). Similarly, in one area where per capita agricultural output seems to have risen (Bombay), R. Kumar (1965:318–330) argues that the benefits probably went largely to the landed peasants and that British rule virtually created marked social inequalities. After the Deccan riots of 1875 the state increasingly protected landholders. Enforced sales of land to meet debts were reduced, and new cooperative institutions were established. But only the relatively wealthy could take advantage of these changes. The rising real output of the twentieth century could thus be a result of the establishment of substantial farmers with access to credit, security of tenure, and so on—probably the very people who benefited most from this growth.

Charlesworth (1978) suggests that in the Bombay presidency generally, patterns of inequality in rural India were accentuated in the early period of commercialization (as the Leninist model predicts), but that the increasing demand for labor for crops like cotton and sugar kept rural wage rates rising in real terms in the 1920s. But in some areas, notably Punjab, per capita incomes may have continued to rise, benefiting the really poor as well as the rest because the distribution of resources was relatively egalitarian and there was sufficient social mobility (Kessinger 1974). But Dharma Kumar (1965), using data on the distribution of landholdings, suggests very little change in inequality in south India over a longer period, from 1880 to 1951. However, other accounts of western and southern India are very different, and "unequivocal answers about the process of economic growth or immiserization" (Tomlinson 1986:11) are still elusive.

Most historical discussions have looked at changes in agricultural or agriculturally dependent incomes under British rule. We know much less about the non-agricultural work force of pre-British times, and the long-term impact of British rule. Habib (1982) argues that under the Moguls in north India the urban population was considerable, perhaps as much as 15 percent of the total. Stable British rule reduced the population which had depended on the urban nobility, and old-established towns, like Dacca, Murshidabad, and Lucknow, decayed faster than the new ones (Bombay, Calcutta, and Madras) grew (Gadgil 1959; Habib 1972). The urban proportion probably began to decline about 1800, until it reached the 9 percent recorded in 1891. Dharma Kumar (1965) accepts that in South India, too, nonagricultural workers may have declined and they were forced back into agriculture. However, since there was still an uncultivated margin of land at the time they did not necessarily become landless laborers.

Within the urban population some categories did begin to grow earlier than 1891, despite the overall decline. There was some steady growth in numbers in the industrial work force from about 1860 onward, with the establishment of cotton and jute textile mills. Morris (1970) argues that even before this the expansion in the domestic market for textiles may have compensated for the loss of export markets and the intrusion of Manchester textiles. Material on real-wage rates for the industrial work force in these new industries suggests stability over a fairly long period, but, as in Europe, conditions for the new urban labor force were often appalling (see below).

The problems of attempting to assess changes in real income are considerable. However, in the period (1860–1920) when per capita incomes were either declining, as Mukherji (1965) argues, or rising, as Morris (1965) and Heston (1982) argue, mortality rates appear to have been fairly stable. But in the period (1920–1950) when even the latter authors accept that income levels probably fell, mortality rates also apparently fell rapidly. A regional analysis is not much more helpful, partly because output data for the princely states are not available. But in areas like central India, where per capita incomes were falling, population grew as fast in the 1920s and 1930s as it did in western India (Bombay-Sind) where per capita incomes were rising (Visaria and Visaria

1983:490, 505). It therefore seems impossible to explain falling mortality rates by changes in incomes.

CHANGES IN LIVING PATTERNS

The changing nature of urban centers and their increasing significance after about 1900 reflect a major change in Indian life brought about by British rule. Sometimes British policy inhibited urbanization—in the aftermath of the Sepoy Mutiny, for example the British operated a deurbanization policy in Delhi as ferocious as that attributed to the Khmer Rouge in Cambodia (Klein 1973). But colonial administrative centers—Bombay and Calcutta are prime examples—grew steadily as did new industrial towns like Kanpur, Ahmedabad, and Howrah. Here mortality rates were high not only because of crowded and unhygienic working and living conditions but also because of problems of water supply and sanitation. Filtered water was introduced by the end of 1869 in Calcutta and made a steady impact on mortality from cholera, dysentery, and diarrhea. Similar waterworks were introduced into other large Indian towns during the next few decades, especially after the 1890s when public-health engineers accepted that the spread of cholera was linked to water supplies (ibid:650). However, drainage systems were slower to improve and death rates in many towns rose after water supplies were improved as malaria, plague, and respiratory diseases flourished in the surplus water and polluted subsoil (ibid:651; see also chap. 3).

Under British rule, the population also became more mobile. People traveled by railway to fairs and religious festivals and were also transported some distance to work and often back again. Short-term movements probably increased the problems of controlling a number of communicable diseases, most notably cholera and plague. The most notable and sizable longer-term movement was of workers in the new tea estates of Assam and Darjeeling and, to a smaller extent, southern India. "Coolie labor" was hired in Chota Nagpur or other parts of central India, taken to Calcutta and thence upriver to Assam in conditions that ranged from little short of murderous in the 1860s and 1870s to merely hazardous by the 1920s (Griffiths 1968). On the estates themselves conditions were appalling, even by local standards, and mortality rates were high at least until the 1940s (Rege 1945). There were comparable losses of life in coal mining (another industry dependent on migrant labor in the early period). Mining and tea were the first industries in which the state insisted on the provision of adequate medical facilities, but there is little evidence that this reduced mortality before independence (GOI 1946).

ENVIRONMENTAL CHANGES INTRODUCED BY IMPERIALISM

The major impact of imperialism on the face of India came in the construction of roads and railways for communication and canals for irrigation. In each case the goal was at least partly developmental, though railway construction was also affected strongly by strategic considerations. In some parts of India these improvements increased agricultural production dramatically and made habitable some areas where previously a shortage of water or poor drainage had made cultivation impossible, as in the canal colonies of the Punjab or the Terai in the foothills of the Himalayas.

But canals and improved communications probably also had negative effects on health and population size—an early case of "development" diseases discussed by Hughes and Hunter (1970) for Africa, but first systematically described by C. A. Bentley between 1907 and 1925 (Klein 1972). Bentley, the director of public health for Bengal noted that some healthy environments of the early nineteenth century were infamous for being malarious by the end of the century. He argued that canals and roadworks obstructed normal surface drainage and that after the monsoon, stagnant pools were ideal for the breeding of mosquitoes. In addition, the labor gangs that constructed these works were a concentrated susceptible population large enough to take the disease with them as they moved on. For the United Provinces (UP) Klein suggests that the deterioration in water supply and drainage laid the foundations for the plague and cholera that ravaged the area in the latter part of the nineteenth century (ibid.). Indeed, as Whitcombe points out, canal construction in western UP was halted briefly in the early 1850s because it was accompanied by a dramatic increase in "fever." Although preventive measures were taken before starting again, for many years districts watered by the Upper Ganges Canal experienced higher mortality levels than neighboring unirrigated districts, probably because of waterlogging. These costs were not foreseen though they were increasingly understood, but the benefits of higher productivity seem to have outweighed the caution of those who stressed the costs of higher death rates.

The changing geography of malaria is the most striking example of a "development disease" in the Indian context. Malaria followed the canals into Punjab in the 1840s as well as in the later developments after 1890; it caused several districts in western and central Bengal and several districts in UP to lose population in the fifty years between 1871 and 1921. Most of these districts had some villages almost totally destroyed by the scourge. Klein (1972) summarizes this pattern as follows:

> The spectacle of a great swathe of territory, highly organised economically, traversed by modern communication, suffering no local wars, and experiencing an extremely high birth rate, yet remaining static in population, reveals compellingly the British inability to effect any dramatic change in the balance between life, economic conditions, and nature. (p. 13)

Apparently south India did not suffer in the same way. The canals in the Madras presidency were on a much smaller scale, with far less water-logging, and evidence of changes in the location of malaria is sparse. Population growth in the south may have been hindered more by emigration (to Ceylon, Burma, the West Indies, and Malaya) than by continuing high death rates.

Social Arrangements To Control Famines

Over and above general attempts to improve agriculture, especially through canal-building, the government of India and the provincial governments made various attempts to mitigate the impact of harvest failure: land revenue assessments could be reduced or set aside when crops failed (though the British may have been less willing to do this than were the Moguls); food grains were imported from surplus areas; and there were other attempts to minimize social disruption and maintain services. In addition, improved communications, especially the railways, helped provide market mechanisms that minimized the impact of food shortages. On the other side of the coin, in some areas pauperization, commercialization and increasing revenue demands from the state may have helped to generate the very problems which these provisions were supposed to mitigate.

Perhaps the most significant move was the use of public works as a famine relief measure. The poor were offered work at rates judged sufficient to sustain them until normal employment prospects returned or until their usual patrons were once again able to support them (Kynch 1985). Official policy limited the numbers and classes of people on relief works, restricting the beneficiaries to the "really" needy (Klein 1984; McAlpin 1983:178). The one major exception was the Bihar and Bengal famine of 1873, when local officials attempted to prevent all famine-related deaths; the cost of this attempt was the main argument used against a repetition (Klein 1984). In addition, varying degrees and quantities of gratuitous relief was provided to those unable to work, though governments were under pressure to limit their total expenditure and were wary of the "demoralizing" effects of charity. A third strand in famine relief was the granting of *takavi* loans with low interest and easy repayments, to allow peasants to employ labor on improvements to their farms (well-digging, etc.). But the government was generally unwilling to intervene in the market for grains, after the expense involved when this was done in 1873, though officials noted how the spread of railways tended to permit private marketing arrangements to reduce local shortages (McAlpin 1983:184–185).

The demographic consequences of these changes are uncertain. Davis estimates 19 million excess deaths in 1891–1901 because of famine by comparing actual population growth in the decade with the average growth of the 1880s and 1900s. However, official estimates of famine deaths in 1896–1901 (the famine years in this decade) were about 5 million. Even recalculating crude death rates to allow for underenumeration only raises this figure by a million or so (Davis 1951:39; Klein 1984:211–212). Sen's method of careful reconstruction of likely mortality has not apparently been applied to the famines of the 1870s and the 1890s, but McAlpin's figures for Bombay for 1891–1901 suggest that famine and plague together account for a population loss of about one million (in a total population of 15 million) with famine accounting for 80 percent of the reduction (1983:80). Since Bombay accounted for between 15 percent and 25 percent of the population affected by famine in this decade, Davis's estimate of 19 million deaths seems extreme. However, British officials generally underestimated the impact of famines by using a too early cut-off date and by ignoring the excess mortality in epidemics which followed most famines.

For Bombay, McAlpin (1983:218) produces the most positive account of the control of famines under imperial rule. She argues that by the end of the nineteenth century famines were indeed a result of abnormal weather conditions rather than pauperization resulting from British rule; and that government arrangements to prevent food-grain shortages, to encourage better transport and irrigation, and then to limit famine-related deaths are the most significant causes of this improvement. However, McAlpin's account ignores the possibility that the social changes under imperialism had weakened the entitlements of the poor, replacing them with a more bureaucratic (but not necessarily less capricious) safety net (Arnold 1985). If the experience of Bombay could be generalized, the famines of the late 1890s and the influenza epidemic and famine of 1919–1920 should be seen as abnormal disasters and should be separated analytically from the earlier ones.

Social Change Under the British

Much has been made in the British and European contexts of changes such as how often and how well people washed themselves, or of changes in human habitation patterns which meant a more distant relationship with animals and their diseases. What evidence is there of similar changes in India?

For rural areas we have very little information; what there is must be used with care, but it does not suggest major changes in living patterns of this kind. Cassen (1978) argues that Indian levels of personal hygiene were probably well above those of medieval Europe, but no one has attempted to assess what part changes in the kinds and prices of soap and its use might have played in mortality decline in India. Similarly for housing, Islam (1978:138), discussing the early twentieth century, notes that figures on occupied houses say nothing about their size, type, or use, but he assumes that fast population growth in a stagnant economy would entail considerable changes in the types of houses to cope with higher densities of population. However, he has no evidence for this claim nor suggestions for ways in which change took place.

Slightly more information is available for urban areas. As in Europe, towns have a reputation for being more unsanitary than rural areas and for having worse housing and diet. Mortality rates were probably higher in urban areas, despite their having a population concentrated in the "productive" age groups and relatively few females (Davis 1951). But differences between the urban and rural areas can be exaggerated. The residential densities of villages in some areas are nearly as high as those of urban slums, and rural slums can be as unsanitary as urban ones.

Overall, then, it is difficult to argue that British rule worsened living conditions by the creation of unregulated towns. Towns grew only slowly, depending mostly on immigration to do so. While they suffered high death rates and bad conditions, differences from the rural living conditions of most of their immigrants were probably minimal. Far from suggesting that urban conditions were bearable, this merely draws attention to the appalling conditions for the rural poor at the time. Since the contrasts in living styles between urban and rural areas are difficult to locate and evaluate, we probably cannot look to urbanization for any evidence of changes in patterns of living during the nineteenth and early twentieth century.

Conclusion

I started this chapter with the conundrum of a population rising because of declining death rates, when most estimates suggest not only no improvement in living standards but, indeed, a decline, caused in part by the rise in population itself. The answer seems to be that mortality decline has two elements: the underlying mortality rate, applying in normal years, and peaks of mortality in years when famine and epidemic diseases operated together.

The declining underlying mortality rate probably dates from the middle of the nineteenth century, and may be due to rising real incomes. The benefits provided by this higher standard of living were possibly sufficient to outweigh the income declines of the 1920s and 1930s. Furthermore, the consequences of the spread of malaria to new areas in north India began to peter out at the turn of the century. In addition, famine policies ensured a minimum income for the poor in times of scarcity, but these and other changes, such as the role of railways in moving grain, did not become fully developed until the last quarter of the nineteenth century. This probably helped reduce the mortality rate in peak years, except for the unusual late famines and epidemics of 1896–1901 and 1919–1920. The two processes working together help to explain why areas that were unaffected by these disasters saw unhindered population growth from the 1870s, within a national pattern of an increase in population growth rates from 0.3 percent or 0.4 percent per year in the nineteenth century, to 1 percent or 1.5 percent per year by the 1920s and 1930s.

I have not so far, however, considered the impact of social arrangements specifically designed to deal with health and disease which Davis (1951:38) believed controlled epidemic diseases at the same time that public disorder and famines were being brought under control. The next chapter, therefore, looks at the nature of so-called indigenous medicine, and assesses arguments suggesting that it lost its ability to contribute to the control of disease as a result of British rule. Chapters 3 and 4 will assess the medical services introduced by the British, and supposed (by colonial apologists) to have caused the decline of epidemic and other diseases.

CHAPTER TWO

Indigenous Medicine and The State Before 1947

Societies have many varieties of healing techniques, explanations of health and illness, and distributions of medical knowledge. The kinds of treatments, the classifications of diseases, and the forms of the division of medical labor are all subject to social and other forces that produce very different results in different parts of the world. These forms, and their historical development in particular, are imperfectly understood. Medical anthropologists give us some understanding of the links between medical and other symbolism, showing parallels, for example, between the structure of religious and medical belief systems and ways of distinguishing healers and their interrelationships; but similar evidence for the past is rarely available.

The major world literary medical traditions are those of Greece, India, and China—all from Eurasian cultural systems described (by Boserup 1970, and Goody 1976, among others) as complex stratified structures and radically different from African or tribal societies. Indeed, one defining characteristic of Eurasian societies is the development of literacy among the elite. Much medical history has been concerned only with the comparative assessment of these literary traditions. Most prominent have been attempts to decide which tradition borrowed from others, and which generated ideas; to assess which tradition has claims to "science," and decide how far core ideas spread.

Medical practice in a stratified society is also stratified as well as distributed along the kind of continua described by Leslie (1976). Healers may be located on a learned folk continuum and on a religious-secular dimension. During individual careers healers may move from one category to another and clientele relate in different ways to the different kinds of healers. The elite sector includes those serving the centers of economic and political power, and they characteristically join the "courts" of local, regional or national rulers. Rulers thus become patrons, with healers maintaining their positions by accommodating their advice to the demands of the patron, and defending their own positions at court by denigrating the claims of others (Johnson 1972). The writings of these healers have been collected and transmitted often by their students and families who have inherited their positions, but their picture of medical practice is inevitably restricted and partial. The healers whose names have survived are those who doctored rulers or perhaps were employed in academies (Ullmann 1978:49), and these men dismissed alternative healers as quacks or "cheats who wander about on the streets boasting in the garb of physicians" (Kutumbiah 1962:liii). Leslie (1976:3) argues that there was a complex reality of bone-setters, midwives, shamans, and so on, but he quotes no evidence to support his plausible view. Indeed, there is very little material available for the period before the mid-twentieth century.

For Indian medicine, two main literary traditions set a general context—*Ayurveda*, associated with Hinduism, written in Sanskrit, and practiced by vaids; and *Unani Tibb* ("the medicine of Greece"), associated with Muslims, written in Persian, Arabic, or Urdu and practiced by hakims. The major Ayurvedic sources consulted by historians of medicine have been the compilations of medical principles and therapies known as the Caraka-samhita and the Susruta-samhita; a third text (the Astanga-samhita, associated with Vagbhata) is sometimes added. Most commentators suggest that these texts took several centuries to emerge and received a fairly fixed form during the first 500 years A.D. For Unani medicine, *The Qanun* of Avicenna has been the main textbook, with commentaries and elaborations published in India in the thirteenth century A.D. and frequently reproduced and further elaborated (Ullmann 1978:52). These classic texts and the commentaries drawing on them are primarily concerned with diagnosis and treatment or to demonstrate an individual author's skill and breadth of learning.

Indicators of the social context within which medicine was practiced have to be winnowed very carefully from such sources. They can provide only tangential evidence on major questions, such as what treatments were available for different groups of the population and which kinds of practitioners provided them in what institutionalized ways.

I am less interested in the techniques of Ayurvedic or Unani physicians than with their social positions (and those of folk practitioners of various kinds) in Indian society from the early nineteenth century onward. Most healers, especially in the literate traditions, were probably male, but I will deal with female healers and women's access to medical care separately, including the impact of British rule on these practitioners. Since the "revival" of Ayurveda (and to a lesser extent, of Unani Tibb) after 1900, its supporters have claimed that its decline in status and scientific standing was due largely to its loss of official patronage under British rule. More recently, Banerjee (1974) has argued that village medicine was similarly destroyed when village economy and society collapsed under the impact of commercialization and alien rule. The validity of these arguments will be assessed in the conclusion of the chapter.

Indigenous Elite Medicine

Ayurvedic medical thought is based on the threefold humors, dosas or dhatus, often translated as wind, fire, and water or as wind, bile, and phlegm. Good health depends on balancing these humors, while disease is a result of imbalance. Castes, individuals, and regions may be dominated by different humors, as individuals may be at different stages of the life-cycle, different times of the day, and different seasons (Jolly 1977:49). Each humor comes in five forms, relating particularly to where it is found. Much diagnosis and treatment consists in determining which kinds of humor are in excess or are insufficient and in remedying this. For example, individual foods have their characteristic qualities, of which the most important are hotness and coldness, wetness and dryness. They can thus be used to counteract imbalances. Other remedies include bloodletting, inducing vomiting, using enemas, or taking in medicines by the nose or in the form of eyedrops. *Susruta* also contains sections describing surgical treatments.

The causes of humoral imbalances are manifold: errors in diet and excesses of everyday life—too much or too energetic sexual intercourse, anger, or exertion, for example. Diagnosis therefore involves investigating all possible causes in taking a history or making a medical examination. Pulse-taking is the most prominent diagnostic tool described. It may be taken in particular places for particular kinds of patients and the pulse's speed and many other characteristics are noted by the skilled practitioner. Prognosis is also important, since practitioners should not treat incurable patients, a position scorned by late-nineteenth century British doctors as unethical. The indicators often seem more mystical (depending on reading omens such as the time the physician is called and by what kind of messenger, etc.) than concerned with apparently practical concerns of etiology and diagnosis.

Hindu and Greek medicine have considerable similarities, and several authors have discussed how one might have derived from the other, or how they might have developed through mutual interaction (Banerjee 1981; Filliozat, 1964; Kutumbiah, 1962). After the seventh century A.D. Arab medicine provided an additional channel of communication and increasing contacts took place with the Chinese. From the twelfth century onward the Muslim invaders of north India brought their own physicians with them, and established secular healing traditions as well as healers associated with the shrines of Muslim saints. The spread of these healers and their typical practices is less well recorded than for Ayurveda, but ideas of humoral balance and interventions to restore and maintain this balance are not very different from those of the vaids. Probably the pharmacopoeia and the therapeutics of both Ayurveda and Unani Tibb changed through the interaction between them, during the Mogul Empire in particular (Metcalf 1985:5).

The final category of medicine often viewed as indigenous is homoeopathy, introduced by British and other European doctors in the course of the nineteenth century. It excited strong passions: the Bengal Medical Association was split by disputes over the reading of a homoeopathic paper. Homoeopathy seems to have appealed to the new urban elite as a "modern" system of medicine which nonetheless did not demand too great a break with traditional ideas, referring (as Hahnemann does) to vital forces and to moral powers (Bhardwaj 1973). How far Indian homopathic practitioners ever practiced a "pure" version of homoeopathy, or adapted to other dominant medical ideas, is unclear. By the 1960s many

homoeopaths merely used the correspondence training as a route
to registration, before using a variety of medical traditions in their
practice (Montgomery 1976).

The classic texts suggest no great restrictions on who might
study medicine:

> The science of life was to be studied by Brahmins, Kshatriyas and
> Vaisyas. Brahmins were to learn it for doing good to all creatures,
> Kshatriyas for self-preservation, and Vaisyas for gain. Susruta asserts that
> some say a Sudra of good family and character may be admitted as a
> pupil. (Kutumbiah 1962:xliv)

Apart from scattered references to monastic or university education in medicine, the study of medicine involved attachment to a
teacher as an apprentice resident in the teacher's household
(Kutumbiah 1962:xlix). This must have placed great pressure on
teachers to admit students of the same or a closely related caste so
as to circumvent difficulties in eating arrangements and other close
contacts. Perhaps for this reason different regions tended to have
dominant medical castes. Vaidyas, a *vaisya* caste, are dominant in
Bengal, but a Brahman subcaste provides most vaids in Kerala
(Zimmerman 1978). Education, according to the classic texts, involved several years memorizing and understanding a text as well
as practical experience before students would be permitted to establish an independent practice. Training in Unani medicine was
also carried out in the "personalistic, informal settings of family
homes and apprenticeship" (Metcalf 1985:4). Again, quite apart
from the need to learn Arabic, this tended to restrict Unani education to Muslims.

Successful practitioners were those who served successful rulers
and, either through regular service or because of some special healing act, were granted an area of land. These grants may have been
supposed to fund specifically medical activities—a dispensary or
a small medical school—or they may have been grants to the man
and his heirs, even if they ceased practicing medicine. On taking
over an area, the British tended to reappropriate these grants unless there were special circumstances. Leitner (1882:152–153) cam-
paigned on behalf of indigenous educational institutions in Punjab.
He mentions a family of hakims in Kalanaur who had previously
run a medical school but were reduced to a mere four or five private students when they lost their *jagir*, (government grant) and a

family of vaids in Amritsar who had lost their jagir but still ran a dispensary.

Not surprisingly, the Ayurvedic texts discuss appropriate behavior of practitioners toward their king. Basham (1976:31) suggests that serving a king would have been the highest ambition of an enterprising vaidya. Both Susruta and Caraka discuss the proper status of a vaid in a king's household, and set out what vaids owed their king (to work for his health and longevity and to refuse to treat those who hate the king or are hated by him) and what they were entitled to in return—protection from competition by quacks and charlatans (Wise, 1845:19).

WOMEN'S ACCESS TO ELITE MEDICINE

The historical accounts imply, as Leslie (1976:3) puts it, that "women were not educated in medicine," and "the perspective of the classic texts was masculine." Learning the secrets of the medical art required a high level of literacy in Sanskrit or Arabic and usually only males were supported in education long enough to acquire this. Apprentices to learned vaids or hakims were almost inevitably young men; and the accounts of practitioners are entirely about men, apart from isolated examples (one female vaid reported by Leitner [1882] in Ambala District, Punjab, for example). Some women were recorded in the early census volumes as vaids or hakims, but many of these were probably widows recorded under the occupations of their late husbands. When most of these cases were excluded (from 1901), the figures are probably contaminated by underenumeration of women whose work was shameful or only parttime. In later censuses the figures are contaminated by those who received training in the new institutions of modern medicine as nurses as well as doctors, and the social process of recording their occupations remains variable and opaque. The fascinating question of the extent to which the wives of indigenous practitioners were also practicing medicine (in association with their husbands or separately), is unanswered.

A subworld of female high-culture medicine may have existed, but it seems unlikely. How far, then, were male "learned" medical practitioners in India able to deal with "women's diseases"? Kutumbiah (1962) notes that the mythical Ayurveda (before the

main texts were written) apparently did not discuss either obstetrics or gynecology, and he infers that obstetrics was at that time
handled entirely by midwives because women would not readily
seek the help of physicians. Charaka and Susruta do include sections on childbirth but largely restrict themselves to instructions for
the preparation of the labor room. A Brahman should be present (to
carry out purificatory procedures) as well as experienced women
who are to act as midwives, but the role of a physician or surgeon
is not discussed. Chattopadhyaya (1977) argues that Ayurvedic
medicine could not throw off Brahmanic control, so the link between Ayurveda and childbirth was probably never strong.

Obstetrics might be a special case, because the impurity associated with childbirth made it an occupation suitable only for un-
clean women. Some parts of gynecology (such as disorders of
menstruation) might be similarly affected. Nonetheless, the classic
texts describe the diseases of menstrual flows and female organs.
But this evidence is inadequate on the role of physicians in actually treating female illnesses. We can say even less about the practice of Unani medicine (probably more widespread in much of
north India than Ayurveda). There may have been thriving male
practitioners whose clientele included substantial numbers of
women, but vaids and hakims have left very few accounts of their
clientele. Western commentators suggest that women from urban
households wealthy enough to consult hakims and vaids would not
do so in obstetric or gynecological cases. But Western observers
were biased and based their comments on cases where they had
been called in at very late stages in a disease.

Women's access to medical treatment was probably most affected
by purdah, or seclusion practices, which not only inhibits women's
access to the public sphere where their modesty might be com-
promised but also limits their access to cash and to legitimate
reasons for leaving their home. A graphic description of late-
nineteenth-century attitudes in north India is provided by Lala
Luchman Narain, who funded a midwifery class in Bareilly (UP)
in 1867: "It is considered indelicate and indecent by us to allow
a doctor to look into a woman's private parts: most of us would
rather let their dear wives and daughters die than allow them to be
examined by a male" (NAI Home, Public 1872:266–267A). Thus
purdah probably seriously restricted the access of "respectable"
women to medical care; male practitioners could diagnose and treat
them only at a distance. However, this may have excluded rela-

tively few traditional diagnostic techniques. Poverty, high fees, distance, and so on, were more important barriers for the great majority of women. Probably only female practitioners would be approached with any ease by women, but this is the category we know least about.

Folk Medicine

Leslie distinguishes between folk healing (bonesetters, snakebite healers, and so on, usually part-time), popular-culture medicine (using patent drugs, popular astrology, and religion, as well as modern science), and homoeopathy, which has, in Bhardwaj's (1973) term, become "naturalized" in India. But these distinctions break down when faced with individuals and groups which not only straddle these categories but also merge into the learned categories, whether indigenous or Western, religious or secular. Thus, as early as 1839 an Indian observer in Bombay described "English doctors" who were from families of vaids but administered English medicine—with no formal education (Leslie 1974:97). Historical data on the numbers involved, categories, patterns of recruitment and careers, are unavailable; these men are almost always dismissed as quacks or charlatans, and serious investigations of their activities are a post-independence phenomenon.

If the census can be believed, most of the female medical personnel were midwives (dais). (For more elaboration on the material in this section, see Jeffery, Jeffery, and Lyon 1985.) Reports about dais appear in official documents in the later part of the nineteenth century, all arguing that the dai was always an illiterate, usually middle-aged or old woman, whose only qualification was her experience. Furthermore, because of the pollution associated with childbirth, dais were predominantly drawn from the untouchable castes. British doctors were adamant that dais, even those prepared to take courses in what passed at the time for modern midwifery, were a danger to their clients, and the records abound in comments on their lack of intelligence, their dirty habits, and their inability to learn new methods.

This evidence about the quality of midwifery is, of course, an inadequate basis for generalization, but it represents almost the only kind available. We do not know the extent to which the dai offered additional services, such as abortions, advice and treatments on menstrual problems, massage, or any other similar services for reproductive disorders. Nor do we know much about the efficacy of their services. However, three arguments can be made. One view is that women's knowledge and referral systems by their very nature would escape historical inquiry, and that oral traditions can develop valuable skills. A second argument would be that the women involved were drawn from such disadvantaged castes, and themselves regarded midwifery as so dirty, that it would be surprising if women took up the occupation willingly, or if they were capable of developing a strong chain for transmitting skills handed down by mothers or mothers-in-law. A third argument (arguably the most plausible) is that female healers in stratified societies are likely to be diverse, and more sophisticated support would be available to wealthier women than to the rest.

None of these arguments, of course, leads to the conclusion that women generally suffered and died without any assistance. The real issue is the extent of their access to public sources of medical advice and the quality of the advice they were able to receive. Household medicines are not insignificant resources, but men and women alike had access to these household remedies whereas men also had much better access to the public sphere when home remedies were felt to be inadequate.

The Impact of British Rule on Indigenous Medicine

BRITISH MEDICAL POLICY

We can only talk sensibly about British policy toward indigenous medicine after 1800. The main aims of the East India Company were trade and later the collection of land revenue. Policy in a wider sense only developed when the company realized that it had to govern increasing numbers of people as a result of its expanding territorial control. However, the actions of some of its employees give some evidence of direct impact on indigenous medicine before 1800. First, some company officials consulted indigenous healers; Crawford (1914) notes a general view in the late-seventeenth century among British officials that local diseases were best taken to local doctors. Second, European doctors were employed as consultants by some members of the Indian elite, either displacing or competing with indigenous healers. Third, some Indians were given training in European medicine either as part of a deliberate expansion in medical services for the army or more informally. Thus "native" doctors attended informal classes at the civil hospital in Calcutta at the end of the eighteenth century (Leslie 1976).

Each of these elements continued into the nineteenth century. In 1814 the Court of Directors in London encouraged its employees to investigate the value of local medicines and medical texts (B. D. Basu 1936:11). The informal training scheme at Calcutta was established on much more substantial grounds in 1822, as a Native Medical Institution (NMI), teaching indigenous and European medicine. The Muslim Madrassa and the Hindu Sanskrit College (both established with European patronage) had already incorporated some European medicine and anatomy into their courses.

These processes of mutual involvement, however, were disrupted by the change in policy in 1835. Macaulay's *Minute* on educational policy argued that European culture should provide the curriculum of schools and colleges. This strengthened opposition to schemes that attempted to mix European and Indian cultures or aimed to restore Indian culture to its presumed glory. The NMI ceased teaching Ayurveda and Unani Tibb. The whole institution was remodeled as a medical school, teaching only European science, for a brief time in English only. In addition, the Bengal government increased its efforts to prevent the local practice of inoculation against smallpox and to insist on the European craft of vaccination (Arnold 1985).

This shift to an exclusion of indigenous medicine did not mean a total ban on its inclusion in government-sponsored education nor on cooperative relationships between the British Raj and indigenous practitioners. As Hume (1977) has demonstrated, for example, in Punjab the provincial government employed hakims in the 1860s and 1870s, usually as vaccinators and health extension workers. The Lahore Medical College taught some hakims and vaids as part of the courses in Ayurveda based in the Dayanand Anglo-Vedic College, and Unani Tibb at the Islamia College, from 1887–1898; the University of the Punjab continued to validate these courses until 1907, when there were very few students (see also, NAI [EHL] 1919; July:26–51 A).

One reason the state displayed tolerance is that its own services

reached a very small section of the population, and very few practitioners had been fully trained in its medical schools and colleges
before the end of the nineteenth century. The 1872 census of Bengal, for example, listed only 3,769 physicians, surgeons, and doctors, but over 24,000 "Gobaidyas" and "Kabirajes" (vaids) and
"hakeems"; and the 1871 census of Madras reported very few Indian doctors trained in European medicine in private practice in
the city. Even in the 1880s, the medical bureaucrats were aware of
the strength of the indigenous groups and plans to introduce medical registration were dropped because graduates from government
colleges and schools were thought to be too weak politically to
overcome the expected hostility from vaids and hakims (Seal 1968).

Medical bureaucrats became more self-confidently hostile to indigenous medicine at the turn of the nineteenth century. The cream
of Western doctors in India—the IMS—was more conscious of its
claims to scientific legitimacy. The number of Indian medical
graduates and licence holders was substantial and they were offering a real challenge to the primacy of indigenous healers in the
major towns, while the growth of a new Indian middle class
provided new financial opportunities for both groups (Jeffery
1979). At the end of World War I medical advisers to the provincial governments asserted that the Indian systems of medicine were
archaic, incapable of advance, and based on unsound principles.
As one put it:

> there is no reason to run away from a frank declaration of our convic-
> tion that Western science includes all that is of any value in the
> Ayurvedic and Unani systems; that it is progressive where they are sta-
> tionary; and that its popularity and prestige are continually on the in-
> crease. (NAI [EHL] 1919; July:26–51 A)

Most of these administrative doctors equated the Indian systems
with quackery and imposture, but they appreciated the political
reasons it could not be said. The director-general of the IMS noted
that the indigenous systems were relatively cheap, with low fees
and low-cost education; but this would not justify diverting funds
from "scientific medicine." However, he recognized the nationalists' support for these systems and argued that their view that the
only reason for the decline of the Indian systems was the effect of
European rule, should be countered by asserting the greater efficacy

of Western medicine (ibid.). But the imperial government was not united in its views. Some of its members wanted to maximize the distance between themselves and the "superstitious mumbo-jumbo" of indigenous medicine. Others, however, lent their prestige to new private medical schools, some of which combined indigenous and Western techniques in integrated courses, in order to "raise" the standard of indigenous medical techniques. In 1916, Sir Pardey Lukis, director-general of the IMS from 1911–1917, spoke on behalf of the government of India:

> The improvement of the training of hakims and vaids is a part of the present policy of Government . . . [because] . . . for many years to come, they will constitute the medical attendants of by far the largest portion of the Indian community. (NAI [EHL] 1919; July:26–51)

In pursuit of this policy, the viceroy opened the "integrated" Unani Tibbia College in Delhi in 1916, perhaps as a sop to the college's founder, Hakim Ajmal Khan, a leading Muslim politician (Metcalfe 1985:7–8). Other requests for symbolic or financial support to indigenous medicine were turned down (NAI [EHL] 1919; July, 26–51A).

The position of vaids and hakims, however, was simultaneously being threatened by Medical Registration Acts, passed in all the provinces between 1912 and 1919, and by a Medical Degrees Act, restricting the use of the title "Doctor." In part these were aimed at private Western-style and homoeopathic medical colleges that had been established in Bengal in the early years of the century. But they also threatened the "integrated" training of indigenous practitioners since Western doctors who collaborated with indigenous practitioners, either in the new colleges or in daily practice, offended the imported British ethical codes and were threatened with deregistration (Steinthal 1984).

The political balance was tipped back slightly toward the indigenous practitioners by the Montagu-Chelmsford reforms of 1919. Nationalist politicians could now implement policies over the opposition of their medical advisers. The British expected the Indian ministers of health and education to try to support indigenous medicine, since the Indian National Congress had begun to pass resolutions in its support. Ayurvedic revivalists tried to reform Ayurveda by bringing up-to-date its use of basic science and its institutional base. Ayurvedic medical colleges and hospitals were established and courses in anatomy and physiology were added to traditional subjects, such as the study of classic texts. They then claimed that historical Ayurveda was superior both to present-day practice and to Western medicine. In 1907 the revivalists established a national representative body called the All-India Ayurveda Mahasammelan, and soon afterward Hakim Ajmal Khan became a prominent leader of hakims on the national political stage. By 1920 both groups were involved in Congress, but modernizers like Nehru supported the spread of Western scientific medicine and Western-style doctors also joined Congress, some (like Dr. M. A. Ansari) rising to senior positions (Brass 1972; Croizier 1972). Congress and non-Congress parties never committed themselves exclusively to one side or the other, as became clear during the 1920s.

The new legislative councils supported "Indian" systems of medicine on both patriotic and economy grounds. However, the ministers were limited by severe financial restrictions, and their impact was further reduced by the IMS, with the support of the British Medical Association, the General Medical Council, and the medical advisers to the India Office in London. Some ministers (in Punjab and Bombay, for example) resisted nationalist pressures and used their limited funds to attempt to bring "modern scientific medicine and surgery within reasonable reach of all," spending only small sums for research into the indigenous systems and for improved training (Indian Statutory Commission, 1928:256–267). As a result, relatively few indigenous medical colleges were given state patronage, the schemes of medical registration continued to exclude those who had not received Western medical training, and the government of India restricted its activities to an investigation into the pharmacopoeia of indigenous drugs.

For a while indigenous practitioners were able to count on support (or at least the absence of overt hostility) from Indian Western-style doctors. When the Indian Medical Association was established in 1928 the early leaders, also prominent in nationalist politics, called for the admission of indigenous practitioners (if they were "sincere") and for a medical registration system which could include them. However, in the course of the dispute over the creation of an all-India medical council, it became clear that international recognition of Indian medical degrees by the General

Medical Council in London depended on a very clear distinction between Western doctors and the rest (Jeffery 1979). By the mid-1930s many of these leaders withdrew their support for indigenous medicine and took up positions in the new Indian Medical Council which excluded indigenous practitioners. Trained indigenous practitioners were first registered in Bombay in 1938 on an entirely separate register.

THE IMPACT OF MORE GENERAL CHANGES

Before 1860 the main impact of British rule on elite indigenous medicine came through the disruption and eventual disintegration of the ruling groups and their courtly life. The most successful indigenous healers would have earned substantial sums and been rewarded by the grant of land rights. The British greatly reduced the size and income of the ruling groups, and elite practitioners suffered along with other occupations dependent on them. In addition, competition from European doctors might also have affected their position. In the nineteenth century indigenous practitioners received little if any patronage from the British rulers, so their position probably declined substantially.

In the period from about 1860 to 1920 the loss of elite patronage was steadily redressed by the growing middle-class market for medical services. Indigenous healers held their own against competition in this market from Western-style doctors, European and Indian. The growth of this market provided the financial support for moves to institutionalize training and provide a clearer pattern of requirements and standards. The elite medical system began to emulate aspects of Western medicine, not merely because the British institutions had higher prestige and state backing but also because market conditions for indigenous medicine permitted this kind of occupational organization (Johnson 1972).

The interwar period showed gains and losses for indigenous practitioners. New colleges began to replace apprenticeship arrangements and several were well funded, especially in Delhi, Madras, and the princely states of Mysore and Hyderabad. Indigenous practitioners also received symbolic support, on the one hand, from special government committees set up to consider policy toward them (summarized in the Chopra Committee Report of 1948). On the other hand, their subordinate position relative to cosmopolitan medicine was reinforced by registration patterns, withdrawal of Western doctors from integrated colleges, and limited patronage from Indian ministers of health. Western-style doctors were trained in increasing numbers, and they formed a much more serious source of competition in private practice in the towns, as well as through a broadening of government medical services.

The position of folk healers probably fluctuated more closely with local economic conditions, benefiting from increasing commercialization when the new settled order led to an expansion of output, and suffering when enhanced revenue demands reduced the surplus held locally. When agricultural incomes, generally, rose (as they probably did in the period after 1860), folk practitioners are unlikely to have suffered. But we have no accounts of changes in the positions, numbers, or types of these kinds of practitioners during British rule.

Two points seem crucial in assessing how the positions of these groups might have changed. First, whatever happened to the village economy (i.e., whether or not there was polarization), their traditional clientele would have remained, providing either the small payments by large numbers of the relatively poor, or the more substantial fees of the landed peasantry. Second, folk practitioners had few competitors. Thus few villages had resident allopathic practitioners before independence or easy access to towns where they were available. The increasing numbers of commercial sources of drugs and other remedies were distributed as much through these practitioners as by their allopathic competitors, and village practitioners seem to have needed a social base within the village to be successful. Any claim that the condition of these male folk practitioners was undercut by British rule must remain, at best, not proven.

In the case of the dais, the state attempted to train them in better techniques and to involve them in the provision of maternity services. However, state training was so limited that it probably made no difference to the quality of care provided at most births, nor is there any evidence that these schemes (or any other changes introduced by colonialism) directly or indirectly undermined or weakened this particular female tradition.

The Decline of Indigenous Medicine

The average social position of the elite vaids and hakims probably deteriorated during British rule, but this does not necessarily mean that the care and services offered also declined or became less "scientific," as the revivalists claimed. I am not here concerned with the arguments about science (see Leslie 1972; Chattopadhyaya 1977; Brass, 1972), but with three plausible reasons for their social decline: the disunity of indigenous practitioners; the active policy of the state; and the perception by clients that indigenous treatments were less effective than Western alternatives.

The weakness of indigenous practitioners as a group was partly due to their own internal divisions. The two main categories were separated by linguistic, theoretical, and religious differences, and the newer group of homoeopaths, strong in Calcutta and Bengal, were uneasy allies. As politics became more communally based in the 1930s, vaids and hakims found it increasingly difficult to act together. Tendencies within each section also led to divisions. Each elite group had a variety of career patterns, usually locally specific, with little agreement about diagnosis or techniques. Often a noted local teacher would prepare his own commentary on traditional texts, and the school that grew up around one teacher would deride and vilify that around another (Leslie 1968:412). In addition, the professionalization of elite groups encouraged them to distance themselves from the others—the folk practitioners or partly trained Unani and Ayurvedic healers. Finally, an ideological split grew between those who wanted integrated teaching of cosmopolitan science and indigenous therapeutics, and those who considered pure indigenous training sufficiently scientific; it was a split that dominated post-Independence debates (Brass 1972).

The modernizing nationalists used one main argument to attack British rule and to defend their own position: that the withdrawal of patronage by the ruling classes led to a decline in the scientific level of most Indian healers. As Leslie (1972) notes, the British were not consistently hostile until the end of the nineteenth century. In the princely states indigenous medicine was not noticeably more "scientific" despite the continuance of patronage. However, elite practitioners depended on small groups of patrons, and the loss of patronage would have had a considerable impact on practitioners' ability to maintain their traditions—which included a large household of students or assistants, substantial fees from a relatively small number of clients, and a generally "cultured" lifestyle. Such establishments may have been necessary for the maintenance of the full range of herbs and more sophisticated treatments. Many British doctors in the late nineteenth and early twentieth century were virulently hostile to healers who had such a position in the major cities, but this hostility suggests the strength of such healers rather than their weakness.

The efficacy of these sources of medical or semimedical advice is difficult to assess. While one can argue that India's high morbidity and mortality rates mean that indigenous treatments were not very powerful, no medical treatments would have made much difference since mortality rates were so closely linked to poverty, famine, and the environment. I do not believe that patients began to use Western medical facilities because they were demonstrably better (though Western doctors always claim this). They were used because they were there, and they seemed to work sometimes. But if efficacy is judged in social terms—whether the ceremony works to reintegrate a society and help patients and their families cope with disaster—the only plausible indicators of efficacy are consultation rates themselves, which makes the argument circular.

British rule thus had a complex impact on indigenous medicine. Elite practitioners probably suffered most through a loss of patronage and the associated status they used to derive from servicing the courts. A decline in their social status may well have affected the more general efficacy of their practice. The impact on the folk sector is more difficult to assess. Most arguments (such as those of Banerji 1974) tend to shade into those about the general impact of British rule in the absence of specific evidence about any impact on healers. We do not know how many folk healers there were before 1800, in which categories they fit; how they earned their living; how they were recruited; and how well they lived. We know very little more about their condition in 1947.

CHAPTER THREE

The Indian Medical Service
and Health Expenditure

> The peaceful and civilising influence of the work done in
> the dispensaries and by regimental surgeons on the front-
> iers of India has been in political importance equivalent to
> the presence of some thousands of bayonets. . . . It is be-
> cause of such unexpected philanthropy that, as conquerors,
> we hold a position in the minds of the people which would
> not otherwise be possible. (General Sir Neville Chamberlain
> in 1887, cited by Crawford 1914:134–135)

The provision of modern health services is fundamen-
tal to those arguments that stress the benefits of British rule in India. Indeed, some authors have considered these services critical
to the decline in mortality after 1921. However, such claims are not
based on detailed examination of actual health-service provision,
for which social groups, at what cost, and with what likely effect.
Moreover, little attention has been paid to the principles apparently
underpinning health policy, indicated either by statements of intention or by patterns of expenditure and provision.

The chief architects of medical policy were the doctors, all male,
of the IMS, which was primarily a military service, maintaining the
health of the fighting forces. It also provided services for European
civil and military servants to help maintain their morale and their
strength in a hostile environment. In addition, health provisions for
the masses were used (in Punjab, for example, as quoted above) to
forestall and respond to demands for some tangible benefits of British rule. The second underlying principle was the desire to spread
"enlightenment," or scientific medicine, as a virtue in its own
right. The third source of dynamism was charity, a part of "mus-
cular Christianity." But these latter two pressures were subordinate

to the structural imperatives of imperial rule: maintenance of order
and revenue. Only when this straitjacket was loosened by nationalist politics and more democratic institutions was a serious effort
made to expand services, but this was hamstrung by new imperatives for the protection of capitalism in Britain and in India—
financial controls retained by the imperial government and reinforced by austerity measures intended to cope with the interwar
depression.

The Indian Medical Service

The origins of the IMS were humble in the extreme
and lie in the provision of ship's surgeons by the East India Company on its vessels bound for India. By 1614 the company had a
surgeon-general who chose, instructed, and equipped men as surgeons until 1644, in spite of frequent complaints that he was corrupt and sent untrained men on the ships (Crawford 1914, Vol. I,
chap. 3). Men were employed to work on one particular ship for
one voyage; later, some doctors were asked to remain in India at
one of the company's warehouses if there was a special request
from the merchants (ibid., chap. 6). By the 1670s, surgeons were
hired expressly for service in India, and over the following century,
the numbers of medical men employed by the East India Company
to tend to their civil employees increased steadily. By 1749, when
the company started to recruit doctors for its new standing army,
it knew of thirty medical men in India.

As the numbers of medical officers grew, a bureaucratic structure
was established in India to organize recruitment and to create a hierarchy of appointments. The civil posts, especially those in the
three presidency towns of Bombay, Calcutta, and Madras, were
reserved for senior doctors, but all were liable for recall to military
employment if the need arose. In 1763 the Bengal Medical Service
was established with 12 full surgeons and 28 mates, but by 1783
the number had risen to 140 (ibid., chap. 14). Surgeons in Madras
numbered 15 in 1767, with 13 assistants, and by 1784 the establishment had risen to 30 full surgeons and 19 assistants. Bombay had
27 members of the Medical Service in 1779. These relatively small
establishments expanded dramatically over the following forty
years, through local recruitment of Europeans and Eurasians, and

by recruitment in Britain. In 1823, 630 officers held covenants (commissioned posts) in the medical departments of the three presidencies. The number of medical officers remained around that level until World War I though the sources are neither complete nor entirely comparable. The complexity of employment patterns is indicated in a survey of staff in northern India in 1876. In Bengal, the North-West Provinces, Punjab, Oudh, Central Provinces, British Burma, and Assam, 229 medical officers were in civil employ (twelve of whom were military doctors holding "collateral charge" of the civil station where they were posted). At least fifty-six were not actually covenanted IMS officers but retired doctors or temporary or warrant officers. These 229 controlled a staff of 245 assistant surgeons and 1,131 "hospital assistants," which included 92 "native" doctors and six so-called passed medical pupils (Papers Showing Progress of Education 1881).

The bureaucratic nature of the service was reinforced by several changes during the first half of the nineteenth century. Medical boards were established between 1785 and 1787, consisting of the two or three most senior surgeons in each presidency, who controlled appointments, discipline, and general policy. Over the next seventy years attempts were made to improve the system's efficiency and to reduce conflicts among its members. In spite of formal commitments to make appointments to the board on merit, whenever the most senior surgeon was not appointed controversy ensued. By the 1820s fixed lengths of tenure were introduced. But Dalhousie, governor-general from 1848 to 1856, was dissatisfied with the state of the service and, on leaving office, he made some recommendations that were followed over the next few years. In particular, the medical boards, with their unclear precedence and responsibilities, were abolished and replaced with posts of director-general in each presidency, assisted by inspector-generals.

Until the 1850s, it was not necessary to have any medical competence or to work mostly in medical activity to be employed as a surgeon. A man's claim to competence was not necessarily investigated, and surgeons who had served on several journeys were allowed to continue even if they had originally been hired in dubious circumstances. Since posts were commissioned, they depended on nomination by a director of the East India Company in London, which was either expensive (the sale of nominations undoubtedly occurred) or required some personal link, thus limiting recruitment to the relatively well-to-do. Not until 1809 was the purchase of appointments made an offense. The directors were unwilling to allow recruitment in India to permanent contracts because they did not want to lose the right of nomination; this made it difficult to expand medical services rapidly during local wars. Nevertheless, local appointments were made, including of men who had served some kind of apprenticeship in the company's hospitals in India.

As medical services expanded and a clear hierarchy was established, more formal arrangements were made to examine the men appointed as surgeons. In London an examining board for the company was appointed in 1773, and in the 1760s and 1770s the Bengal and Madras governments resolved that all assistant surgeons be examined on appointment, though they could not reject men duly appointed by the directors in London. The London Corporation of Surgeons and its successor bodies granted certificates of competence which were a basic qualification for service with the company from 1745 onward, but the first clear statement of regulations for admission date from 1822. The first competitive examinations for entry to the IMS were held in 1855 and continued (with a break of five years from 1860 to 1865) until after World War I.

One attraction of service in India was the income that could be made outside the formal job of surgeon to the company. Surgeons' pay was not high relative to that of the other civil appointments, and the surgeons had to find other ways to supplement their incomes if they were to retire handsomely to Britain. In company hospitals in the eighteenth-century soldiers had to pay for hospital services, and surgeons were paid for each patient they treated over and above their salary. They had private medical practice, probably treating mainly nonofficial Europeans and the families of officials, but also including "native gentlemen" or members of the Mogul or other Indian courts.

Nonmedical work was also potentially lucrative. The range of nonmedical work included holding other positions (notably that of postmaster) in the early nineteenth century. Several surgeons made (and sometimes lost) small fortunes in banking, trade, or land ownership and management. IMS officers in military posts were barred from commercial speculation in 1824, but as late as 1838 a leading surgeon took it for granted that surgeons in civil posts would spend a large part of their time in commercial activities. In 1841 the surgeons in civil posts were also barred, though it took at least ten years before the prohibition was enforced (Crawford: ch. 25).

Officers in the IMS bore military rank and could serve as regimental surgeons or in civilian positions. Toward the end of the nineteenth century a new recruit to the medical service usually spent at least the first two years as a subordinate doctor with a regiment or in an army hospital. The rest of his career would involve moves into and out of military service, depending on choice and the posts available. Officers were liable to recall from civil duties if the army required them, but from the Mutiny until 1914 this power was rarely used.

The tension between civil duties and military obligations resulted in various schemes for the division of the civil and military services or the amalgamation of the Army Medical Department (for British troops) and the IMS (for European and "native" soldiers employed by the government of India). From the first time that the issue was seriously discussed (in 1766) to the last (in 1935) the considerations remained the same, even though the work required of the two parts of the IMS varied considerably during this period. The primary concern was to have European medical officers in case of war; the secondary concern was to ensure that recruitment of Europeans to the "ruling" services—the Indian civil service, the police, and the army—would not be inhibited by the absence of European medical advice, especially for service wives.

The first concern required enough doctors in India for calling up at short notice. In India, authorities were convinced of the need to provide the war reserve by having far more doctors under their control than was needed for normal military work in peacetime. But the only way to employ such doctors and to make the service attractive was to allow them civil opportunities. Before the 1840s and 1850s, civil work was reckoned to be less medical than commercial or administrative, and medical experience was to be found primarily in military work. In the latter part of the century the balance swung the other way and the civil work included the management of district, police, and jail hospitals, provision of medico-legal services, the organization of vaccination and other sanitary work, and the superintendence of the local jail (Crawford 1914, I: 293–294) as well as private medical practice to supplement the various sources of official income. Not surprisingly, most doctors applied for a transfer to civil employment as soon as possible and looked forward to steady progression through the more distant districts up to provincial headquarters or into clinical positions in the medical colleges and schools.

Nationalist critics of the IMS latched onto its military nature; the numbers of doctors transferred to civil duties reflected the state of military, and not civil, needs. Recruits had to meet military standards (for example, as horse riders). This became important politically after World War I, when the balance between European and Indian doctors on each side became a delicate issue. Furthermore, the careers of individual doctors might be seriously upset by military concerns: Ronald Ross's researches into the role of mosquitoes in the spread of malaria were interrupted by postings away from his laboratory. However, this was a general feature of official employment and not confined to the military. Thus, in looking for the limitations of the IMS, its character as handmaiden to the imperial state (as an inducement to recruits to the other services) and the orientation characteristic of Western medicine in general at this time are more important than its military origins or hierarchy. Most members of the IMS saw their careers in terms of access to lucrative private practices, and providing medical care to the imperial services as a prime function; it would be surprising if such men took public health or sanitary reform very seriously.

By 1860, then, India's Medical Service had most of the characteristics of a formal bureaucracy. Appointments were made on merit, and the examinations were open to Indians as well as Europeans. However, because examinations were held only in London, access by Indian candidates was restricted and only 55 had entered by 1913. Several early Indian recruits resigned after a short career, some of them feeling unwelcome among other members of the IMS or among other officers—a criticism increasingly voiced during the 1920s and 1930s. At least for European doctors though, promotions were based on seniority. Positions were well defined and were expected to take up most of the time of the employee, whose recompense was largely fixed in the form of a regular salary though it could still be supplemented by private medical practice, especially in the larger towns. By this time, too, as chapter 4 demonstrates, the responsibilities of the members of the IMS were much broader than merely the treatment of sick employees of the Crown.

The changing nature of the IMS in this period can be gleaned from the summaries of qualifications and medical schools attended provided in Crawford's *Roll of the Indian Medical Service*. In the early years, the men who reached the top (usually with few formal qualifications) often remained for many years. By the 1860s seniority rules and promotion to higher positions partly by qualification, meant that senior men occupied the top positions for only a few years before retiring. As the century went on more top positions were created, as new provinces were established, sanitary commissioner posts were added to those of inspectors-general of hospitals; and posts of professor at the major medical colleges were regarded as of equal status. The character of the IMS thus changed quite substantially.

The impact of changing patterns of medical education in Britain after about 1820 is fairly clear, though complicated by lack of information on the earlier recruits and by the years used by Crawford for grouping his data. Before 1800 at least half the recruits had no qualification at all, and only 6 percent are known to have attended a medical school. From 1800 to 1860 most recruits had a diploma from the Royal College of Surgeons in London, usually gained before joining the service, but sometimes acquired during leave in England; one in six had an Edinburgh degree. After 1860 London medical schools provided at least one-third of all recruits, another 30 percent had been to the Scottish universities and 17 percent attended an Irish school. In addition, after joining the service recruits acquired a wide range of degrees and diplomas, including those given by the Indian universities.

The social origins of recruits also changed. In the first half of the nineteenth century one-third of all recruits were born in Scotland, one-third in England, and nearly 10 percent in India (with European surnames). In the last half of the century the Irish-born recruits (22 percent) outnumbered the Scots (18 percent), the share of the English-born remained about 30 percent, but 25 percent of recruits were born in India, including 6 percent with Indian names (Crawford 1930:648–649). Throughout this period, for those where information is available, roughly one in six were the sons of doctors, one in seven the sons of clergymen, and the rest largely drawn from the military, other professions, business and trade, or from the land (13 percent) (Crawford 1913, II:650–651). Other information on the backgrounds of recruits is very limited.

Unfortunately, we do not know whether recruits to the IMS differed from those who established themselves in Great Britain in practice or joined the growing Poor Law medical service. In the later nineteenth century, service in India was apparently preferable to service with the British army, since those qualifying in the common competitive examinations chose the Indian Medical Service over the Army Medical Department when they had a choice. This probably reflected the attractions of private-practice possibilities in India that were unavailable to doctors serving in the British army or navy (ibid., II:527–529).

A final indicator of changes in the IMS is in the "hazards of membership." For those recruited before 1838 for whom information is available, more than half had their careers ended by death (usually from disease) or by illness; another 10 percent or so resigned or were dismissed, and only one-third or less reached normal retirement age still in service. For those recruited in 1839–1860, half retired in the normal way, and two-thirds of those recruited in the thirty years after 1865 reached fifty-five or fifty-eight and retired (table 4).

The IMS declined during the twentieth century as opportunities in India became less attractive and employment prospects in Britain improved. The government was pressed by nationalists and their supporters to open the civil posts of the IMS to the independent medical profession—those trained in the Indian medical colleges and schools who had not taken up official employment. In 1907 more Indians were drawn into the management of the Indian government with recruitments to the imperial councils under the Morley-Minto reforms. Although fierce rearguard actions were fought in India and in London to reduce the impact of these changes, they created a climate of uncertainty about long-term prospects. In addition, recruitment of doctors for India was hit by the competition of improved health insurance schemes in Britain. The number of British applicants to join the IMS fell very rapidly.

Then the overall size of the IMS declined after 1919. The number of senior medical positions it held by right was steadily reduced as a result of the devolution of power to elected ministries in the provinces. The proportion of its recruits who were Indian rose. In 1913 only 5 percent of the service was Indian, but during World War I considerable numbers were inducted on temporary commissions and stayed on afterward. A minimum quota for Indian recruits was established in 1919, and by 1938 their share had risen to 37 percent of the civil posts. A more important reason for this

TABLE 4
ANALYSIS OF "FINAL RESULTS"

"Final result"	Year of recruitment				
	1652– 1763 %	1764– 1800 %	1801– 1838 %	1839– 1860 %	1865– 1896 %
A. Service ended by death or injury					
Killed in action	3.0	1.0	1.2	2.2	0.4
Suicide or violent death	1.4	2.0	1.1	0.7	2.5
Died while serving	49.8	59.7	51.8	40.2	24.5
Invalided out	0.0	1.7	1.9	0.3	0.7
TOTAL GROUP A	54.2	64.4	56.0	43.4	28.1
B. Resigned or dismissed					
Resigned	12.8	3.7	2.7	4.1	3.3
Dismissed, etc.	7.3	6.2	6.2	3.0	0.7
TOTAL GROUP B	20.1	9.9	8.9	7.1	4.0
C. Retired	25.7	25.7	34.7	49.5	67.0
TOTAL KNOWN CASES (N)	(240)	(784)	(1639)	(1108)	(991)
Unknown (N)	(119)	(88)	(7)	(0)	(0)

SOURCE: A reworking of the analysis in Crawford (1930:652–653).

rise was a shortage of European applicants. The threatened loss of some of the senior posts under the 1919 reforms was a major reason for the problems of recruitment of Europeans to the IMS after World War I. The main drawback of this situation as the Indian government saw it, was the likely deleterious effect on European recruitment to key military and civil services. Europeans were unwilling to serve in small district towns if the only medical advice available for their wives was from an Indian doctor (Jeffery 1979). The IMS, then, was easily cast as a willing accomplice in attempts to retain European control over medicine as part of wider imperial concerns: as an "imperial" service, the IMS remained under the control of the government of India, not the provincial governments

which might be controlled by nationalists. The consequent un-
popularity of the IMS in nationalist political circles undoubtedly
accounted for the decision in 1947 to abolish it as an independent
service, and to give local governments in independent India full
control over their medical civil servants.

The history of the IMS, then, can be viewed in three stages. Prior
to 1860, the service was organized in an ad hoc way, recruiting its
members (some with very little medical training) from a range of
backgrounds. Its formal organization was unclear and the careers
of its members were as much nonmedical (in trade, etc.) as medical. This pattern changed around the middle of the century, as
medical training was institutionalized in Great Britain and recruitment depended on recognized medical qualifications. The organization became highly bureaucratic and its members increasingly
self-confident about their medical abilities and concerned to spread
their knowledge and services to the Indian population. This pattern gave way at the beginning of the twentieth century, as the
numbers of Indian recruits began to increase, the service was involved in political disputes, and the power of its members was increasingly threatened by doctors who were outsiders—in private
practice and in official employment. In the next sections I will consider in more detail the changing patterns of medical expenditure
heavily influenced by the members of the IMS.

Patterns of Health Expenditure

It is difficult to establish a clear picture of health expenditures
prior to the 1860s. Indeed, one indicator of how the Indian government became more fully bureaucratic is its reform of accounting
practices in 1867. Before that, most health expenditures were classified as military—the employment of doctors by the Indian Medical Service and their hospital subordinates, primarily for European
and later for "native" troops, though others also received some
benefits. Even as late as the 1900s, military medical expenditures
took nearly 40 percent of all health expenditures (see table 5).
Control over these expenditures was increasingly decentralized as
the nineteenth century went on. Until the 1860s the presidency
governments in Calcutta, Bombay and Madras were, with the
government of India, the only significant financial bodies. The

TABLE 5
CENTRAL AND PROVINCIAL GOVERNMENT HEALTH EXPENDITURES

Category	1870–79	1880–89	1890–99	1900–09	1910–19	1920–29	1930–39
				Decade			
			Rs millions (annual averages)				
Civil medical ⎫	6.2	7.3	11.6	14.1	23.0	{ 35.1	39.4
Civil sanitary ⎭						17.0	17.6
Military	4.2	5.5	7.1	8.2	6.3	n.a.	n.a.
Total health	10.4	12.8	18.7	22.3	29.3	n.a.	n.a.
Gross revenue expenditure	560.0	760.2	938.5	1131.3	1440.8	2175.6	2104.9
(% Health)	(1.8)	(1.7)	(2.0)	(2.0)	(2.0)	n.a.	n.a.
(% Civil health)	(1.1)	(1.0)	(1.2)	(1.2)	(1.6)	(2.4)	(2.7)

SOURCE: *Statistical Abstract for British India*, relevant years.
NOTE: Military medical expenditures are not separately recorded after 1919. "Health" includes medical and sanitary expenditures.

Mayo reforms of 1870 established municipalities on a firmer footing, and district and other local boards for rural areas date from the end of the 1880s. The municipalities saw health matters as one of their major concerns, and spent up to a quarter or more of their very small budgets on sewage removal ("conservancy"), water supply, dispensaries, and so on, more than did the provincial and imperial governments (see table 6). The district boards controlled even smaller amounts of money, despite the much larger populations for which they were responsible, and spent only around 10 percent of their total budgets on "sanitation, hospitals, etc."

These institutions of local government were not particularly democratic; civil servants often constituted a sizable proportion of council membership, and they nominated some of the other members. The process of democratizing these institutions followed policies at provincial and national levels—the reforms of 1907 (Morley-Minto), 1919 (Montagu-Chelmsford), and 1935. These changes were accompanied by steady increases in the numbers of provincial units—from the original three presidencies to over a dozen substantial units by the 1930s. After 1900, municipal politics were brought into prominence in the larger cities by the growing nationalist movement and, for most regions, the 1919 reforms were crucial in widening the area of participation. But even in the 1930s the chief medical advisers to all these levels of government were most likely to be members of the IMS—district medical officers or civil surgeons for district or local boards and most municipalities, and administrative medical officers for the provinces.

Civil health expenditures before 1919 increased steadily in money terms, but remained a fairly constant share of the revenue expenditures of the different levels of government. After 1919 health expenditures of central, provincial, local, and district boards rose substantially in money terms, and more rapidly than the growth of other revenue expenditures. In the municipalities, the growth in health expenditure was slower than that of total expenditures. Taking all levels of government together, health expenditures as a proportion of public expenditure rose from about 4.2 percent in the 1910s to 5.5 percent in the 1930s.

Table 7 summarizes these changes, taking account of population growth and changes in prices. Problems with these calculations include some possible double counting (provincial governments subsidized local government institutions, but this probably came from

TABLE 6

MUNICIPAL HEALTH EXPENDITURES

Category	1870–79	1880–89	1890–99	Decade 1900–09	1910–19	1920–29	1930–39
				Rs millions (annual averages)			
Water supply	1.1	3.5	5.1	5.7	10.4	23.0	17.2
Drainage	0.8	1.4	2.2	4.2	6.3	9.8	8.3
Conservancy	4.5	4.4	7.4	10.9	14.8	25.8	24.7
Hospitals, etc.	} 1.7	} 1.2	} 2.2	3.3	} 4.5	8.2	9.5
Vaccination						3.1	3.8
Sanitary					} 1.8		
Plague	—	—		1.0	0.7	0.4	0.4
Other	—	—	0.4	1.8	2.7	5.3	3.8
Total	8.1	10.5	17.3	26.9	40.3	75.5	67.7
Gross Expenditure	29.7	38.6	59.2	91.0	165.4	367.7	385.1
% 'Health'	(27.3)	(29.2)	(29.2)	(29.5)	(24.4)	(20.5)	(17.6)

SOURCE: *Statistical Abstract for British India*, relevant years.

NOTES: "Sanitary" appears as a separate category from 1915/1916 and the figure for the period 1910–1919 is an average of five years only. The periods covered in the other cases are financial decades beginning 1 April 1880, etc., and ending 31 March 1890, etc. "Health" includes medical and sanitary services.

TABLE 7
Per Capita Civil Health Expenditures: Current and 1870s Prices

Category	1870–79	1880–89	1890–99	1900–09	1910–19	1920–29	1930–39
				Decade			
			Rupees (annual averages, per capita)				
Central/provincial	0.03	0.04	0.05	0.06	0.10	0.22	0.21
Municipality	0.04	0.05	0.08	0.12	0.18	0.32	0.25
Local board	0.00	0.00	0.01	0.02	0.03	0.06	0.08
Total	0.07	0.09	0.14	0.20	0.31	0.60	0.54
(Current prices)							
Price index	100	87	116	129	201	271	160
Total	0.07	0.10	0.12	0.15	0.15	0.22	0.34
(1870s prices)							

SOURCES: First three columns from tables 5 and 6; Population figures for British India derived from Davis (1951), taking the average of adjacent census years; price index from the wholesale prices index in Reddy (1972:172–173), with the 1948–1949 base translated into a decadal average, based on 1871–1872 to 1879–1880, as 100.

a separate budget head); the price index used may not reflect changes in the costs of items in the medical budget; and the population deflator used is that of the total population when, for some purposes (e.g., for municipalities), the population covered by that form of institution might be more meaningful.

One addition factor complicating an assessment of changing priorities is the 1920s and 1930s world recession. The dominant economic philosophy demanded that budgets be balanced, and this placed the most severe restrictions on any expansion of expenditures and also led to a decline in prices. It is thus difficult to assess how democratic participation changed expenditure priorities toward health matters, since price changes may exaggerate the impact. But the changes seem large enough to suggest that they reflect real increases, so that "real" per capita expenditure rose about 50 percent between the 1910s and the 1920s, and by the same amount again by the 1930s.

The new form of government, introduced by the 1919 Government of India Act, probably had a major effect on the size and distribution of public expenditure. Under this act, and despite the objections of medical civil servants, large areas of health policy became the responsibility of provincial governments and were transferred to the control of elected ministers. The British government argued that *something* had to be transferred to the ministers, and there was little chance that ministerial control of public health could threaten imperial interests. The political disputes generated by this decision focused on attempts by the IMS, the BMA, and the GMC to stop Ayurvedic and Unani medicine from getting official support (see chap. 2 above) and to establish an Indian medical council to ensure a continuing powerful role for the imperial government (Jeffery 1979).

After 1919, then, public-sector health expenditures increased in money, in real and proportionate terms. Ministers may have seized upon the opportunity to use a commitment to public health as a means of demonstrating their "scientific" outlook. But it may be misleading to suggest that the reforms were the cause of this increase. Ministers did not have a prior record of any interest in implementing improved health services, so they may not have initiated the expansion, merely serving as instruments of plans laid down by civil medical services before World War I. Alternatively, since so few departments had ministerial control, the British may have diverted some resources in their direction to ensure the success of the reforms and to provide sufficient attractions to the politicians willing to give the new system some measure of credibility. A clearer answer to these questions must await a more detailed investigation of policy making in the provinces during the interwar period.

Conclusion

In this chapter I have argued that the IMS, as a fully bureaucratic institution, was clearly established by the 1860s and dominated medical policy making without any challenge until World War I. After the 1919 reforms, and with a much enlarged Indian membership, the collective character of the IMS changed, but it retained most of its influence. Major constraints on the way it was organized were its role both as a military reserve and as part of the welfare services provided for European civil servants and military officers; these were its main bargaining counters. Take away the lucrative civil medical positions, and recruitment from Britain would wither away; take away British doctors from India and the Indian civil service, the Indian army and the Indian police would complain; and these were the backbone of imperial rule. The orientation of the IMS reflected these priorities; there was little interest in expanding medical services for the mass of the civilian population, and public health measures (sanitary work) played no part in career advancement for ambitious doctors. But this does not mean that these were the only concerns affecting medical policy. Chapter 4 looks more closely at the implications of IMS domination in the three main areas of medical policy—medical education, sanitary policy, and the provision of medical services.

CHAPTER FOUR

Medical Education, Public Health, and Medical Services

The three legs of medical policy in India under the British were (in order of prestige) medical education, medical services, and public health. By 1860 the general outlines of provisions in each sector were established in a formal bureaucratic pattern that lasted for 60 or more years and retains significance today; but the changes made in each sector after 1920 had the greatest impact on the provision of postindependence medical services.

Medical Education

I shall deal only with the education of doctors, despite the risk of reinforcing a doctor-dominant view of health care, because of the difficulty of outlining the development of training for other kinds of medical staff. Certainly, classes were held for several grades of doctors and also for compounders (pharmacists), sanitary inspectors (from the end of the nineteenth century in Madras, later elsewhere), nurses, and later health visitors, and for indigenous midwives, or dais (see chap. 9). Few doctors were then assisted by more than one or two trained staff members. Information on these courses, the numbers attending, and the destination of the students is scarce and reflects the assumption that medical education was the most significant.

Educational provisions responded to changes in Britain (in the organization of medical knowledge, the social interests of different groups in imperial government, etc.), and also to wider political changes in India (the growth of Indian participation in government and the rising involvement of Indians in higher education, in particular). Prior to 1860 medical education in India, as in Britain, differed little from apprenticeship systems, outside one or two centers where a scientization of medicine had begun. Between 1860 and 1914 medical education was controlled—the student body was drawn from restricted social origins and the Indian Medical Service had virtually unchallenged sway over the terms of the education it provided. Indian medical schools and colleges were probably not too different from those of Europe; the time lag between the IMS man's education and the education he passed on to his Indian students was probably of little significance. By the 1920s, though, medical education in India was caught between conflicting pressures of nationalism and a swiftly changing, increasingly scientized European medicine. Student numbers expanded dramatically, control over the kind of education offered became a significant political issue, and Indian medical education became increasingly outdated (Jeffery 1979). The key decisions taken in this period include the phasing out of the training of a subordinate level of doctor, and the exclusion of indigenous medicine from the medical education of Western doctors. I will discuss the circumstances of those decisions at the end of this section.

After 1860, when the Indian universities were established, medical colleges must be distinguished from medical schools. Recruitment to the medical establishment was regularized, formal qualifications gained a central place, and the distinctions between grades became more marked. Increasingly colleges prepared students for university qualifications which permitted entry to the IMS or (after 1892) to the Colonial List of the General Medical Council in London. College graduates could thus practice in the United Kingdom and register for examinations held by the British royal colleges. Schools provided only shorter courses aimed at employment in the subordinate medical services. For a time, some medical colleges and schools shared premises, and college staff may have been involved in teaching junior classes, but this became uncommon. By the 1930s, those with college degrees were called graduates, while the holders of school qualifications were called licentiates, which is the current usage. However, before 1914 the most common university medical degree was the licentiate in medicine and surgery (LMS), so I will not use these terms.

The Portuguese in Goa were probably the first to teach medicine and surgery of the Western kind in a systematic way in India (Jaggi 1979b:24–26). They established a three-year course in 1801 and extended it to four years in 1821. Until 1812, the only equivalent medical education in British India was the training of assistants by surgeons on an apprenticeship basis. Some of these assistants were later recruited to the subordinate (uncovenanted) medical service (Crawford 1914, 2:103–105). In 1812 these schemes were extended and formalized by attaching European and Eurasian boys to hospitals in Calcutta and Madras for training as compounders and dressers (ibid.:106–108). These arrangements were designed explicitly to provide recruits for paramedical positions for the East India Company's army, both native and European.

In 1822 medical education in Calcutta was raised in status and changed in quality by the establishment of the Native Medical Institution (NMI). There was some general expansion of education provisions by the company at this time. The directors in London had no great enthusiasm for the NMI, expressing hostility to the cost of paying for a supervisor and comparing the new arrangements unfavorably with the system still in operation in Madras, where the company merely permitted an apprenticeship system (*Asiatic Journal* 1826). Originally, the maximum number of students at the NMI was twenty, but this number grew to fifty in 1826. They received a stipend during training and were taught in Urdu or Sanskrit. European texts were translated into these languages and also used at the Sanskrit College and the Madrasa, where classes of theoretical medicine had been supported by the company since their establishment (Jaggi 1979b:28–29; Hartog 1936). Only one European doctor worked at the institution, assisted by a Bengali pandit and other assistants, and dissection—the touchstone of modern medical education at the time—was carried out only on animal bodies.

The NMI was among the educational institutions caught up by Bentinck's reforming zeal when, as governor-general, he introduced "utilitarian" principles into aspects of the East India Company rule (Stokes 1959). Bentinck established a committee which complained that institution students were not admitted according to a single standard; tuition, period of training, and examination were inadequate; and practical anatomy was nonexistent. After disputes, the committee resolved that in future English should be the medium of instruction and only European science should be taught. The institution and the medical classes at the Madrasa and Sanskrit College were abolished in January 1835 and replaced by the Calcutta Medical College. The new orientation was clear; the course would cover "the principles and practice of the medical science in strict accordance with the mode adopted in Europe" (Crawford 1914, 2:436). However, some vernacular medical education (without instruction in indigenous theories of medicine) restarted in 1839, with teaching in Urdu and later in Bengali. Similar courses were introduced in Madras in 1835 and in Bombay in 1845, including vernacular classes for training compounders, native doctors, and subordinate medical staff (ibid.: 446–450).

Training for inferior levels was slowly removed from the medical colleges. The Calcutta Medical College transferred the Urdu classes to Agra and to Lahore in the 1850s, and the Bengali classes to Sealdah in 1873. Madras Medical College removed the vernacular classes three times, in 1857, 1882, and finally in 1903. Bombay transferred its vernacular classes in 1878–1881 to Poona, Ahmedabad, and Hyderabad (Sind). The colleges used these transfers to gain respectability with British medical authorities; Calcutta Medical College had already been reorganized in 1845 for this reason, and Madras courses were recognized by the Royal College of Surgeons from 1856 (Crawford 1914, 2:chap. 43). When Calcutta, Madras, and Bombay universities were founded in 1857, the medical colleges became their medical faculties. In 1892 Indian universities giving medical qualifications (including Punjab, after 1882) all received recognition from the General Medical Council in London. The council did not insist on inspecting the medical colleges but were apparently persuaded that Indian and British standards were comparable. In order to maintain this, the Indian colleges periodically raised their entrance requirements. Recruitment to medical schools then increased and, by 1900, several medical colleges in Calcutta, usually homoeopathic in orientation, recruited from those excluded from the official colleges.

University status did not make an immediate difference to the medical colleges. At the start the numbers taking the university qualifications were small: only ninety-nine passed the final licentiate examination in medicine and surgery at Calcutta in the ten years from 1856 to 1867, and two passed the BM degree examination in the same period (Reports 1870:58). In Bombay two or three students passed the final LM examinations each year in the mid-1860s, while only two candidates received Madras University medical qualifications between 1857 and 1868 (ibid.:61, 100). In addition, considerable tensions remained between the military medical authorities (who controlled appointments to senior medical college and medical school posts) and the educational authorities. For example, the education department in Bombay complained in the 1860s about the Grant Medical College where senior appointments suited the requirements of the medical administration, not the criterion of scientific ability—and the medical storeskeeper declined to give lectures in materia medica, so there were none (ibid.:394)!

During the nineteenth century the numbers of medical colleges and schools and their pupils grew, but not steadily. Tables 8 and 9 show the figures for the most accessible years (those of the Quinquennial Reviews of Education) but they do not show the extent of fluctuations in numbers. Sixteen schools were opened between 1853 and 1900, but three of them closed in the same period. Lahore became a medical college with the founding of Punjab University in 1882, and King George's Medical College, Lucknow, opened in 1912. A period of rapid growth during World War I was followed by decline in the 1920s, partly in response to pressures exerted by the General Medical Council in London (Jeffery 1979).

Figures for passes in final examinations, however, underestimate the impact of medical education. The heads of the medical schools and colleges saw this as an issue of the quality of their students. In Madras in 1867, for example, thirty-two graduated from "inferior" departments, but sixteen were "dismissed for incompetence" (which suggests the military character of the institution); and in Calcutta, 124 passed the first licentiate in medicine and surgery examination between 1860 and 1868, out of 317 candidates (Reports 1870:55, 444, 417). Many of those who failed at one attempt probably did not succeed later. But these failures are only part of the story. Many students did not complete the course; some were removed for nonpayment of fees, but some left for other reasons. For example, during the 1870s the principal of the Madras Medical College complained that several students studying for the licentiate (LMS) or the bachelor of medicine, bachelor of surgery (MBBS) left without attempting to complete the course, some to go to England to complete their studies (Sanitary Commissioner's Report 1876).

TABLE 8

STUDENTS REGISTERED AS ATTENDING MEDICAL COLLEGES: SELECTED YEARS

University	1866–67	1876–77	1886–87	1896–97	1906–07	1916–17	1926–27	1936–37
Calcutta	139	176	172	468	425	1100	1616	1470
Bombay	18	286	276	279	679	703	618	1244
Madras	8	143	138	82	195	207	586	1016
Punjab	–	47	68	238	243	232	488	545
Allahabad	–	–	–	–	–	137	254	504
Delhi	–	–	–	–	–	30	67	138
Patna	–	–	–	–	–	–	154	266
TOTAL	155	652	654	1067	1542	2511	3783	5183
of which:								
European/Eurasian			26%	9%	10%	4%	2%	3%
Native Christian			10%	6%	8%	6%	6%	6%
Muslim			2%	6%	4%	7%	12%	11%
Hindu-Brahman		} 43%		72%	23% }	25% }	75%	72%
Non-Brahman					37% }	50% }		
Parsi			17%	6%	16%	6%	2%	2%
Other			2%	–	1%	3%	3%	6%
Final university qualifications:								
Candidates	30	–	–	154	404	512	1525	1549
Passed	22	–	–	76	168	329	558	566

SOURCE: Quinquennial Reviews of Education, relevant years; Reports 1870; Moral and Material Progress 1876–1877.
NOTES: "Students" excludes those attending other classes attached to the medical college. Final university examinations were predominantly for the LM, or LMS, until 1914, when most students took MBBS examinations (Bachelor of Medicine Bachelor of Surgery). In 1876–1877 and 1886–1887 Madras figures may include some school pupils.

TABLE 9
Pupils at Medical Schools: Selected Years

Province	1866–67	1876–77	1886–87	1896–97	1906–07	1916–17	1926–27	1936–37
Bengal	278	862	793	1,482	1,845	1,119	2,282	2,409
Bombay	?	?	123	203	307	512	441	850
Madras	113	?	204	423	318	600	881	920
United Provinces	–	76	125	253	314	679	351	420
Punjab	–	84	143	333	394	513	772	1,324
Assam	–	–	–	–	[a]	178	[a]	
Bihar	–	[a]	[a]	[a]	[a]	257	387	212
Orissa	–	[a]	[a]	[a]	[a]	[a]	[b]	150
Central Provinces	–	?	–	–	–	55	247	266
Sind	–	–	[c]	[c]	[c]	[c]	[c]	147
Other	–	–	–	–	–	–	296	301
TOTAL (British India)		1,022	1,388	2,694	3,178	3,983	5,637	6,999
Princely States:								
Hyderabad					65			
Central India					?			
Final examinations:								
Candidates					690	–	1,693	3,547
					549	–	898	1,961

SOURCE: Quinquennial Reviews of Education, relevant years, except for 1866/1867 figures, from Papers 1870; and 1876/1877 figures, from Statistical Abstract 1878.

NOTES: These figures sometimes include pupils registered in courses at private aided and unaided institutions, in some years including homoeopathic, Ayurvedic and Unani schools. Burma is excluded throughout.
[a] Totals included in Bengal.
[b] Total included in Bihar.
[c] Total included in Bombay.

Similarly, in Calcutta in 1872 only 8 percent passed the examinations, while the remainder left to practice without any formal qualification (*Indian Medical Gazette* 1872). In other words, the numbers of successful graduates is probably the lower estimate of those who gained enough medical education to establish a medical practice, either directly or after more training elsewhere. An upper limit might be provided by dividing the number of college students registered in each year by five; and of school students by four (see fig. A). Those leaving without passing the final examinations had several career options, since they could take up appointments in princely states or set up in private practice. There were no constraints on prescribing or on the operations they might carry out. Unfortunately, we know nothing about these "MBBS failed."

The main expressed intention behind the establishment of medical education was to supply subordinate medical staff for government service, but the impact of the training was much broader, for colleges and schools alike. The medical colleges had, almost from the start, interpreted their role much more widely than just "providing subordinate medical staff." Medical colleges accepted substantial numbers of privately funded students in addition to those on stipends who had to serve in subordinate medical services

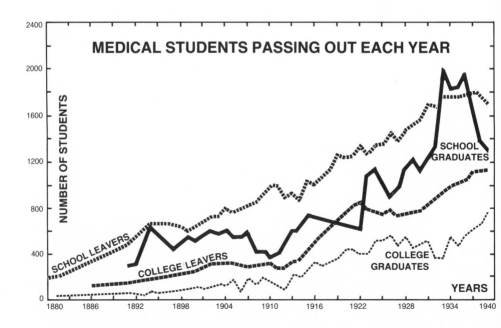

if requested. As early as the 1880s, these private students established practices in the major towns and competed with European doctors for the private market. Thus, of 142 graduates of the Grant Medical College, Bombay, between 1870 and 1881, over half were in private practice in 1882 (Gumperz 1965:234). Moreover, the medical college professors encouraged their better students to gain British qualifications or to compete for entry to the IMS. In 1845 a professor at Calcutta Medical College took four students to England to complete their medical training and one of them joined the IMS at the first competitive examination in 1855. Medical college graduates were likely to go to Britain for higher qualifications when they were ambitious, and the medical colleges seemed proud of such achievements however unpopular the Indian member of the IMS might be with European civil servants.

The training of private practitioners was also part of the role of the medical schools. More of their students were on government civil or military stipends; in some periods the numbers admitted to medical schools reflected the posts available. Entry was cut back when a surplus in the numbers of students appeared likely, compared with available posts, as in Punjab in 1871 (Kerr 1979:296). Even so, private students were common, especially in Calcutta. The Bengali department of the school section of the Calcutta Medical College was regarded as the major source of independent medical practitioners from about 1865, receiving most of its income from their fees (Reports 1870:65, 452).

By 1900 the spread of employment of those leaving medical schools was as wide as of the college graduates (*Quinquennial Review* 1908:160). Substantial numbers of graduates had established themselves in private practice in the main towns. They took patients away from the hakims and vaids as well as from government hospitals and dispensaries. This latter was undoubtedly unintended, but at least some senior members of the IMS accepted it as an inevitable (and desirable) result of their medical education policy:

> The object (of medical education) was not merely to secure a constant supply of subordinate medical officers for the Government service but also to raise the standard of medical knowledge and encourage the practice of medicine and surgery on established scientific principles. That private practitioners possessing the necessary qualifications should be able to compete successfully with public medical charities, is a satisfactory result. (Bengal Administration Report 1885:306–307)

When these same men began to threaten the private practice of IMS members as well, the objections were more substantial, and the IMS jealously prevented Indian doctors from claiming the prestige associated with being attending doctors at major hospitals. However, IMS exclusiveness began to break down after 1919 as it became Indianized. Until World War I medical college students were recruited from a relatively narrow social background, with Christians (often European and, later, Anglo-Indian) and Parsi students (in Bombay) providing a disproportionate share of the student body. Only sporadic evidence is available before the 1880s. In the 1840s roughly one-third or one-quarter of the Calcutta Medical College students were Christian (Commercial Tariffs 1847–48. 360–364; Returns 1852). In the 1860s, one-quarter of the Calcutta students were Christian and some of these were either European or Eurasian. As table 8 shows, these groups were still substantial as late as 1916–1917, with a peak around 1911–1912 when they amounted to 15 percent of the student body, with native Christians accounting for only 3 percent and Europeans or Eurasians making up 12 percent. Parsis were heavily overrepresented in terms of their share in the general population or in other forms of higher education, with Parsis accounting for one in six students in the 1880s and again in the early years of the twentieth century.

In the medical schools these groups were never so dominant. In the colleges, as in the schools, Hindus were the largest group, but those classified as Brahman were much fewer than the rest, in contrast with the other sectors of higher education. The share of Muslims only began to approach a due proportionate level in the 1920s and 1930s, when the reservation of places for Muslims began to have some impact. The overrepresentation of Indian Christians and of Parsis was stable until World War I, and suggests "both the strong symbolic value of the degree as an index of Westernization and the strong identification of these groups with Westernization in this particular form" (Gumperz 1965:228).

Medical education expanded rapidly during and after World War I and the proportion of the ethnically similar groups dropped dramatically. This may have been one reason for the changing attitudes of British medical authorities to the issue of Indian medical standards in the 1920s and 1930s. The GMC in London began taking more interest in the quality of the qualifications it registered after 1907, when it warned that midwifery training needed improving. In 1920 the Indian universities were asked for more details of their arrangements, and their unsatisfactory replies resulted in 1921 in a threat to remove recognition. The Montague-Chelmsford reforms of 1919 had given the area of medical education to the provincial governments, for elected ministers, though retaining control of medical standards for the central government. The GMCs threat enabled members of the IMS to maintain their control over the medical colleges, reduce the number of students admitted, toughen up the conditions for passing examinations, retain more of the lucrative medical college jobs than they might otherwise have done, and control ministers who wanted to change the pattern of medical education in their provinces. The number of medical undergraduates, which had nearly trebled between 1908 and 1922, dropped steadily until 1927, only rising above the 1922 level in 1934. The pass rate in the MBBS examinations dropped from over 50 percent in the period 1915–1921, to under 40 percent from 1925 up to World War II.

Although midwifery training remained inadequate—the basic problem was a shortage of midwifery cases in the medical college hospitals—the GMC continued to recognize Indian colleges (apart from Calcutta for a few years after 1924) until 1930. It then refused recognition until an Indian Medical Council was established (in 1933) which was able to negotiate retrospective recognition (in 1936) for most graduates in the intervening period. The rhetoric was that Indian graduates who wished to practice in Britain should meet British standards, but the implications were to affect the patterns of medical education in and for India thereafter. Medical schools were excluded from the terms of the Indian Medical Council, and this fueled campaigns for them either to be closed or upgraded into colleges.

These pressures were reinforced by the world recessions immediately after World War I, and again after 1929, severely restricting government expenditure, reducing employment opportunities in the public sector and increasing competition in the private sector. Reports on unemployment in Punjab and in the United Provinces in the 1920s and 1930s claimed that only 15 percent to 20 percent of doctors in private practice were making a decent living. Graduates began taking jobs that required only a school qualification. The clinching example came in 1938 when 995 licentiates and 428 graduates applied for two poorly paid posts in Aden.

In the 1930s these trends resulted in a major attempt to disman-
tle the "two-tier" system of medical education in India. Where possible, it was proposed that medical schools should be upgraded and
courses lengthened to turn them into colleges; elsewhere, schools
should be closed. This policy was supported by representatives of
school-educated doctors, who hoped to gain the benefits enjoyed
by college graduates; by British members of the IMS, who considered that this policy could blunt criticism from London of the ambiguous position of Indian medical education; and by nationalists,
who felt that the second tier implied second-class care and gave
other countries reasons for mistrusting Indian qualifications. Opponents felt that school-educated doctors were more suitable for a
poor country, being cheaper to train and, because of their lower social origins, more willing to work in rural areas or in unpopular
specialities such as public health (Jeffery 1979). As I shall show in
chapter 9, these debates have recurred in the postwar period. By
1938, the decision to destroy the medical schools had been taken
in principle; the intervention of the war prevented its full implementation for another fifteen years.

The political nature of these disputes and their consequences for
the lower level of medical personnel tend to distract attention from
how medical education in India was diverging from European developments. Indian medical colleges remained on the London pattern, where eminent clinicians dominated. The rising role of
laboratory medicine in the other European centers was reflected in
India when a Pasteur Institute was opened in Kasauli and the King
Institute in Madras. But these institutes had little organic relationship to the medical colleges and were in themselves a "piecemeal
and ad hoc response to sudden epidemic emergencies" (Ramasubban 1982:32). In the interwar period, medical research was hit by
the cuts in public expenditure and never developed an autonomous
tradition or career structure.

In terms of comparative colonial history, India is a striking exception to the general rule that "natives" were excluded from the
benefits of higher medical education. Medical education at all
levels came early and was widespread. The doctors trained in the
medical colleges and schools were the backbone of the government
medical services and, by 1900, they also provided a substantial
number of private medical practitioners. We know very little about
the services they offered; we cannot simply assume that they practiced what they were taught or what they were ordered to do. Some

collaborated actively with indigenous practitioners until the 1920s, when the "ethical codes" of the Registration Acts made that risky (Steinthal 1984). Others were accused of ceasing to practice Western medicine under the stress of making a living. However, those in government service were part of a structure which was intended to provide curative and (after 1865) preventive services.

Medical Services

The East India Company began to set aside special houses for sick employees in the seventeenth century, but not until the end of the eighteenth century were separate provisions made for the native indigent sick in Calcutta, Madras, and Bombay (Jaggi 1980:75–88). Separate provisions were made on employment and racial grounds, though in some places nonofficial Europeans might be allowed access to hospitals designed for civil servants. In general hospitals, some wards for Europeans and Eurasians were separated from those for the rest of the population. Medical theory in the early nineteenth century advocated removing the sick from their homes and localities on the basis that patients in hospitals were more obviously under medical control and observation (Arnold 1985). But dispensaries were cheaper, more popular, and often attached to the new hospitals. The Calcutta Medical College had a hospital of its own, and used several local dispensaries for teaching purposes in the 1830s.

These facilities were slowly extended beyond the presidency towns. In the 1830s dispensaries were opened, primarily for outpatients but with some inpatient beds and operating facilities. In 1838 Lord Auckland, then governor-general, sanctioned an increase in government dispensaries in Bengal and established them more formally, specifying the grade of doctor in charge and the total cost (Rs 250–300 per annum) government was prepared to bear; any additional funds were to be found from native contributions (Sykes 1847). By the early 1840s the seventeen dispensaries in most of the major towns in the Bengal presidency treated approximately 100,000 cases annually. Madras was slower to act. Apart from two dispensaries in Madras Town (one dating from 1828, the second from 1837), there was little growth before the mid-1840s. In 1848 fewer than 50,000 outpatients were seen, with a government expenditure of Rs 29,000 (Medical Reports 1850).

However, subsequent growth was much faster in Madras and Bombay than in Bengal, and the Punjab government acted even more decisively to establish medical facilities for the general population. In Punjab, the government was "deeply sensible of the benefits which dispensaries are likely to confer on our poorer subjects" (Punjab 1849–1850 and 1850–1851:151), but it also appreciated the benefits to government:

> The munificence of this Government charity [dispensaries], conferring such tangible and widespread advantages, will doubtless be appreciated by our new subjects. (General Report on the Administration of the Punjab Territories for 1851–1852 and 1852–1853: 200)

It opened 33 dispensaries, treating over 70,000 cases a year by 1855 (ibid.: 1854–1855; 1855–1856:113). This pattern continued right up to 1939. Use rates per 100 population were highest in Punjab and, later, Baluchistan and the North-West Frontier Province. Rates were lowest in Bengal and in the United Province. Of course, use rates tended to rise in times of epidemic or famine and, since these were not national calamities, they affected interprovincial comparisons. Further, numbers were sometimes inflated, either to keep a dispensary in existence or to demonstrate the assiduous work done by the dispensary doctor (Bengal Sanitary Report 1880). They say nothing whatever, of course, about any benefits from a visit, and we cannot distinguish between multiple visits by a small number of people and occasional visits by a much larger number. Nevertheless, the interprovincial pattern is fairly stable and represents different levels of medical provision as well as different degrees of use of Western medicine. Use rates nationally show a steady rise, from about four in 1881 to eleven in 1911, and twenty-six in 1939 (Jeffery 1985).

Initially these facilities were restricted to the major towns, but dispensaries spread with the devolution of government after 1880. Thus in 1881 one-quarter of all outpatient attendance in Bengal was accounted for by Calcutta hospitals and dispensaries; this had declined to 13 percent by 1891, and to 6.5 percent in 1901, though Calcutta still dominated the inpatient totals. The establishment of municipalities after 1870, and district and local boards after 1890, resulted in a steady increase of expenditure on medical matters and the creation of more dispensaries.

Detailed records were kept of the patients seen, and particularly of the operations carried out. Surgery was regarded as the main field where Western medicine outperformed the indigenous systems, and it also had the highest prestige among British doctors. Dispensary reports carry glowing accounts of the surgical skills of particular doctors, and the army claimed that on the borders, particularly in the North-West Frontier, the fame of individual surgeons brought in patients from a wide distance.

MEDICAL SERVICES FOR WOMEN

Men greatly outnumbered women and children as patients, and yet women and small children were obviously suffering high levels of morbidity and mortality which the existing clinics were unable to deal with. The state showed little interest in this disjunction, but prominent individuals and the medical missionaries made this a major concern. Viceroys' wives seemed to feel obliged to raise funds to improve the position of women in India. Lady Dufferin established a fund in 1885 to provide medical aid to the women of India; Lady Curzon established a fund to train indigenous midwives in 1903; Lady Chelmsford established a league to train lady health visitors (LHVs) and fund maternal and child-health work in 1920; and in 1924 Lady Reading established a fund for the women of India, which paid for a hospital in Simla and a training college in Delhi.

The main proposals for improving medical services for women were that women doctors should be employed and women encouraged to enter medical education; women's hospitals and wards were to be established, staffed by women; and subordinate female staff, notably health visitors and indigenous midwives, were to be trained and employed. The first two of these were seen as of particular benefit to the respectable classes, because secluded women could not consult male doctors (National Archives of India, Home, Medical 1887: 32A). By the 1920s, female doctors in the United Provinces were making more than 7,000 visits to *parda-nashin* and other women in their homes (cited in Civil Hospitals and Dispensaries, Uttar Pradesh, relevant years). These visits obviously benefited the relatively wealthy in urban areas; poor women were offered female dispensaries and improved midwifery through trained dais, both of which depended on women doctors.

The first female doctor employed in India was an American missionary, Clara Swain, who arrived in 1869. The missionary sector continued to provide more female medical care than did the state. Private hospitals under women doctors were opened in Madras in 1884 and in Bombay in 1886 (Balfour and Young 1929: chap. 2). The first female doctor to be employed by government was probably Elizabeth Beilby, who started a women's hospital for the Lahore Municipal Committee in 1885. Thereafter the Dufferin Fund employed European female doctors more regularly and began to build hospitals. The numbers employed grew very slowly and in 1907 the government was asked for more support for salaries to be increased and careers to be properly organized. A Women's Medical Service was established in 1914, with an annual grant from the government of India. Salary scales and conditions of service remained much below those of the IMS. By 1928 there were forty-four doctors in the Women's Medical Service, compared with 750 men in the IMS at the time.

Women were first admitted to medical training in India in 1875, when Mary Scharlieb and three others were admitted to the Madras Medical College and gained a school diploma three years later. Women were admitted to degree courses in the 1880s, despite the objections of the medical college staff (Jaggi 1979b:93–110). In Calcutta, women students were all provided with scholarships and the Dufferin Fund also prompted municipalities to provide scholarships for women to be trained in medicine. The numbers of female medical students rose steadily, but the proportion of women to men was always very low. The scope of female medical education expanded when female medical schools and, in 1916, the Lady Hardinge Medical College for women in Delhi were opened, but as late as the 1920s fewer than twenty women a year were receiving higher medical qualifications (MBBS or LMS) in the whole of India, and under fifty were graduating from medical schools (Quinquennial Reviews, relevant years). Their numbers grew in the 1920s and by 1937 475 women were studying in medical colleges, and 964 in medical schools, nearly 12 percent of medical students (Quinquennial Review 1936–1937).

Until the 1930s, most women doctors were Indian Christians, Europeans, or Eurasians. In 1926–1927, nearly two-thirds of those at female colleges and schools were from these groups, though this had declined to one-third by 1936–1937 (Quinquennial Reviews, relevant years). Female doctors were always expected to be solely concerned with women and children and not to challenge male dominance of providing medical care for males or most general surgery and medicine. Balfour and Young (1929:43–45) tactfully discuss some of the disputes over precedence as members of the IMS attempted to control women's hospitals as well as their own.

Female dispensaries, staffed only by women, were first established in North India in the 1890s. A major limitation to their expansion was the number of female doctors. In 1920 only seventy-six medical women were employed by government in the whole of the United Provinces; ten years later there were 108 (Balfour and Young 1929:168; Civil Hospitals and Dispensaries, Uttar Pradesh 1930:13). The available data show much lower consultation rates for women than for men not only as inpatients (well below male levels) but also as outpatients. Around 1,900 consultations by women at hospitals and dispensaries were rarely above 50 percent of the level of consultations by men. The figures available for children suggest that girls (aged 12 or less) were taken for consultations about 60 percent as often as boys. In some cases women were represented at the clinic by a male relative, and the woman herself would not attend (Balfour and Young 1929:34). Consultations at female dispensaries raised female rates, but the number of female dispensaries was never large enough to make a substantial difference (Kynch 1986; Administration Reports, relevant years).

It is difficult to keep track of attempts to improve midwifery in India by training local midwives. The earliest example from North India is a course held in Amritsar from 1866, still going in the early 1880s when nine or ten were being trained every year. A class was established in Bareilly in 1867, and a Lahore class, founded in 1876, was expanded in the early 1880s (NAI, Home, Medical 1887:76–83 A). But these attempts were not widely copied. In Bengal the medical establishment offered little support and the classes, run by men, could have given little practical instruction because there were no maternity cases in the hospitals and dispensaries. It is interesting that the civil surgeon in Bareilly favored midwifery training because it might help reduce infanticide. The Infanticide Act three years later heralded a far more intensive intrusion into matters regarded locally as private, family affairs than was ever considered for purely medical purposes. The most direct attempt to obtain access to maternity cases was a proposal to pay women to attend hospitals to have their babies, but this was to provide teaching cases for the dai classes and for medical students, rather than to reduce the neonatal and maternal mortality rates (UP 1881:312). The scale of dai training ebbed and flowed, along with the length of the courses and the financial attractions offered. Before World War I, between four and five hundred dais received certificates every year for successfully attending courses in the United Provinces but in the 1920's fewer than fifty a year were under training (UP, relevant years). Moreover, even its proponents admitted they had little success in training dais and even less success in supervising them once trained (Balfour and Young 1929:128–140).

Crucially, the impetus for much of the maternal and child welfare work done in India came not from the state apparatus but from private funds raised by leading British women. The state contributed funds to these schemes, but its commitment was limited. A fierce rearguard action was needed to save the Women's Medical Service from financial cuts threatened by the Inchcape Committee in the 1920s (Balfour and Young 1929). The state was far more bothered by the GMC requirements for maternity cases for medical students than by evidence of maternal and neonatal mortality and morbidity (Jeffery 1979).

By 1947 an infrastructure of health services existed for women; there were female dispensaries, staffed by women, in the district headquarters towns, and some women were trained for nursing positions, again generally staffing clinics in the larger towns. But there had been no concerted effort to improve the medical services for rural women. The attempts to train dais were obviously sporadic, urban-based (since they depended on female staff to do the training), and had little impact on how children were delivered in most of the country. Given the small number of medical graduates practicing in rural areas, the even smaller number of female graduates, and a probable absence of women providing Western drugs as pharmacists, Western medicine probably made little impact on women under the British.

Public Health and Sanitary Policy

Before the 1860s sanitary arrangements for the civilian population were discussed only sporadically. For example, in 1810, when some Dacca citizens proposed local improvements, such as the removal of filth, or the repair of wells and drains, the governor-general rejected the proposal out of hand (Ahmed 1980:134–135). By 1823 the governor-general allowed the surplus from town taxes to be spent on urban improvements; but in Dacca, at least, most effort went into widening roads, draining marshes, and clearing land for (among other things) a race-course (ibid.:147–148). Efforts depended on the individual officials appointed to improvements committees, all of which were abolished in 1829 as a measure of economy (ibid.:159). More concern was shown for the health of the army; for example, after 1835 medical officers were encouraged to submit details of the climate, geography, and medical statistics of districts in order to guide military campsites and cantonments to healthy places (Ramasubban 1982). However, one measure of civilian preventive medicine predated the 1860s: vaccination against smallpox was supported with fluctuating energy and attempts were made to eradicate the indigenous practice of inoculation (Arnold 1985).

Preventive health measures in India are usually dated from the Royal Commission appointed to inquire into the sanitary state of the army in India, which reported in 1863. This commission was established, in part at least, because the deaths of British soldiers from disease during the mutiny greatly exceeded those from injuries received in fighting. It reported that the health of the army could not be separated from "the sanitary condition of the 'native' population" close by, and that "well-considered measures of water-supply, drainage, paving, cleansing, and general constitution in these towns would be attended with most beneficial results to the health of the troops quartered near them." All the native towns had some system of cleansing and dealing with human excreta and other nuisances; nonetheless, the commission concluded, there was much more to be done (Sanitary Commission 1865:77, 81; Statistical Abstract 1870:53). The priority of sanitary work was thus based on military arguments, and it retained this basis for the rest of the nineteenth century. Sanitary policy was restricted to towns and military areas because the remit of the commission was to consider improvements for the towns "in proximity to military stations" (ibid.: para. 35). A classic example is the Contagious Diseases Prevention Acts, designed to protect soldiers from venereal diseases and totally unconcerned with civilian sufferers (Ballhatchet 1980).

The government of India implemented the proposal of the commission's 1863 report for sanitary commissions in each presidency with advisory, but few executive, powers. These sanitary commissions were replaced two years later by a single sanitary commissioner each and, by 1868, one for each of the provinces. For twenty years little was achieved, partly because sanitary officers were subordinated to medical ones, and partly because sanitary concerns were restricted to official circles. In addition, technical disputes about the relationship between sanitary measures and medical science hindered the implementation of policy, especially with respect to the role of clean water in preventing cholera (Farrell 1973; Jaggi 1979c; Hume 1984).

The IMS was unconvinced of the need to separate sanitary from medical work. In 1866 Gordon argued that the sanitary commissioners would unnecessarily limit the functions of army medical officers, and the *Indian Medical Gazette* also waged a fierce war against the appointment of Major G. B. Malleson, a layman, to be head of the Bengal Sanitary Department (Jaggi 1979c:98–99). Indian authorities had little training in epidemiology as was then understood in Britain, which helped to render the sanitary commissioners' work almost valueless. For example, in the 1870s the Bengal sanitary commissioner was attacked in the London press for apparently doing little beyond collating vital statistics which he was unable to analyze to any effect.

Further criticisms came from international concern with cholera. In 1866 an International Sanitary Conference in Constantinople concluded that India was the source of cholera epidemics, and that the Indian government had failed to control them. The measures proposed to deal with cholera were progressively implemented for the army and cholera mortality dropped to three deaths per 1,000 in the 1870s. But when medical men came to deal with civilian cholera, they hid behind "Orientalist" excuses: Indians were inferior, and one sign of their inferiority was their relentless attachment to superstition, which made it impossible to tamper with religious customs such as pilgrimages, widely agreed to be a major route of cholera transmission (Ramasubban 1982:21–23).

Sanitary commissioners were expressly excluded from any concern with the cantonments and the European civil lines themselves; these remained the responsibility of the army (Harrison 1980:173). Increasingly, towns had local municipal committees, with some elected members. Initially, these committees focused mainly on conservancy—the removal of feces from residential areas. In Allahabad in 1870, 280 sweepers were employed to collect sewage and 90 drivers to remove it for burial. In Calcutta in 1867, a municipal railway was built to deal with the transport problem (ibid.:182–183). But the financial limits of these committees prevented them from making much impact on sanitation. Thus, in 1883, when Ranchodlal Chhotalal, the first nonofficial Indian to be made chair of the Ahmedabad Managing Committee, proposed better water supplies and drainage, better hospitals, and more planning controls over housing, his vehement opponents attacked the increased taxation needed to pay for the proposed improvements (Gillion 1968:136–138). Eventually, in 1891 an improved water-supply scheme was implemented; but it was not until 1903, after the municipality was ordered by the Bombay government to take the advice of experts, that the drainage scheme was completed. Similarly in Allahabad, the water-supply scheme first mooted in 1883 was in operation by 1891, but a drainage scheme for the extra water supplied was not started until 1913 (Harrison 1980:186).

This delay in providing drainage systems (common throughout Indian towns because of the extra expense involved) meant that introducing clean water supplies actually seems to have increased mortality rates. In six north-Indian towns, recorded death rates in the five years following the introduction of filtered water supplies were higher than in the five years before (Klein 1973:651). The surplus water probably formed stagnant pools, ideal breeding grounds for mosquitoes, thus increasing the spread of malaria, though deaths due to dysentery, cholera, and diarrhea probably did decline.

In the late 1880s Florence Nightingale pressed the Indian government to improve sanitary arrangements in the villages which had been almost totally ignored. No rural agency existed to implement the rules established for village sanitation. Decentralization only reached the provinces in 1872, under Lord Mayo's reforms, and larger towns were given some autonomy in 1882, with the Ripon reforms. A new extension of local government was set in train with acts in Bombay (1889) and other parts of the country designed to promote district authorities for whom sanitary measures would be a primary concern. Training in hygiene and sanitation was expanded and, over the next ten years, graduates were brought into sanitary work.

Activity, however, was severely restricted by the shortage of funds available and by the limitations policymakers believed were caused by the "ignorance, prejudices, callousness, and superstitions of the people" (Harvey 1895:5). This blaming of the poor and sick for their own conditions may have allowed some doctors to escape the responsibility for eradicating the real causes of high rates of morbidity and mortality. But some doctors advanced more sophisticated arguments, suggesting that European methods of disease control were inapplicable in India, because of social (e.g., caste) and environmental (e.g., the monsoon) barriers (Arnold 1985:6). Clearly, medical administrators were uneasy about their record in sanitary work, particularly when challenged in international settings with responsibility for cholera which emanated from Bengal (Jaggi, 1979c:103). However, they were undoubtedly right to argue that implementing sanitary improvements throughout rural India would be beyond the financial limits of Britain, let alone of the Indian government. Funding problems were probably exacerbated by linking sanitary reform to local governments with even less adequate sources of finance than the towns had.

Attempts to intervene in the provision of water, the control of sewage, and other aspects of everyday village life would probably have led to great hostility and little success. Vaccinators had to deal with frequent rumors of the dangers of the treatment and general hostility, partly because they were also trying to eradicate inoculation which was a much more accepted form of smallpox prevention (Arnold 1985:8). The response to plague measures after 1896 reinforced this view. Sanitary measures, based on little understanding of village life, would probably have been unsuccessful, though this does not justify the pathetic attempts that were actually made. Expenditures on preventive medicine were always small, relative to overall public or to medical expenditure. Probably only water supplies and some vaccination programs made any marked impact on morbidity and mortality before World War II.

Yet medical administrators appreciated the links between providing sanitation and a population's health, especially in urban areas where collective arrangements for waste disposal, water supply and drainage were major concerns. As in Europe, town planning until 1900 was almost entirely a matter of sanitary provision, fueled by demands from the wealthy for protection from diseases of the poor. In India this took on a racial form, with attempts to protect Europeans—civilians and the military—from native diseases. This is obvious in the reports of the sanitary commissioners, but its most notable results lay in the separation of city from cantonment and in other attempts to place physical barriers between Indian and European. The Royal commission deplored these efforts (Sanitary Commission 1865:79), but they accorded with theories of contagion through bad air (Harrison 1980:174; King 1966). Thus, conditions in European areas were much better than in Indian areas; roads were paved and swept, water supply and drainage was quickly improved to a higher standard, and there was infinitely less crowding. But sewage removal arrangements in the European areas differed little from those in the rest of the city, at least during the nineteenth century, and provisions for Indians living there (servants, traders, etc.) were possibly even worse than in the towns (ibid.:182).

After 1900 improvement trusts were established in many larger towns and Patrick Geddes, among others, was asked to advise on the development of urban areas—prompted partly by a concern for the appalling conditions in the slums. The trusts had power to control only new building, beyond the city limits. Attempts to improve working-class housing ran into overwhelming opposition from powerful slum landlords as well as the municipal committees, for whom they were too expensive. Despite Geddes's propaganda, it was only in Hyderabad (where the nizam gave considerable support) that there was any substantial attack on unsanitary conditions (Meller 1979:347).

The other impetus to urban renewal came from plague epidemics. Plague was probably common in India before the British arrived and its association with rats was known (Anstey 1936:72). But it apparently disappeared from India in the early nineteenth century before being reintroduced from China through Bombay in 1896. Since its signs are distinctive and it generated such horror and official inquiry, deaths from plague were probably recorded fairly accurately. If so, the estimates of some 15 million plague deaths in British India and 18 million in the princely states, between 1896 and 1921, cannot be far off the mark (Census 1921:350). The disease spread quickly to most parts of the country, speeded by railways, trade, and commerce. The urban poor suffered most and then, panic-stricken, escaped into rural areas, taking the disease with them; Europeans were almost immune.

The vital point to note here is that plague reappeared in India when control and prevention measures were understood, and yet the response of the authorities was almost totally ineffective. The Bombay authorities took drastic action; sufferers were compulsorily removed to hospital, the infected were segregated, premises were evacuated, a sanitary cordon was attempted around affected areas, and travelers were medically inspected. These measures were inadequately explained and few people accepted the rationality of what was proposed. Some resisted openly; traders rejected bans on exports or the movement of goods, millowners rejected steam cleansing, while Jains and others destroyed rattraps. Others concealed infected people and then dumped their dead bodies anonymously in the street, escaped around cordons, or refused to leave infected areas for fear of theft from their unprotected houses (Klein 1973). When pushed too far, they rioted.

Western medicine's arrogant self-confidence and its failure to deal with the plague is well exposed by the medical authorities' compromises with Indian opinion. Originally, the authorities wanted all patients to be treated by Western doctors, but they were forced to accept instead the use by patients of hakims and vaids. They also had to deny that plague inoculation would be made compulsory (Arnold 1985:10–11). By 1900 the sanitary commissioner noted, the plague epidemic was treated as a political emergency, not as a matter of public health, and he argued that this was because the idea of public health was alien to the sympathies and traditions of the people (Annual Report of the Sanitary Commissioner 1902:117–21). Dealing with the threat to trade and social order became paramount: treatment and control measures had to follow behind these imperatives, and the imperial government withdrew from active attempts to prevent the spread of the disease, merely responding to calls for medical services (Klein 1973).

Public health in India thus has to be seen as a qualified failure. Even in the towns most directly amenable to British influence and action the conditions of life of most inhabitants remained appalling, with very high mortality and morbidity rates in the worst areas. Only European areas enjoyed the benefits of civic concern. This racial distinction and the much more pronounced role taken by the state in Indian towns, provide the main points of difference between the Indian and British experience. Despite having a more centralized, active, and interventionist government than in Britain and one which attempted to draw on British experience, India gained remarkably few benefits. Capitalist development and the rapid unplanned increase of the urban population led to slums, overcrowding, and urban squalor in India just as in Europe.

Conclusion

It makes little sense to see imperial medicine in India solely as either social control or humanitarian concern. The picture is more complex. Both aspects are important and were often closely intertwined. Issues of social control were paramount in setting the structural context within which the Indian Medical Service worked. When issues of general policy were discussed, the IMS undoubtedly pointed to its role in keeping the troops healthy, the civil servants content, and the masses convinced of the benefits of British rule. But these arguments were weak. The troops were not particularly healthy, and the British army in India, served by the Army Medical Department under the War Office, was more crucial to the defense of British interests in India than the IMS under the India Office. The indigenous masses were not, in fact, desperate to accept Western medicine. They used dispensaries and accepted training in Western medical schools and colleges in enlightened self-interest, rather than out of a commitment to Western science or imperial rule. The problems with vaccination and plague control brought home how alien Western medicine remained to most of the Indian population.

But the structural context and the alien nature of British rule and provisions explain neither why medical services became part of the symbolic justification for imperial rule nor the form they took; they form a set of shifting boundaries within which members of a bureaucratic structure acted according to their own view of the purposes of imperial rule, the proper role of medicine, and their own preferred careers and activities. Imperial stability was compatible with many possible health policies, ranging from virtually nothing to a successful rural health service.

In addition, none of the policy innovations went unchallenged nor were policies ever applied rigorously. In particular, uncertainties remained in the relationship with indigenous medicine until the end of British rule. The quest for a common ground continued although official policy was to exclude indigenous practitioners entirely from the government ambit. Another example was the training of personnel, especially for rural services. The Medical Degrees and Medical Registration Acts from 1912 to 1919 seem intended to force India into a "professional" model for health-services delivery. But the 1920s saw a flowering of attempts to use local people as the bottom tier of the medical and sanitary services. Schemes for village nurses and for schoolmasters as medical workers were not merely proposed but were implemented by British doctors working within the government (McGuire 1929; Hooton 1928). Such experiments were welcomed in the *Indian Medical Gazette* in December 1924, which pointed to comparable experiments with government assistance in the voluntary sector. The Rockefeller Foundation supported a similar project in Travancore (Tampi 1931).

The imperial impact on health in India was thus contradictory. Changes in famine policy and food distribution helped reduce mortality; increasing numbers of men (and, later, women) were trained in medicine according to international standards of the time; hospitals and dispensaries attracted considerable numbers of patients; and issues of disease prevention and public health provision were addressed as never before. But equally, the impact of many measures was restricted to a small sector of the population, first, to the European civil and military servants and their families, later to Indians with access to urban facilities. Therefore, even if nineteenth-century medical services had been beneficial, the mass of the Indian population could not have benefited. Preventive campaigns were never fully pushed through; vaccination and, more powerfully, plague control, demonstrated the failure of British health policy to come to terms with local society. Health measures, per se, probably had little influence on mortality and morbidity, but they did establish a framework (of personnel, ideas, institutions) that permitted more substantial postindependence provisions, whose impact is more noticeable.

Ramasubban argues that this pattern was a "colonial mode of health care," characterized by segregation and by provisions for the enclave sector which kept pace with "metropolitan" developments. The rest of the population "missed going through the period of sanitary reform which swept through most of Europe in the nineteenth and early-twentieth century" (1984:107). This view is too sweeping. First, nobody thought segregation could be complete and the interests of colonialists were linked with those of the Indians who surrounded them. Indeed, the most substantial urban improvements (in water supply and drainage) were designed to improve the living conditions of Indians. Second, provisions (hospitals and dispensaries and places in medical schools and colleges) soon outran the needs of the army and the European civil population, and this was regarded with satisfaction, not alarm. Third, the most effective European sanitary reforms were also largely urban; many rural areas in Europe were without centralized water supply, drainage, or refuse disposal for many years. To blame the colonial government for not transferring urban solutions to a largely rural India is to underestimate the problems involved. And fourth, the role of public health in Europe is overstated by this view, since rising living standards and changes in personal hygiene were largely independent contributors to the changes in the level and kinds of morbidity and mortality experienced by the European population. We should not dismiss these arguments as self-interested excuses merely because they were made by the imperialists themselves.

The failure of the colonial government to make a substantial impact on morbidity and mortality in India, then, depended on factors outside its control as well as on the constraints imposed by the nature of that government. Most prominent among the problems faced by health policymakers was the poverty of the Indian population (not all caused either by the depradations of British conquest in the eighteenth century or by commercialization and the sustenance of landlordism in the nineteenth). The diseases of the poor were (and are) difficult to treat and, with the technology of the time, difficult to prevent. In addition, the tax base for raising revenue for public solutions also was limited. The imperial government did not, of course, place sanitary reform or medical services high on its list of priorities; but in some ways they were given higher priority in India than in Britain. In Britain the government tended to leave medical provision to charitable or voluntary hospitals; medical education to independent medical schools; and sanitary reform to urban councils. In India all these were seen as the proper concern of the imperial government.

A further problem arose from the radically different understandings of the rulers and the ruled of the causes of disease and the consequences of some aspects of the environment. This was most marked for plague, but it was also true for sewage disposal, water supply, and antisepsis. Some nineteenth-century views put forward on these issues may now seem wrong, and they might have made little difference if they had been widely followed. But the proposed solutions encountered real technical problems (e.g., for water closets or water purification) and they were ill-adapted to the local economy and society—which helps to explain the hostile reception they received. The commitment to implement such policies may have been weak and the constraints (financial, political, or administrative) set on health policies were undoubtedly considerable. But it remains uncertain how much difference would have been made by any conceivable historically available alternative structures or commitments.

Basically, the colonial state was not a totally integrated structure. The political processes within the state were not all closely defined by the need to reproduce the colonial structure. Other pressures had an impact on medical policy: the perceptions of medical bureaucrats, the requirements of meeting some of the demands made by the rising political classes, demands in the market for medical services and education, and the need to defend the state from accusations of exploitation. After independence, the alien rulers were replaced by Indian rulers, albeit ones often rebuked as no less alien in thought, speech, and action that many of the British. The extension of liberal democratic institutions and changes in the nature of the international environment had consequences for state structure and medical policy after 1947.

PART II:

Health Policy in Independent India

Introduction to Part II

The impact of independence in 1947 was much less substantial than political rhetoric suggested. Nationalist policies were focused on gaining power and removing the British, and there was no agreed-upon program for social and economic change beyond this. Ideologues in Congress—Gandhians and Socialists alike—had ideas about creating a new society, but most leading members of Congress wanted to operate the levers of power in a government in ways not radically different from the British in the decade or so before they left. As Maddison (1972) put it, Congress was a party of "step-in-my-shoes Nationalists."

Furthermore, the circumstances of independence made it difficult to consider long-term goals. Congress politicians gained power in the provinces in 1946 and nationally in 1947. However, the normal problems of making and implementing policy were exacerbated by the massive upheavals caused by partition, which diverted resources and attention to refugee problems and the maintenance of public order. Not until 1950 did Home Minister Patel manage the accession of the princely states to the Indian Union and deal with the major rebellion in Telengana and minor uprisings elsewhere. Inevitably, the new governments had to rely on the essentially colonial civil service—sometimes the very individuals who had imprisoned their new leaders during the Quit India Movement five years previously.

Nonetheless, independence does mark a step in the metamorphosis of the Indian state. The changes of 1907–1908, 1919, and 1935 foreshadowed the Independent Union of India and the implications were followed through in the 1950 constitution. The franchise was extended to the whole of the adult population, all government action was subjected to the Indian Parliament through elected ministers held responsible to the House of which they were members, and the governor-general was replaced by an elected president. India is that rare case in the postcolonial world of a state that has retained all the liberal-democratic institutions it inherited on independence, but developed new forms of political process, as the implications of a rural electorate, organized largely in factional terms, have worked their way through. (See chapter 7 for how this has affected health policy.)

Here I will sketch out three of the other key features of the postindependence state in India: the changing role of the world economy; the management of the federal political structure; and the role of the state in the economy and in planning.

India In A World Economy

The British had dominated those parts of the Indian economy most closely linked to export markets and imported goods and no sharp break occurred after 1947. The Indian government did not nationalize these assets wholesale, nor did British capitalists carry out a massive disinvestment, though some of both happened (Lipton and Firn 1976). Furthermore, little new investment by British or other companies occurred before the 1960s. Partly this reflected domestic economic policy to protect Indian industries. Indian foreign policy also stressed balanced links with the dominant world powers and left some American companies uncertain about the climate for investment in India. However, India's international position weakened dramatically in 1958, when its foreign-exchange reserves ran very low, and again in 1964–1965, when bad harvests, the 1962 war with China, and the 1965 war with Pakistan depleted stocks still further. The United States government used this opportunity to encourage a devaluation of the rupee and shifts in policy on foreign investment, agriculture, and population control.

The new patterns of foreign investment were very different from the older, imperialist ones (Kidron 1966; Alavi 1965). New investments were in industrial manufacturing, in the expanding areas of the economy, were technologically more advanced, more profitable, and served the internal market rather than an export market. Foreign companies leaped over tariff barriers to establish production operations within India. Controls introduced in the 1972 Foreign Exchange Regulation Act reduced the equity shares of foreign corporations, and companies such as International Business Machines (IBM) and Coca-Cola withdrew. Since the early 1970s multinational corporations have generally preferred collaboration agreements with Indian companies, with low foreign capital input.

Indian academics have been relatively unwilling to explain these changes in terms of "dependency" analyses (Blomstrom and Hettne 1984). Discussions of the state have focused on local class alliances and the implications of changing production relationships in agriculture (Thorner 1983). In part, this is because the Communist party of India has muted its criticisms of Congress in order not to damage Moscow's relationship with the Delhi government, but it also reflects the relative unimportance to India of foreign trade, foreign capital, and foreign aid, compared with other "peripheral" capitalist societies. Short periods of crisis have left the government particularly weak, but India is not an export-oriented economy. An import-substitution policy has kept imports to about 10 percent of national income or less. The indigenous capitalist sector was relatively well developed before 1947, having benefited greatly from the war economy, and it maintained strong links with the Nationalist movement which, in turn, protected it after 1947. In 1981–1982, after the increase in foreign investments, only about 10 percent of total value added, in manufacturing and mining, was controlled by foreign firms (Bardhan 1984:44). In some years foreign aid has provided a substantial share of Plan expenditure, but India has rarely had to borrow from the International Monetary Fund (IMF), and now has a relatively low level of international public debt, with substantial reserves created by foreign remittances.

Management Of A Federal Polity

The Government of India Acts of 1919 and 1935 established a federal system of government which the new government of India accepted with little amendment. The structure was altered slightly by the inclusion of princely India, and then (in 1956 and the early 1960s) the states were reorganized along linguistic lines and their number was reduced. The constitution of 1950 made little change in the formal division of functions and financial powers, but in practice, power has become concentrated in the hands of the central (or Union) government. This can be seen in the control of the central government over state-government finances through the mechanisms of the finance commissions, which make five-year distributions of tax revenues, central government control over the Reserve Bank of India, the lender of last resort to state governments, and the Planning Commission. The states have complained about their weakness, because the final arbitration of awards rests with the central government.

The political aspects of these relationships have changed through time. Before 1964, the Congress party held power in most of the states almost all the time. Within Congress, the core of nationalist politicians from the independence movement, dominated by Western-educated groups, especially lawyers, had considerable local autonomy. Since then, several changes have concentrated power in the hands of the prime minister. Indira Gandhi, in particular, used her patronage during her disputes with the Congress "old guard" which split the party in 1969–1970 and again in 1975–1976. The political "emergency" of 1975–1977 represents an extreme form of centralized power or "emergency regime" (Rudolph and Rudolph 1981) but not an aberration. Chief ministers of states now know that their positions depend on the central government and the prime minister no matter what their local support may be.

The central government has become less willing to tolerate political and administrative diversities (Dua 1981:272–273). The other consequence is that state governments have experienced increased demands from local pressure groups. Patrons within the party press for resources or jobs, contracts, and so on, to be distributed in particular ways, and local opponents of chief ministers can ask for his or her removal by the prime minister. The central government, by contrast, is more susceptible to pressure from foreigners wanting contracts and support than from pressure from within the country. The result has been increasingly populist. Policymaking has reflected a desire to meet interest group demands, often through an expansion in the role of the public sector, rather than for ideological coherence or overall rationality. Myrdal (1968:895–900) called this a "soft" state, one which places few demands on its citizenry, and attempts to offer services, employment, and other benefits without, for example, establishing a centralized tax system or a political structure that can call upon individuals in the way epitomized by Communist China. The campaigns to "eradicate poverty" (Mrs. Gandhi's 1971 slogan) or the "20-point program" (to legitimate the emergency, and revived by Mrs. Gandhi when she returned to power in 1980), did not envisage direct attacks on class privileges or the mobilization of individual resources. Land reforms are the obvious example of this tendency. Despite the abolition of *zamindars* (the largest landholders) very little land has been appropriated or distributed to the actual farmers.

The State, The Economy, And Planning

The government has also expanded its role in economic decision making, by introducing detailed controls and using Plans to provide an overall coherence to the economy. Industrial Policy Resolutions of 1948 and 1956 gave the state a commanding role in the economy, reserving key areas (power, heavy industry, capital goods) for the public sector. Later came the nationalization of financial centers—banks and insurance companies. The numbers employed in the public sector have risen substantially in the organs of government and in public-sector industries, services, and financial institutions. In ways like these the government has attempted to achieve the goals of the five-year Plans.

The imperial government undertook very little direct planning, but the various planning proposals put forward before World War II by academics and industrialists bore some fruit in the programs introduced after 1942 to convince Indians both that the British expected to win the war and that it would be better for India if they did. A postwar Reconstruction Committee that made plans for the situation after the war grew into the Planning and Development Department. Specialized committees drew up plans for the five years following the war in the context of a fifteen-year perspective plan (never actually produced). A wide range of topics was covered by these committees, including the role of the state in reducing glaring inequalities of wealth and the control of major industries. In 1945 the Second Report on Reconstruction Planning was produced, which Hanson considers foreshadowed all the fundamental objectives and methods used in the five-year plans of the 1950s (Hanson 1966:38).

The Planning Commission, established in 1950, provided the central government with a capacity to affect health and other policy in matters that were, constitutionally, solely for the states, because it has controlled most of the uncommitted funds. In recognition of this power, the Planning Commission was under Nehru's direct control and it has remained near the center of Indian political life ever since, except for a few spells when planning fell into disfavour, especially the "Plan holiday" years 1966–1967 to 1968–1969, and under the Janata Government of 1977–1979. The First Plan (1951–1952 to 1955–1966) did little more than list existing projects and was not adopted until two of the five Plan years were already over. The later plans have played a substantial role in public-sector expenditure patterns. The First Plan explicitly rejected total nationalization, while the Second Plan, with its emphasis on heavy industry, stressed that the public sector should grow faster than the private sector, in line with the Industrial Policy Resolution of 1956 and the nationalization of life insurance companies and the Imperial Bank of India. The Second Plan foundered in 1958, because of a poor harvest and a balance of payments crisis, and was only rescued by considerable foreign assistance. The Third Plan (1961–1962 to 1965–1966) continued most of the emphasis of the second, with greater dependence on foreign assistance.

Planning was seriously challenged, however, during the Third Plan when the 1961 census revealed that the population was growing at 2.1 percent per annum whereas the Plan framework assumed only 1.2 percent. (Maddison 1972:114). In 1965 formal planning ceased due to the war with Pakistan, and a consequent cut in United States assistance, and a severe drought. For the next three years only Annual Plans were produced. The Fourth Plan (1969–1970 to 1974–1975) had a much lower profile and gave more emphasis to rural development. In retrospect, other difficulties can be dated from the mid-1960s, such as the failure of state operations to make profits for reinvestment and the absence of an internal market for its goods (Toye 1979). The third "crisis of planning" arose in 1972–1973, when the rising price of oil imports and another poor harvest raised the rate of inflation dramatically. The delayed

Fifth Plan only existed in draft form for several years. In 1977 the new Janata government attempted to replace the five-year planning sequence by rolling Plans in a longer perspective. Mrs. Gandhi's return to power in 1980 restored the position of the Planning Commission nearer to the center of power and the five-year planning process was resumed. The Sixth Plan for the years 1980–1981 to 1984–1985 was finally published in 1981, and the Seventh Plan in 1986.

Most discussions of the planning process in India have focused on the overall context and the problems dramatized by the crises of planning (for example, Streeten and Lipton 1968; Bhagwati and Desai 1970; Cassen 1978; Frankel 1982). The Planning Commission's power has depended on its closeness to the prime minister; while Nehru took a considerable interest, his successors have been less involved. Raising the resources for the Plans has not been the task of the Planning Commission but of ministries of finance at the center and the states. Thus the Planning Commission has had a limited ability to determine the patterns of public sector expenditure, while its planning for the private sector has been even more difficult to implement. The Plans' optimism about the volume of resources that would be raised and about the external environment, led to exaggerated estimates of growth in national income. The major determinant of growth in the economy—the productivity of agriculture—has received less attention than it deserves.

The catalog of criticism is almost endless. Specifically relevant to health sector planning is the weakness of concern for distributional aspects of development. Until about 1970 planners presumed that the benefits of increased economic output would inevitably trickle down to the mass of the poor. The assumption has come under increasing attack (e.g., Chenery et al. 1972) and alternative planning strategies have been proposed. One of these, concerted land reforms to attack the institutions that generate poverty in rural India, has not been seriously considered either by the Planning Commission or by the rest of the government of India. Instead, the response since 1971 has been the Minimum Needs Program, a basic-needs strategy to raise the priority of providing basic social services—health, education, housing and social welfare—for the mass of the population. I shall consider the details of health in the Plans in chapter 6.

The Context of Health-Policymaking After 1947

The context of health-policymaking after 1947 is set by two major influences—the report of the Health Survey and Development Committee, known by the name of its chair, Sir Joseph Bhore, and the activities of the Central Council of Health.

The Bhore committee was part of the World War II planning apparatus described above and published its four-volume report (GOI 1946) which, in the tradition of British committee reports, gave a detailed analysis of available data, evidence of expert witnesses, and recommendations produced by a secretariat. However, alternative proposals were also available, emanating from the Congress party itself. Congress established a National Planning Committee (NPC) in 1938, under Nehru's prompting. Nehru's socialism was essentially Fabian and involved national planning for a mixed economy, but his more radical ideas were ground down in the intense politicking of the first years after independence and his interest in the NPC seems to have evaporated. The committee report on public health (NPC 1946) was shorter, less well argued and costed, and drew on far less detailed analysis of the existing situation than the Bhore Report. Without a supporting secretariat or any political power base within the Congress party it disappeared with very few traces. Thus the Bhore report provided the framework for most health decision making.

In many areas the two reports overlap and show their common reliance on a perspective on rural health which had been developed under the League of Nations Health Organization and implemented in different degrees in Yugoslavia and Nationalist China (Lucas 1982). Both looked toward a socialized system of health services in which public health provisions dominate and eventually replace private medical practice. Bhore's phrasing was very similar to the Beveridge report, which foreshadowed the National Health Service in the United Kingdom, that "no individual should be unable to secure adequate medical care because of inability to pay for it" (GOI 1946; II:17). Both reports also supported insurance-based services for industrial workers, but accepted that this was impractical for the mass of the Indian population in the foreseeable future.

Both reports pointed to nutrition and general living standards as the major determinants of health, and argued that preventive measures should be most important. Both saw the integration of preventive and curative services provided by full-time salaried workers as the way to achieve this, and both called for government doctors to lose their rights to private practice. The importance of rural provision was also common ground: in Bhore's words, "it is the tiller of the soil on whom the economic structure of the country eventually rests" (ibid.: 4). Bhore also accepted that services should be as close to the people as possible. Both proposed a system of health centers in the villages linked to larger units at district level, though the details of how many were to be provided for a given size of population differed. The Bhore report was much more specific about desirable staffing levels over a thirty- to forty-year period, and also suggested a strategy for the shorter term, the first ten years. Both reports called for a substantial increase in public investment in health matters but stressed that a shortage of trained personnel would be a major constraint.

Finally, both reports emphasized health education—to change the habits of mind and ways of life of the mass of the population—and the need to engage villagers' cooperation in the work. The Bhore report cited an article by Henry Sigerist in arguing that Soviet-style health committees, as at Singur in Bengal, were a desirable model for India.

There are two main differences. First, Bhore advocated campaigns against specified diseases, particularly malaria, tuberculosis, venereal diseases, and leprosy, whereas the NPC report was silent on this issue. Second, clear differences emerged over the priority categories of personnel for training and the proper role of semitrained villagers and indigenous medical practitioners. For Bhore health assistants could relieve medical men (*sic*) of some of their curative and preventive duties, but he saw no role for the part-time health workers, who were the cornerstone of the NPC proposals (see chap. 9).

Both sets of proposals, then, envisaged much more conscious planning for health services than in the British period. But health-policymaking after independence was constrained by essentially the same federal structure as that created by the Montagu-Chelmsford Reforms of 1919 and slightly amended in 1935, a structure giving primary responsibility in health matters to the states. The center only kept control over international aspects—quarantine etc.—and over a limited range of all-India matters, including the regulation of standards of medical education (to permit medical personnel to practice throughout the country) and the control of communicable diseases.

Before independence, however, the central government could influence health policy in the provinces through the IMS officers heading the medical administration. But during the interwar period the IMS had become so unpopular with Congress that it was abolished in 1948 and not replaced by an alternative all-India service. Thereafter, central government had to rely on the financial incentives offered through the Plans, and on persuasion through informal channels, and through the Central Council of Health (CCH) which consists of health officials and ministers and meets annually to discuss health policy. The council grew out of the less formal and infrequent meetings of the Central Advisory Board for Health which was replaced in 1946 by conferences of health ministers. After the third conference in 1950, the Central Council of Health was established, with membership of the central government and all the states and chaired by the central minister of health. In the 1970s there was also briefly a Central Council of Family Planning, but this was later combined into the Central Council of Health and Family Welfare.

Each state is usually represented at CCH meetings by a minister, some generalist civil servants from the health ministry, and their main technical advisers from their health directorates. They are supplemented by a changing body of observers, usually including representatives from other cognate ministries, the president of the Medical Council of India, a representative from the Planning Commission, someone from major international agencies (WHO, UNICEF) and, during the 1950s and early 1960s, people from U.S. aid agencies, not only the U.S. government but also the Ford and Rockefeller Foundations. The agenda is largely set by the Central Health Ministry, though states can propose items. However, the council's second meeting established that the conclusions or motions passed by the CCH were only advisory and the states would not regard them as binding (GOI [CCH] 1954). This exposed the center's weak position, which has led some, including the Health Survey and Planning Committee (GOI 1962:46–46; 463–476), to reiterate calls for an all-India cadre of medical administrators to replace the IMS.

The Framework of Part II

Dealing with health policies that emerged since 1947, the guiding themes again will be drawn from critiques of health services in the Third World which are concerned to explain the inappropriateness of health services through a political economy of policymaking. Nationalist opponents of colonial rule have long made such criticisms and, since 1965, they have become increasingly common in discussions of health-service delivery in the Third World as almost the orthodox position (e.g., Bryant 1969; Morley 1972; Djukanovic and Mach 1975; Newell [ed.] 1975; World Bank 1980). From this perspective, too little is spent on health, while urban, curative, tertiary services receive undue support. For example, the UNICEF/WHO joint study (Djukanovic and Mach 1975:15,18) argued:

> Owing to the high cost of sophisticated equipment and other requirements, it tends to absorb, for the benefit of a minority of the population, a substantial share of limited resources . . . curative services and, more generally, personal services, tend to receive undue emphasis. . . . In many developing countries over half the national health budget is spent on health care in urban areas, the home of no more than a fifth of the total population.

These arguments rest largely on material gathered from Africa and Latin America (e.g., Frankenberg and Leeson 1972; Navarro 1974; Segall 1972; Doyal 1979), but writers have tended to assume that this picture also applies in India. Thus Cassen, in the most substantial discussion of India's population in a social and economic context yet, argues that

> India's health system shares several features of the pattern of health services in other developing countries [including] a large share of health budgets devoted to major hospitals in urban centres and a consequent relative neglect of the rural health infrastructure. (Cassen 1978:201)

Other aspects of India's health services have been vigorously attacked by Indian commentators; indeed, it is hard to find anyone with a good word to say about them. Only government and official publications dwell on the positive side of the medical history since 1947. One critical source summarizes the strengths of the Indian health system as follows:

It is obvious that there are several achievements to our credit, such as reduction in mortality rates or increase in expectancy of life at birth; the expansion of medical research and education; the expansion of the health care services including especially the establishment of the Primary Health Centres; the excellence of our specialised institutions; the control of communicable diseases like smallpox, cholera, plague and malaria; the provision of MCH services on a larger scale; the initiation of a family planning programme; and the investment of far larger funds than at any time in the past. (Ramalingaswami 1980:5)

It then argues that the weaknesses of the system are greater still. However, as with many of the critical discussions the report does not develop a theoretical account of the mismatch between health needs and health services. The criticisms are specified in the following terms:

1. Health services are not integrated with wider economic and social development;

2. Virtually no impact has been made on basic aspects of disease prevention and health maintenance, such as nutrition and environmental sanitation;

3. The most vulnerable social groups remain largely excluded from health services, whether vulnerability is indicated by poverty, age, sex, geographical isolation, or other factors such as occupation which increase the levels of disease and illness;

4. Health education is virtually nonexistent; and

5. The goal of participatory involvement remains a chimera.

In the words of the joint Indian Council for Medical Research– Indian Council for Social Science Research study (ibid.:6):

The imported and inappropriate model of health services is top-heavy, over-centralised, heavily curative in its approach, urban and elite oriented, costly and dependency creating. The serious shortcomings of the model cannot be cured by small tinkerings or well-meant reforms.

Some Indian critics have been heavily influenced by Ivan Illich, who has tried to move away from a doctor-centered approach to health services and to return health to the people. Others have assumed that the health services being offered are desirable, but they are not reaching the groups that need them most. Thus, for some people (Srivastava 1975) modern medicine itself is the culprit, while for others (Banerji 1983) the capitalist nature of Indian society distorts the potential contribution of scientific medicine. The Ramalingaswami report attempts, not very successfully, to bridge these divisions while remaining within an administrative framework which calls for yet more programs without providing an account of how the failures of past programs are to be avoided. In Rifkin's (1985) terms, it remains within a "health-planning" perspective in which economic and social rationality tempers the application of a medical model but does not radically challenge the top-down perspective of planners.

Some, however, have argued that the mismatch between health needs and health services can be explained through understanding the political economy at national and international levels (e.g., Navarro 1975; Doyal 1979; Banerji 1974; Zurbrigg 1984). These writers argue that health services in India, as elsewhere in the Third World, articulate poorly with people's health needs because the colonial system was racially skewed and focused on curative services in the interests of larger colonial interests—particularly social control. In addition, dependency relationships were established; models of health care were borrowed wholesale, despite being unsuited to local conditions. The class structure within medicine and which medicine served did not disappear overnight with the end of colonial rule but continued to subvert attempts to change. The established medical profession maintained its rewards and its access to a world market and its class links helped to perpetuate the imbalances that characterized colonial medicine. International aid and operations of multinational companies reinforced these tendencies. As a result, while the rhetoric changes the contemporary reality is one in which the mortality and morbidity experiences for the mass of the population have changed little since independence.

A simplified form of this general argument provides the structure for what follows. The picture that unfolds demonstrates that the Marxist questions are worth asking, but that the answers given by most Marxists have been too simplistic. In particular, Marxist accounts imply an almost functionalist integration of those different layers of the state distinguished by Alavi, whereas these layers are in reality disarticulated. The class interests of doctors mesh with those of the Indian ruling classes, but the complexity of the Indian state, and how it is integrated into the world economy, means that Indian health policies cannot be read straight off from those interests.

CHAPTER FIVE

Health Care and Development in Postcolonial India

Many Third World societies have experienced substantial declines of mortality since World War II, at much lower levels of living, and much more quickly, than in the historical experiences of developed countries. Mortality rates in poor countries seem more responsive to improvements in living conditions than to other changes; yet over this period, living standards, at least as measured by conventional indicators of economic growth, have not improved dramatically and sometimes have been stable or declined. The availability of powerful techniques to attack the transmission of many of the common diseases of poverty, such as malaria, cholera, and smallpox may be crucial. In industrialized countries these diseases gave way to the more general improvements in living standards, hygiene, and environmental health provisions, such as protected water supplies. However, the possibilities provided by disease-specific health policies may be limited by poverty (Ruzicka and Hansluwka 1982).

The available evidence suggests a steady decline in mortality in India since 1947 despite the slow fall in its major component, infant mortality. The expectation of life at birth has risen, but life expectancy at age five has risen more decisively still. Mortality might continue to fall over the immediate future. Yet poverty indicators show no overall decline (despite a rise in per capita national income); inequality in consumption has not noticeably fallen; unemployment has risen and so has landlessness; and indicators of nutritional status remain poor. Indicators of specific infectious diseases show dramatic declines (especially malaria and smallpox, but also plague and cholera) so it is tempting to conclude that specific disease-control programs have caused the decline in mortality. Yet this conclusion flies in the face of most assessments of Indian public health provisions, which point to their urban, curative bias and to the inadequacies of single-disease programs in improving public health.

First, I shall consider evidence of changes in mortality rates, and then morbidity and causes of death, especially infant and child deaths, for different groups in Indian society. I shall then look at material on social and economic development in India since 1947, with particular emphasis on evidence of the differential impact of such changes on men and women, on different regions, on urban as against rural populations, and on different economic groups. Finally, I shall briefly assess some explanations for these patterns. The statistics of mortality, nutrition, and living standards improved around 1970, so much of the discussion concerns the period since then. Throughout I assume that health services respond to a (distorted) disease reality, but they also modify that reality, though rarely in a direct and clear-cut way. Patterns of health and illness do not result from the impacts of health services alone, but must be seen in terms of changes in the social and physical environment, living standards, and patterns of living.

Mortality Since Independence

Clearly, mortality has declined in India since independence. But is the timing of this decline accurately represented by the official estimates? Does the decline in infant mortality follow that of general mortality? Has the position of females deteriorated relative to that of males? How has mortality declined in different parts of India? And what can explain the different patterns of mortality decline?

GENERAL MORTALITY

The simplest measure of mortality, the crude death rate, has declined from 27 per 1,000 population in 1941–1951 to 16 or 17 per 1,000 in 1971–1981, and 12 per 1,000 in 1981–1983 (Ruzicka 1984:14; Jain and Adlakha 1984:51). A more sophisticated indicator of mortality decline is life expectancy at birth; official estimates suggest that this has risen from about thirty-two years in 1941–1951, to fifty years in 1971–1981. These estimates were derived from the censuses and (for 1970 onward) from the Sample Registration Scheme (SRS), and they have different weaknesses. Calculations using the census make assumptions about how people wrongly state their ages or the ages of their children or parents. The 1941 and 1951 censuses have additional problems because of deaths and migration during partition. Visaria (1969) argued that the life expectancy figures based on the 1951 and 1961 censuses overestimated life expectancy at birth by as much as four years; Dyson (1979) similarly cast doubt on the 1961 and 1971 calculations. Such uncertainties account for the different figures for mortality decline in table 10.

INFANT MORTALITY

The major component in high mortality rates in India has always been the high level of infant mortality, and considerable

TABLE 10
ESTIMATES OF MORTALITY DECLINE

Changes in crude death rate	1941–50 to 1951–60	1951–60 to 1961–70	1961–70 to 1971–80
Registrar-General	– 17%	– 17%	– 20%
Visaria (1969)	– 5%	– 27%	
Ambannavar (1975)	– 12%	– 21%	
Changes in life expectancy at birth:			
Males			
Official life tables	+ 9.4 years	+ 4.5 years	+ 4.3 years
Visaria (1969)/Dyson (1979)	+ 5.3 years	+ 9.4 years	
Females			
Official life tables	+ 8.9 years	+ 4.1 years	+ 5.3 years
Visaria (1969)/Dyson (1979)	+ 5.3 years	+ 7.7 years	

SOURCE: Ruzicka (1984:14); Verma (1983). For 1961–70 to 1971–80 the figures are derived from the Sample Registration Scheme.

doubt has been cast on the rates estimated by intercensus comparisons (see table 11). A particular problem is the peculiar pattern of female-male ratios; it is unlikely that female rates rose above male rates for the first time in the 1970s, and more likely that this can be explained by the inferiority of the census-based estimates compared with those from the SRS. The intercensus estimates seem to have been supplemented by data from the National Sample Survey (NSS), which probably took insufficient account of underreporting of deaths, especially infant ones. Further, the evidence from small-scale studies such as the Khanna project in Punjab or from the SRS indicate that male death rates up to age ten are lower than female death rates, especially in the populous northern states that dominate the all-India figures. Finally, SRS estimates of infant mortality rates are higher in 1970–1975 than official estimates for 1961–1971, but the recorded crude death rate in this period fell, so the IMR almost certainly also fell, since it is such a major contributor to the overall death rate. Thus the apparently uneven decline in IMR from 183 in 1941–1951 to 132 in 1970–1975 may be misleading because the estimates for the 1960s (and earlier) may be too low: Dyson (1979), for example suggests 156 for females and 146 for males (see also Visaria and Visaria 1981; Visaria 1985).

TABLE 11
OFFICIAL ESTIMATES OF INFANT MORTALITY RATES

	Rural			Urban			Combined		
	male	female	total	male	female	total	male	female	total
1941–50	–	n.a.	–	–	n.a.	–	190	175	182
1951–60	–	n.a.	–	–	n.a.	–	153	138	146
1961–70	–	n.a.	–	–	n.a.	–	130	128	129
1972–73	141	152	146	86	87	87	132	141	136
1974–75	145	143	144	77	81	79	134	129	133
1976–77	135	146	139	79	82	81	125	135	130
1978–79	131	137	134	74	73	73	121	126	123
1980–81	–	–	122	–	–	63	–	–	112
1982–83	–	–	114	–	–	65	106	104	105

SOURCE: Ruzicka 1984:18; Visaria and Visaria 1981; Visaria 1985; Government of India 1985a. The first three rows are derived from intercensus calculations, possibly using survey data from 1958–59 and SRS data from 1968 onwards; the remaining rows are averages for the two years quoted, and are derived entirely from SRS estimates.

Other problems of consistency among different indicators remain. Censuses show very similar population growth between 1961 and 1971 and between 1971 and 1981—yet fertility had almost certainly declined substantially. Using two national surveys, Jain and Adlakha (1984) estimate that the crude birth rate fell by between 8 percent and 14 percent from 1972 to 1978, while the SRS figures produce an 11 percent decline (*Sample Registration Bulletin* 1982). If fertility declined but mortality did not, population growth must have been lower after 1971 than before. Either mortality rates have fallen more since the mid-1960s than official estimates suggest, or the 1971 census undercounted the population by more than did either the 1961 or 1981 censuses or both. Jain and Adlakha (1984:52) suggest that population growth was probably higher in 1961–1971 than previously thought (not 2.2 percent but perhaps 2.4 percent per year) and population growth between 1971 and 1981 was less (not 2.2 percent but perhaps 2.0 percent per year). They note an additional complication: if the number of births has dropped, the significance of infant mortality in total mortality must also have declined.

To summarize, mortality probably declined between 1945 and 1955 at much the same rate as during the previous twenty years. The rate accelerated between about 1955 and 1965, but in the next ten years mortality may not have declined at all. Mortality decline has since resumed, with the SRS recording crude death rates (CDRs) in 1981–1984 as 10 percent lower than those in 1975. Infant mortality rates seem to have dropped more slowly, and were possibly as high as 200 in the 1940s, 160 in the 1950s, 150 in the 1960s, 140 at the beginning of the 1970s, and about 115 at the end. Fluctuations, annually or in two- or three-year cycles, prevent any meaningful analysis of shorter periods.

REGIONAL VARIATIONS

These patterns of mortality and mortality decline are not common to all parts of the country. Dyson and Moore (1983) pull together a variety of indicators to suggest that different "demographic regimes" characterize different parts of the country. Crudely, north India has high fertility and high mortality (and high excess female mortality); in south India the reverse is the case. Dyson and Moore argue that these patterns correspond to differences in women's status which can be traced to different systems of kinship and inheritance, leading, for example, to higher rates of female education and marriage at a later age in south India. Not all the links between these variables are clearly understood, but historically, mortality rates were lower in many parts of south India than in the north, and the north shows no sign of catching up. Kerala's rural death rates are half the national average, while the rates for Uttar Pradesh are 30 percent above the all-India figures. No clear pattern of mortality and mortality decline by states emerges in the data for the 1970s, the earliest period for which reasonably reliable figures are available. In general, the states of the center north (Uttar Pradesh, Bihar, Madhya Pradesh, and Rajasthan) have high rural death rates (14.5 per thousand or over in 1982–1984), and the rates for Bihar and Madhya Pradesh dropped only about 10 percent over the previous twelve years. At the other end of the continuum Kerala, Punjab, and Maharashtra had rural crude death rates of 10.5 per thousand or under in 1882–1987, with over 20 percent declines since 1970–1972 (*Sample Registration Bulletin* June 1986).

High poverty rates, low literacy rates, and poorer general social infrastructure help to explain the high mortality rates in the center-north, and their slow decline. But states with low mortality rates include some very wealthy ones (Punjab, Haryana, and Maharashtra) as well as Karnataka and Kerala, which are much poorer. In addition, Maharashtra, Kerala, and Karnataka have high levels of inequality, indicated by their high proportion of poverty, compared with Punjab and Haryana. Other health indicators (such as nutrition data) correlate poorly with levels or speed of decline of mortality, at least in the 1970s. Thus the variations in the decline in mortality rates by states cannot simply be understood in terms of conventional measures of income and inequality. Comparisons of changes in infant mortality display similar regional patterns, though Dyson's estimates show some very surprising features, such as low figures for Bihar and very high ones for Gujarat. As table 13 shows, the rate of decline in infant mortality rates varies substantially with the decline in Kerala being the fastest from an already low level.

TABLE 12

CHANGES IN CRUDE DEATH RATES FOR MAJOR STATES
1970–1972 TO 1982–1984

	CDR 1982–84		1982–84 as % of 1970–72		1982–84 as % of all India	
	rural	urban	rural	urban	rural	urban
South						
Andhra	11.5	7.4	68	72	86	94
Karnataka	10.5	6.3	74	80	79	80
Kerala	6.5	6.9	71	88	49	87
Tamil Nadu	12.9	8.1	76	92	97	103
East						
Assam	12.8	8.0	71	82	96	101
Orissa	13.7	9.1	74	83	103	115
West Bengal	11.8	6.9	n.a.	73	89	87
West						
Gujarat	12.7	8.5	75	71	95	108
Maharashtra	10.3	6.9	71	74	77	87
Center-north						
Bihar	14.5	8.0	90	84	109	101
Madhya Pradesh	15.8	8.9	87	82	119	113
Rajasthan	14.3	9.3	81	97	108	113
Uttar Pradesh	17.4	10.7	76	79	131	135
North-west						
Haryana	10.5	6.7	88	81	79	85
Punjab	9.8	6.5	79	71	74	82
All-India	13.3	7.9	76	80	100	100

SOURCE: *Sample Registration Bulletin*, June 1986.

VARIATIONS BY SEX

The Indian subcontinent is one of the very few
regions where women have tended to die younger than men, and
most indicators of mortality by sex suggest that between the 1940s
and the 1970s females did not benefit as much as males from the
decline in mortality (e.g., Indian Council for Social Science
Research 1975). For example, the all-India sex ratio (the number of

TABLE 13

INFANT MORTALITY RATES FOR MAJOR STATES
1968 TO 1982

		c. 1968		1972		1978		1982		1982–72	
		male	female	male	female	male	female	male	female	male	female
South:	Andhra	133	113	123	108	129	93	84	75	68	69
	Karnataka	117	106	107	88	82	67	73	56	68	64
	Kerala	75	62	64	61	38	40	32	28	50	46
	Tamil Nadu	142	128	122	121	107	99	82	83	67	69
East	Assam	149	128	149	124	130	105	106	96	71	77
	Orissa	192	179	126	136	128	139	140	124	111	91
	West Bengal*	78	79	n.a.	n.a.	83	73	90	81	n.a.	n.a.
West:	Gujarat	193	222	134	122	114	123	113	110	84	90
	Maharashtra	119	123	100	103	81	69	71	69	71	67
Center-north:	Bihar*	88	93	n.a.	n.a.	92	95	107	118	n.a.	n.a.
	Madhya Pradesh	151	151	152	161	141	128	142	124	93	76
	Rajasthan	199	229	111	137	124	134	96	98	86	72
	Uttar Pradesh	210	259	186	220	154	180	142	152	76	69
North-west:	Haryana	79	86	80	111	101	119	92	95	115	86
	Punjab	110	125	108	130	104	101	78	73	72	56
All-India		146	156	132	148	120	131	106	104	80	70

SOURCE: 1968 figures are by Dyson 1979; 1972 and 1978 figures are from Registrar-General 1983; 1982 figures are from Government of India 1985a.
*Bihar and West Bengal are regarded as particularly unreliable, both for 1972 (Sample Registration Scheme) and for the 1978 special survey. The last two columns express the 1982 figures as a percentage of the 1972 figures.

females per 1,000 males) declined from 946 in 1951 to 935 in 1971. Almost all state sex-ratios declined, including states with high ratios (Kerala, Orissa, and Tamil Nadu) and some with low ratios (Uttar Pradesh, Rajasthan, and Madhya Pradesh). Rates for the Punjab, Bengal, and Assam rose. The 1981 census produced a higher sex ratio; some have argued that the trend has now changed (Sen 1986), though some have suggested that the 1971 figure was an underestimate, so the trend may still be downward. The intercensal estimates of life expectancy at different ages (tables 10 and 14) support the view that the relative position of women worsened from the 1940s to the 1960s. Since then, some evidence suggests that the trend may indeed have changed. The 1971 to 1981 life expectancy figures for women are 5.3 years higher than those for 1961–1971; the equivalent figures for men are only 4.3 years. According to some methods, female life expectancy may now have caught up with that of men. The SRS figures for infant mortality (table 13) show that in the southern and western states male rates are only slightly below (or even above) female rates, whereas in the northern states, female rates are considerably above male rates. From 1972 to 1982, the national figures show a decline in excess female infant mortality, with most states, including the largest ones, sharing this pattern. The 1982 figures are the first to show higher male rates, though the difference is very small (Government of India 1985a).

Morbidity and Causes of Death

AMONG INFANTS AND CHILDREN

Infant and child mortality is by far the largest source of death. In the 1970s about 30 percent of all deaths recorded by the SRS were of infants (i.e., under the age of one), and another 20 percent of children under the age of 5 (GOI 1983:43). This varies somewhat by state, with Kerala at one extreme, where only eighteen percent of all deaths are of infants, and Uttar Pradesh at the other, with infant deaths 38 percent of all those recorded.

Infant mortality can be divided into two major groups—neonatal (within the first month of life) and postneonatal mortality (after the first month but within the first year). In India, evidence on neonatal mortality is derived from special local studies (such as at Khanna

TABLE 14
Life Expectancy of Males and Females in India, 1941–51, 1961–71, and 1970–75 at Selected Ages

Age	males			females			% age Increase c. 1946 to c. 1972	
	1941–51	1961–71	1970–75	1941–51	1961–71	1970–75	male	female
0	32.5	46.4	50.5	31.7	44.7	49.0	55	55
10	39.0	48.8	53.8	39.5	47.7	54.2	38	37
20	33.0	41.1	44.8	32.9	39.9	45.6	36	39
30	26.6	33.3	36.0	26.2	32.0	37.5	35	43
40	20.5	25.9	27.6	21.1	25.4	29.3	35	39
50	14.9	19.2	19.8	16.2	19.7	21.3	33	31
60	10.1	13.6	13.4	11.3	13.8	14.3	33	27

SOURCE: For 1941–51 and 1961–71, Ram & Schultz (1979); for 1970–75 *Sample Registration Bulletin*, XVI, 1 (June 1982).

and Narangwal in Punjab) or from the less reliable (but national) SRS. For the 1970s the latter suggests that neonatal mortality accounted for over 50 percent of infant mortality rates in urban and rural areas alike in each year (Visaria 1985:1,354). The one exception was Punjab: in 1970–1972 only 20 percent of infant deaths were recorded as neonatal, though the 1976–1978 and 1982 figures reflect the national picture.

Most neonatal mortality results either from genetic defects or from infection or injury received at the time of delivery. Reduction of neonatal mortality is limited by the existence of a hard core of congenital malformations, but in poor countries that limit is very far from having been reached. Neonatal mortality can be affected most by improving mothers' health during pregnancy and the quality of midwifery services. The Khanna study suggested that neonatal deaths were largely a result of tetanus or septicemia, because the cord was not cut or was not tied in a sterile way (Wyon and Gordon 1971). A study in eastern Uttar Pradesh in 1973 agreed that tetanus was probably a major cause of neonatal death (Simmons et al. 1982), and a survey in 1981 suggested that about 40 percent of all neonatal deaths nationally were because of neonatal tetanus, ranging from over 70 percent in rural Uttar Pradesh to 17 percent in Maharashtra and Gujarat.

Inoculating the pregnant woman against tetanus (whereby the child is also protected) and ensuring more hygienic conditions at delivery are both strategies that have been attempted, though with very low priority before 1977. States with high rates of immunization have lower tetanus rates, but they are also states where birth attendants are more likely to come from the immediate family or be trained, rather than untrained dais. The data are not sufficient to allow the significance of these two factors to be distinguished (Gopalan 1985:160; Visaria 1985:1400–1401).

A second cause of early infant mortality is the poor nutritional status of the mother. Gopalan (1985) summarizes some of the scanty information on maternal nutrition. Complications during pregnancy and delivery and low birth-weight babies who are less likely to thrive are closely related to maternal weight and height. Using a weight cut-off band of 38 kilograms (83 lbs.), and a height cut-off of 145 centimeters (just under 4 ft. 8 in.), Gopalan suggests that around 20 percent of women of reproductive age are badly at risk in pregnancy. However, variations by state do not conform with expectations: Kerala, with its low infant mortality rates, has more at-risk women than does Uttar Pradesh. Probably this is because Uttar Pradesh women give birth more often. Higher parity children are generally at greater risk partly because older women in all the states are lighter than younger women. Some of this may be due to nutritional improvement over the past thirty years since older women are typically shorter. Further, childbearing itself is a significant nutritional drain on women who start the process undernourished. They breast-feed their babies relatively successfully but at the cost of their own long-term survival, though there are regional variations.

Such factors can be expected to lead to high maternal mortality rates. The evidence is very poor, but a commonly accepted estimate is that from 1970 to 1972 about 400 women died for every 100,000 live births (ibid.:164), around forty times the level in Western Europe. Karkal (1985:1,835) quotes higher estimates, of between 500 and 800. Estimates of regional, age, parity, and social-class variations do not seem to exist, though one study suggests that the maternal mortality rate in Greater Bombay was still around 150 although nearly all births take place in medical institutions (ibid.). A proxy for maternal mortality is differential age-specific mortality rates. During the reproductive years, female mortality rates are higher than male rates; in 1980, in Uttar Pradesh and Madhya Pradesh, they were twice the male rates for ages fifteen to thirty (Gopalan 1985:162). Kerala is unusual; there female mortality rates are lower than male rates at all ages, which is the pattern in most of the rest of the world.

Maternal nutrition, then, affects infant and child mortality, not just in the first month of life (small babies are less likely to survive the traumas of birth) but also later, when mortality tends to relate closely to infection and nutrition, often working in combination. The most common fatal infections among infants are pneumonia and bronchopneumonia, which account for up to 25 percent of infant deaths in some years (Mitra 1978:176–177; Arora et al. 1979:296). The link with nutrition is especially obvious in diarrheal and parasitic diseases, which may account for another 15 percent of infant deaths, and a larger share of deaths of children aged one to five (Arora et al. 1979).

Measuring children's nutritional adequacy and estimating the extent of malnutrition have been hotly debated in India since 1975

(Payne 1984). This debate has considerable potential policy significance, since Indian estimates of the poverty level are based
partly on the income required for a nutritionally adequate diet. One
point at issue is whether mean figures for nutritional requirements
(in, for example, calories) should be used. If they are, at least 40
percent of the Indian population is in "absolute" poverty, apparently unable to obtain enough food to maintain themselves. Yet
people do stay alive in these circumstances, so it has been suggested that the mean figures are unrealistic. People have very variable abilities to maintain themselves on given food intakes; and
since distribution is not equitable within the household, few
receive the "mean" amount.

Individual variation is obviously crucial, since people of similar
ages, height, weight, and patterns of activity may have very different nutritional needs. If this is recognized, and estimates of minimum requirements are reduced, estimates of absolute poverty can
also be reduced, since some of those absolutely poor under the first
procedure can actually obtain enough food for their own
metabolism to maintain them relatively stable. That is, some people may be "naturally" small, and this could be a beneficial pattern of adjustment rather than owing to inadequate nutrition which
weakens people and makes them more vulnerable to infection and
early death (Cassen 1978:98). But this alternative procedure underestimates the numbers not receiving a nutritionally adequate
diet, since some of those in wealthier households nevertheless do
not receive enough food for their requirements; and others with
enough food are not well nourished because disease weakens their
ability to use the food they eat or because their diet is unsatisfactory, or they are well nourished during some seasons but not in
others.

This debate is, ultimately, rather arid. Nobody denies that very
many, perhaps most, Indians do not have enough to eat and, as
Banerji (1982) argues, they know that themselves. However, two
points do emerge from the more detailed evidence. Children under
the age of two are likely to be undernourished even in families with
adequate purchasing power. Studies in Tamil Nadu, Punjab, Kerala, and Calcutta provide evidence for this (Cassen 1978). First, the
combination of late weaning, unsuitable weaning foods, and weanling diarrhea (diarrhea accompanying the shift from breast milk to
a mixed diet) probably accounts for this finding. Second, a large

proportion of Indian babies have birth weights low enough to suggest that they start their lives malnourished (about 25 percent below 2,500 grams) because their mothers are undernourished and do not eat enough in the last few months of their pregnancies to allow their fetuses to grow adequately (ibid.:104).

Which nutritional standards are appropriate for assessing Indian children? Some argue that international standards are too strict, while others argue that international standards should be used since affluent Indian children's growth accords with these standards. But whichever standard is chosen, undernutrition of children is widespread in India, with one estimation of 85 percent of all children under five (Gopalan 1985:160). The extent of severe undernutrition varies by state: Uttar Pradesh seems one of the worst, with one study showing 14 percent of all children severely malnourished (ibid.). Gopalan argues that this undernourishment is generally a result of inadequate breast-feeding caused by the poor nutritional status of mothers; poor Indian women rarely use commercial alternatives even in the major cities and their surrounding areas.

Female babies and young children get even less, proportionately, than do boys. The greatest differences are usually found in north India, where sons are valued much more highly than daughters. Thus, one study in Uttar Pradesh found 58 percent of boys malnourished (by an international standard), compared with 70 percent of girls. Even in Madras, where preference for sons is usually considered weaker than in north India, one study showed that 70 percent of boys but 80 percent of girls were undernourished by an Indian standard (ibid.).

The infections that in combination with poor nutritional status are often fatal in children, are diarrhea and dysentery, and diseases such as measles (Scrimshaw et al. 1968). Donoso (1979) suggests that weaning diarrhea peaks in the second six months of life but continues at a high rate until about the end of the third year. Using Khanna and Narangwal data, he suggests that most mortality occurs in children from 6 to 18 months, and that about 1 million children in India die every year in this way (ibid.:105). Malnutrition does not cause these deaths directly, but malnourished children (especially those in unhygienic conditions) are more vulnerable to illness and, once ill, to death.

AMONG ADULTS

As in most poor countries (except, apparently, China [World Bank 1985]), infectious diseases constitute the major causes of morbidity and mortality among adults and children alike. The format in which "cause of death" is returned from states and union territories has reflected this focus. Mitra (1978:148) points out that the "meaningful, operational, and classificatorily significant" categories are cholera, smallpox, plague, dysentery and diarrhea, respiratory diseases, fevers, accidents and injuries, and all others (which are occasionally further classified to distinguish whooping cough, diphtheria, and maternal deaths). Since some diseases, such as smallpox, have declined in significance, causes such as cancer or heart disease should become more prominent, but information on the epidemiology of these diseases in India is elusive. The Model Registration Scheme, which reports on a sample of some 20,000 deaths a year, is more sophisticated, but many deaths are not classified beyond a very general category (fevers, cough) and some distinctions seem implausible given the problems of data collection involved (Cassen 1978:108).

Since high mortality in India has been seen in terms of separate major infectious diseases, preventive health campaigns were also planned along separate lines. The major killers of the British period were plague, cholera, smallpox, malaria, and tuberculosis, with influenza an occasional mass killer as in 1918–1919. Plague was causing very few deaths even before 1947, and influenza has not received special attention, but each of the others has formed the focus of single-disease campaigns similar to those used by the British (most notably, for smallpox). But it was the campaigns against malaria, particularly those run by the WHO, USAID, and the Rockefeller Foundation in the 1930s and the 1940s which provided more detailed models, since these agencies were crucial in providing funding and technical support to the Indian campaigns of the 1950s and the 1960s. The literature describing these diseases in India assumes a clear relationship between disease-related mortality and morbidity and these individual disease-control programs. I shall briefly describe these programs in turn, though a more general discussion will be provided later on.

Cholera. Cholera has been concentrated particularly in certain parts of India—West Bengal, Orissa, Bihar, and eastern Uttar Pradesh in the east, Tamil Nadu and Andhra in the southeast, and Assam in the northeast. This pattern hardly changed from 1900 to 1965, with twelve districts in these areas responsible for nearly 40 percent of all reported cases between 1954 and 1964 (Mitra 1978:152–153). In the late 1960s, some new focal areas developed (especially in Maharashtra, Gujarat, and Kerala) with some declines in the older focal areas. Some mechanisms of the spread of cholera from its "home" in the Ganges delta have been undermined since 1947, partly by strong controls over pilgrims attending religious fairs (vaccination is nominally compulsory and water supplies have been greatly improved). The numbers reported dying from cholera are now possibly under 0.5 percent of all deaths, or less than 60,000 per year (Cassen 1978:84). Mitra suggests that cholera is now less virulent, though the reason is unclear. However, because cholera can be transmitted from individuals who may harbor the disease for a month or more with no symptoms, it cannot easily be excluded from an area, and often returns in flood or famine situations. The basic conditions for its transference—unsanitary water supplies and food-handling conditions—have been unaffected by the cholera control programs. However, the rural water-supply schemes, which have been a feature of the 1980s, may make some impact.

Smallpox. Smallpox mortality was low by 1947, though the disease was still common. Smallpox came in periodic waves which, during the early twentieth century, became farther and farther apart and lasted for shorter periods. After 1947 this general trend continued, with only 1950–1951 and 1957–1958 recording relatively high levels. Vaccination operations continued to reduce the incidence of the disease, but vaccination was not compulsory nor sufficiently widespread (e.g., for children) to prevent new outbreaks. Vaccination was stepped up after 1962–1963, with the creation of a Smallpox Eradication Program. However, its record was indifferent until much more substantial international assistance was provided through WHO after a smallpox outbreak following the 1971 war with Pakistan. The new strategy involved focusing all efforts at cordoning off smallpox enclaves and covering the population there, rather than spreading the effort throughout the country (Basu et al. 1979). The apparent increase in the numbers of cases from the 2,700 in 1971 to the more than 30,000 in 1974, probably reflects improved reporting mechanisms (Mitra 1978:160). This was apparently the last flourish, for no new cases have been reported since July 1975.

Malaria. In the 1940s about 75 million people suffered from malaria every year, with about 800,000 deaths a year (5 per 1,000 population). This excludes those who died from associated complications, such as pregnant women or those weakened by malaria, who more easily succumbed to something else (Dutt et al. 1980:320). Pyrethrum had been used to spray breeding areas and house sites before World War II and after 1946, DDT began to be used. In Bombay state an estimated 500,000 cases a year were being prevented by 1949. WHO ran demonstration projects elsewhere in the country and, in 1953, a national organization was established for malaria control with WHO and USAID assistance. In 1958 the apparent success of these campaigns and changes in WHO strategy led to greater efforts and a new goal, eradication.

These programs increased reporting of fever cases, were able to make a better estimate of how many cases were due to malaria, and they also collected other data on malaria morbidity. These data suggested a steady decline in malaria cases, a decline that continued until 1965 when very few cases and hardly any deaths were reported. Since then, the numbers of malaria cases have risen steadily, and more rapidly since 1975. Until recently, mortality from malaria has risen much more slowly, but increasingly reports suggest that more cases of malaria are leading to death (Gill 1985).

Several factors contributed to the apparent failure of the eradication program. In 1965 (the year when lowest morbidity was reported) DDT supplies were interrupted. The United States government reduced its aid because of the Indo-Pakistani war that year, and two poor harvests gave food imports a high priority, so foreign exchange was scarce. Supplies were further disturbed by health-budget cuts (while defense expenditure rose) and by the disruption to trade through the Suez Canal after 1967.

But the Health Ministry had its own problems. Preventive campaigns were difficult to sustain in the face of apparent success. Harrison (1978:241–246) graphically describes the problems of ensuring effective work from the lowest category of staff. Spraying must be done conscientiously, but it was much easier to avoid locked houses, unwilling villagers, and villages that were inaccessible just in the season when spraying was most required. Blood slides must be collected routinely, accurately and quickly assessed, and new cases treated before they spread the disease to others. But the funding constraints were tight. All workers had large areas or populations to deal with, no allowance was made for staff illness, desertion, or recalcitrance, and managers were continually pressed to wind down the campaign for budgetary reasons. While control of malaria probably has quite wide margins of error, these considerations probably meant that in several areas pockets of malaria remained, some on the borders with Pakistan where comparable antimalarial campaigns were not being waged.

By 1965 most areas were in a consolidation phase, the special campaigns were wound down, and the policy focus shifted to population control. Antimalarial work was passed to normal health services, but the rural health program was lagging well behind the desired pattern (Dutt 1980:321; Sinha 1976:946–947). Malaria returned but was not recorded, and remedial measures were not undertaken. In 1965 three substantial zones still contained untreated tracts and the disease has since spread out from them. Antimalarial activity since 1970 has been additionally hindered by problems of resistance to DDT and exacerbated by the use of DDT for agricultural purposes. But DDT resistance was not the cause of malarial resurgence though it now hinders control programs (Chapin and Wasserstrom 1983).

Tuberculosis. In 1947 tuberculosis was probably second only to malaria as a cause of death. While malaria mortality has dropped sharply, the level and virulence of tuberculosis does not seem to have changed very much. It is mainly an adult disease, and for those over fifteen it may cause as much as 50 percent of the deaths attributed to "cough" and at least 10 percent of all adult deaths, according to the Model Registration Scheme data (Mitra 1978:178–179; Cassen 1978:107–109). The Khanna study data suggest that tuberculosis was the third most important cause of death after diarrhea and pneumonia, which are more important for children (Wyon and Gordon 1971).

In Europe tuberculosis probably declined because of improved nutrition and spreading immunity, but neither is having much impact in India yet (Cassen 1978:88–89). Poor nutrition, dense housing, and migration patterns that help to spread the disease have not been affected by the single-disease campaigns that have dominated public health in India since independence. The National Tuberculosis Control Program shows no signs of success. The mainstay of the preventive and protective activity has been the BCG (bacille Calmette-Guérin) vaccine, which may be almost useless. Tuberculosis control requires that cases should be discovered and should complete a long course of effective treatment. However, TB sufferers are generally treated for cough in the first instance. They often fail to complete the full course of anti-TB treatment because they feel better long before it is completed. Thus they relapse and transmit the infection to others. Treatment at home, however crowded or unsanitary, can be effective (as Fox demonstrated in the 1950s), but ensuring completion of treatment remains an intractable problem. Finally, the treatment is anyway probably only about 75 percent effective. The control of TB in India is unlikely to be imminent.

Other diseases. Other diseases that contribute significantly to mortality are probably digestive diseases (diarrhea, dysentery, gastroenteritis) and respiratory diseases (pneumonia, bronchopneumonia, and bronchitis). The Khanna study reported heart disease and cancer among the "top ten" causes of death, but these causes are absent from national estimates, or estimates more recent than the 1950s. No assessment of the quantitative significance of these other causes of death is available. Some 6 percent of adult deaths could well be from violence or accidental injuries (Cassen 1978:108), while accidents probably account for a substantial part of young male and female adult mortality; women seem particularly vulnerable to "aggravated" accidents. Many of these accidents would better be recorded as murder or suicide, linked to pressure on young married women to provide more dowry from their parents or brothers for their husbands' families. In urban Maharashtra about 25 percent of all deaths of women aged 15–44 were accidental, of which "burns" was the major subcategory (Karkal 1985).

Despite these exceptions, the main causes of mortality in India remain those infectious and water-borne diseases characteristic of poverty. Reducing the significance of some diseases (like smallpox and malaria) as causes of death has not markedly altered the broad outlines of morbidity and mortality, because the living conditions of the mass of the Indian population have not changed.

Social and Economic Development

The living standards of Indians have been much discussed on the basis of relatively poor data. Table 15 suggests a qualified optimism. National income has risen by at least 2.2 percent per annum (the rate of increase of the population), so that at constant prices, average per capita incomes in 1983 were about 60 percent higher than those of 1950. Official figures are probably underestimates, because "unaccounted for" and "black" incomes may have grown proportionately since 1950 and now add a further 20 percent or so. The amount of food available in the country per head is rising (if the "right" years are used for comparisons) and indicators of basic nonfood consumption (domestic electricity, largely urban, and cloth) have also risen. On the other hand, a slightly different set of indicators will show that the proportion of the population living below the poverty line is stable or increasing, that unemployment, poor housing, and other indicators of poverty show no improvement, and that the lot of India's poor is deteriorating in other ways as well, even if the inequality of income in India is less than in many comparable countries.

The economy is still heavily dependent on agriculture and successful crop seasons lead to higher economic growth, and vice versa. Agricultural output has risen rapidly in some crops (notably wheat), more slowly in others (such as rice), and shows no growth trend for others (like the pulses). Taking all sources of food grains together (making allowance for government stocks, imports, and exports but not for changes in private stocks), per capita availability has risen by about 12 percent between 1950 and 1982. However, the situation has fluctuated, and the peak levels reached in 1961 and 1978 have not been sustained. More important, the availability of pulses (which are nutritionally very significant in the diets of the poor) is now little more than half its earlier level.

Estimates of the distribution of increased incomes and consumption are derived largely from successive rounds of the National Sample Survey (NSS). The classic studies using this source date from 1970 and draw on survey results from 1956 to 1957 onward. The most recent figures are from the 1977–1978 survey. It should be possible, then, to describe what has happened to the Indian population over this twenty-year period and answer three ques-

TABLE 15

INDICATORS OF NATIONAL INCOME, AGRICULTURAL OUTPUT, AND CONSUMPTION

	1950–51	1955–56	1960–61	1965–66	1970–71	1975–76	1980–81	1981–82	1982–83	1983–84
Net national product (Rs. bill) (1970–71 prices)	168	200	244	273	345	402	475	499	511	551
Per capita incomes (Rs.) (1970–71 prices)	466	508	559	559	633	664	700	715	721	749
Index of agricultural production (1967–70 = 100)										
rice	56	70	88	78	107	125	137	137	120	154
wheat	38	48	61	58	132	160	201	207	237	252
pulses	82	97	112	88	104	115	96	104	106	117
Net availability per head										
Food grains (grams)	395	431	469	408	469	453	454	454	436	478
of which cereals		361	400	360	418	402	417	415	397	436
pulses		70	69	48	51	51	37	39	39	42
Domestic electricity (KWH)	1.6	2.4	3.4	4.8	7.0	9.7	13.5	15.1	17.0	18.2
Cloth/cotton (meter)	11.0	14.4	13.8	14.7	13.6	12.6	11.0	10.2	9.9	10.8
Man-made (meter)	n.a.	n.a.	1.2	1.7	2.0	2.0	3.7	4.3	3.7	4.0

SOURCES: *Economic Survey* (1982–1983):77, 80; Bardhan 1984:92; Tata 1982:46, 52; Cassen 1978:257; Government of India 1985b (105, 108, 122).

tions: has the distribution of income become more or less equitable? Has the population below an appropriate poverty line increased or fallen? Have the incomes of the poorest groups risen or fallen in absolute terms? (Cassen 1978:237).

This material seems to pose more problems than it solves. Income information from surveys is never very reliable; then the sample is not representative, especially at the top and bottom of the ranges; estimates in current prices need to take account of price changes, which have not affected all income groups equally; and different indicators tend to give different results (ibid.:238–241). Only relatively large changes in indicators would constitute convincing evidence to answer the questions posed above, but most changes seem to be small. For example, the poorest 20 percent of the population apparently had about 7 percent to 8 percent of incomes and consumption in 1956–1957 and in 1975–1976 (ibid.:240; Bardhan 1984:1–2). One indicator (the Lorenz ratio) of the degree to which rural consumption is concentrated among the relatively wealthy, fluctuates between 0.28 and 0.32 between 1956–1957 and 1977–1978, using NSS data in current prices (Cassen 1978:240; Gupta and Datta 1984:635). Similarly, some estimates suggest that 40 percent of the population was below a poverty line of Rs 15 per head per month (in 1960–1961) prices in 1960–1961, 1972–1973, and 1977–1978 (Cassen 1978:241, 243; Bardhan 1984:2). For the whole country, the only simple conclusion is that there is no clear evidence of change one way or another. There is little agreement, for example, about the impact of new agricultural technologies on income inequalities or the level of poverty, particularly in wheat-growing areas, let alone on the likely changes suggested by any emerging trends.

Examining regional variations may help to understand what is happening. Much of the improvement in income levels can be accounted for by rises in a few states—notably Punjab, Haryana, Gujarat, and Maharashtra. In the central-north Hindi heartland of Uttar Pradesh, Bihar, Rajasthan, and Madhya Pradesh, per capita income levels in the 1970s probably declined by about 35 percent (Bardhan 1984:93). The mechanisms of change in levels of income or wealth inequalities are, however, poorly understood (ibid.:94). In any particular year the states which have experienced relatively fast agricultural growth tend to have lower poverty rates than the agriculturally more stagnant ones. However, poverty rates in states with faster agricultural growth rates are not falling faster than in those with slower growth rates (Bardhan 1984:5). Thus Punjab and Haryana have poverty proportions of only 12 percent and 23 percent respectively, in 1977–1978, but these rates are not tending to decline (Tata 1982:11). Cassen's conclusion seems as valid now as it was in the mid-1970s:

> It seems that wherever one looks it is difficult to find any evidence of a trend of improvement for the poor. Their fate in rural areas . . . is bound up most importantly with the magnitude of the harvest and in urban areas . . . with the slow progress of manufacturing and service trades employment. The data on expenditure, income distribution, wages, prices and employment do not show any very distinct trend. (Cassen 1978:249)

This conclusion is based largely on estimates of income and consumption. In some respects, however, the poor may now be better off because of infrastructural investment and special government programs. Since 1971, when Mrs. Gandhi's Congress party won an election campaign on the promise to "eliminate poverty," Plan expenditures are claimed to have shifted toward providing the population with the ability to meet their minimum needs. Undoubtedly, progress has been made in the provision of physical amenities in Indian villages. The first economic census, carried out in 1977 in most of India, lists the numbers of villages with basic amenities within, or close to, their borders: Some 93 percent of villages have drinking water within the village for at least part of the year; 33 percent have electricity for at least some of the time; and banks, credit cooperatives, fair-price shops, buses and schools, roads and post offices are increasingly available to villages (Economic and Political Weekly 1985:615–616). Some of the benefits of this "overhead consumption" (as Cassen calls it) will have gone to the poor. While we know that they are relatively disadvantaged (for example, in access to schooling) we do not know whether this disadvantage has increased or declined over time.

Special programs designed particularly to benefit the poor date from the 1970s. They include small farmer development agencies, projects for marginal farmers and agricultural laborers, a crash scheme for rural employment, and the drought-prone areas program. They were either short-lived or replaced in 1980 by the Integrated Rural Development Program. These programs were designed to increase incomes or production and any impact should have shown up in the NSS data. Nutrition programs which put food into the mouths of small children and their mothers might have effects on the poor which are not measured by income or consumption expenditure data. The amount of food imported and transported to feeding centers throughout the country since 1947 is impressive, but only since 1970 have nutrition programs been an integral part of the Plan process.

The government of India recently claimed that poverty has decreased as a result of its antipoverty programs. The mid-term appraisal of the Sixth Five-Year Plan concluded that it could anticipate the results of the 1983 National Sample Survey and that 57-million people had crossed the poverty line in 1980–1982 (GOI 1983:8). This claim presumes that the expenditure on special poverty-alleviating schemes would all have accrued to the poor, but this conclusion has been strenuously denied (Sundaram and Tendulkar 1983, 1984). As with other schemes supposed to benefit the poor, there are leakages. Much of the expenditure never reaches the supposed beneficiaries. Bureaucrats and politicians, able to control access to these benefits, and those who are not really poor also end up with some of the benefits. One estimate is that about 15 percent of those benefiting from the Integrated Rural Development Program were already above the poverty line, with the figures for some states (notably Assam and Punjab) reaching above 33 percent (Rath 1985:241).

What is the net result of increases in national income, the spread of social infrastructure, and government programs designed specifically to relieve poverty? Most indicators of income and consumption suggest fluctuations, with no discernible trends. Indicators of unemployment suggest some deterioration, and those of productive wealth, particularly landholding, also suggest that more people are landless or own insufficient land to sustain themselves now than at independence.

Thus poverty, in the strict sense of the ability to purchase a defined basket of goods, has probably not increased. But insecurity of access to the resources necessary to do so probably has increased, and dependence on the state for subsidized employment or credit has become increasingly common.

Conclusion

Mortality has continued to decline since independence, though it has not fallen steadily, for mortality fell relatively little, if at all, in the decade around 1970. It has not fallen equally for all age groups, though if official estimates of infant and child mortality before 1970 are corrected upward, the variation by age becomes less significant. Mortality has fallen more in states that already had low mortality rates than in those with higher ones. Male-female differentials seem to have worsened until about 1970, perhaps because men received more of the early benefits from improved medical services, but now seem to be narrowing. These declines cannot easily be explained by reference to the increase in per capita income, since there is no evidence of this having benefited the poorest sectors of the population.

Two factors might help to explain the apparent paradoxes of substantial declines in mortality, stable or declining per capita food-grain availability, no change in the proportion of the population below poverty level, and little reason to believe the general health services provided by the state have been very effective. First, protection from famine has probably continued to be effective. Several measures, all flawed because they "leak" and leave the very poor in vulnerable and insecure positions, probably do prevent the poor from starving to death. Second, public health measures may have been more effective than they have usually been credited for, an argument that will be assessed in the chapters that follow.

CHAPTER SIX

Health Plans and Expenditures 1951–1984

On the face of it, health planning has stressed preventive and public-health programs with a rural bias. This emphasis is reflected in all the Plan documents, to a greater or lesser extent. All the Plans call for a rural bias: rural areas "should receive much greater attention" (GOI 1952:197); they are "the most urgent need to be met in the Second Five-Year Plan" (GOI 1956:534); the expansion will reach "progressively larger number of persons, especially in the rural areas" (GOI 1961:653); rural areas will be the "emphasis" (GOI 1968b:309) or the "accent" (GOI 1973:234). Similarly, a preventive bias was urged. In the First Plan "additional resources should be concentrated on preventive work rather than curative facilities" (GOI 1952:197); in the Third Plan they were to receive "increased emphasis" (GOI 1961:651); and in the Fifth, minimum public health facilities were the "primary objective" (GOI 1973: 234). The need for many more paramedical or nonmedical personnel to supply such services received a more muted and changing emphasis. Early proposals saw their rapid expansion as "necessary," and the Second Plan was most forthright about the need for "accelerated and sustained action" on ancillary training if "even elementary services are to reach the mass of the people in any adequate degree" (GOI 1956:538). But the Third Plan merely "recommended" a new scheme for medical assistants, the Fourth Plan talked only of doctors, and the Fifth Plan of raising the quality of training, career paths, and so on. The most notable schemes for extending paramedical training—for multipurpose workers (a kind of feldsher) and community health workers (1977)—were introduced outside the normal process of Plan construction.

The general image of Indian health planning is the reverse of this picture. For example, Cassen (1978) concludes that public sector expenditures in health are concentrated in large urban hospitals; and a large number of Indian critics, both from within and without government, have made similar claims (Ramasubban 1984; Banerji 1981; Srivastava 1975; Ramalingaswami 1981). I do not wish to claim that all is well with health policy in India, but in this chapter I shall argue that public sector health expenditures have been somewhere between these two positions. The reason both positions can be held is that relatively little has been published which sets out the parameters of actual government health-sector expenditures in India.

Most discussions of the pattern of health expenditure in India have gone little farther than noting the size, and trends through time, of proposed Plan expenditures, and interstate variations in total per capita expenditures (e.g., Ramasubban 1984). Proposed Plan expenditures give some insight into the priorities for new spending, but some health expenditures are in one Plan but not the next, so trends drawn from Plan proposals alone are misleading and proposals are not uniformly implemented. Detail on the total actual Plan expenditures or the pattern of state expenditures (including non-Plan spending), has remained elusive. The most readily available sources are the Five-Year Plans; these deal in "outlays," or proposed expenditures, and offer only a haphazard record of actual patterns in the previous Plans and they say nothing whatever about non-Plan expenditures, which are hidden in the budgets and accounts of the individual states.

This chapter addresses two sets of questions: One, How much is spent by central and state governments on health-related sectors; and how does this relate to Plan and non-Plan expenditures? Two, How far are Indian health-sector expenditures skewed in favor of curative health services in urban areas?

The Planning Commission and government accounting agencies use a fairly consistent set of categories. I shall use the following terminology: "health" will refer to their categories of "medical" and "public health"; "health-related" will include the Plan categories of "health," "family planning" (or "family welfare"), "water supply and sanitation" and, where possible, "nutrition."

Public-Sector Health Expenditures

No single source provides a clear picture of how much is spent by government on health-related topics, partly because of the many different agencies involved. Health is formally the responsibility of the twenty-two states, which, in 1981, ranged in size from a population of over 110 million (Uttar Pradesh) to less than one million (e.g., Nagaland). The central government also has some health functions (medical standards, family planning, quarantine, etc.) and provides health services in the Union Territories (the capital, Delhi, and some other small territories). Health services may also be provided by local government bodies, predominantly urban but in some states rural as well, and by several ministries other than Health and Family Welfare.

The Ministry of Labor is responsible for most social insurance schemes. Some are covered by legislation, like the Plantation Labor Act, while other employers run their own schemes. Some are restricted to individual industries, either in the private sector (e.g., plantations), the public sector (e.g., coal mines), or for government servants (such as the Central Government Health Scheme). However, the largest scheme, the Employees' State Insurance Scheme (ESIS), serves employees from many industries and covers over 7 million workers and 21 million of their dependants, or some 4 percent of the total population. Another large scheme covers 7.6 million railways, employees and dependents (GOI 1984:146, 246). The development of facilities for industrial workers often proceeds quite separately, with duplication of urban medical services (Jeffery 1976), and although the ESI Commission is usually represented at CCH meetings, it has only recently taken any interest in public-health matters (Singh 1983).

Nutrition services are the responsibility of the Department of Social Welfare. Prior to 1971 nutrition had a very low profile within government, and even since then it has proved difficult to identify nutrition expenditures. Food aid was regarded as a famine-prevention measure rather than a feature of routine government services. When nutrition services became more significant, as part of the Minimum Needs Program of 1971, they were still provided by Education ministries (which include social welfare) through school meals or feeding programs. The current attempts to integrate nutrition and maternal and child-health services, particularly in the

Integrated Child Development Scheme (ICDS), do not seem to have resolved the problems of coordination between the Social Welfare and Health ministries.

Plan and Non-Plan Expenditures

All government expenditures are divided into Plan and non-Plan categories. The Plan covers most new, developmental expenditures (but is not the same as "capital"), whereas the non-Plan category covers most routine activities (but is not identical with "revenue"). Plan expenditures have generally included all those on preventive campaigns (smallpox, malaria, etc.), family planning, and some water supply and sanitation. In other parts of the health budget, only new developments have been paid for from the Plan budget with recurrent costs becoming part of the non-Plan budget at the end of the relevant Plan.

Table 16 brings together data on actual Plan expenditures and total state and central government health-related expenditures. It shows that the Plan has only recently accounted for more than 60 percent of this total. The proportion of government expenditure spent on health-related subjects has risen steadily, by 50 percent over the last thirty years, and its share of national income has risen even more, by 250 percent. These increases can also be seen in the rise in per capita expenditures in constant (1960–1961) prices. These general rises, however, hide very different patterns for the different sectors.

The three financial categories of Plan expenditures are those paid for entirely by the central government and disbursed by its own agencies; those paid for (in whole or in part) by the center but disbursed by state governments; and those funded and disbursed by state governments. Family planning has always been a completely centrally funded area, as have been the campaigns against communicable diseases before the Fifth Plan. On the other hand, nutrition and water supply and sanitation have always been largely state-funded. The pattern of outlays (proposed expenditures) by these categories has changed from Plan to Plan; in health, the role of the center increased from the Third Plan to the Sixth Plan (Table 17). For example, in the annual allocations during the Fifth Plan the centrally funded sectors were given priority, so that in the

TABLE 16

PUBLIC-HEALTH-RELATED EXPENDITURE

	First Plan (1951–56)	Second Plan (1956–61)	Third Plan (1961–66)	Plan Holiday (1966–69)	Fourth Plan (1969–74)	Fifth Plan (1974–79)	(1979–80)	Sixth Plan[a] (1980–85)
Total expenditures:								
Plan	980	2,163	3,565	3,133	11,566	23,450	7,290	74,175
Non-Plan	933	1,410	3,024	3,342	8,552	17,630	5,261	31,664
Total	1,913	3,673	6,589	6,475	20,120	41,080	12,551	105,839
Plan percentage	(51)	(59)	(54)	(48)	(57)	(57)	(58)	(70)
Annual per capita expenditures				Rupees				
Current prices:								
Total	1.0	1.9	3.0	4.4	4.7	13.3	19.0	30.0
1960–61 prices:								
Total	1.4	2.1	3.6	2.7	3.6	4.2	4.9	5.0
				Percentages				
Share of total government outlay								
Health-related	2.7	2.6	2.9	3.1	3.8	3.9	4.2	3.9
Proportion of national income								
Health-related	0.42	0.62	0.76	0.80	1.04	1.19	1.42	1.52

SOURCES: Plan documents (GOI 1956, 1961, 1967, 1968a, 1973, 1978b, 1981a, 1983); Reddy 1972:218; Barnett 1977; GOI 1986.

[a] Sixth-plan total expenditure figures are still subject to minor revisions. These figures are not strictly comparable and the classifications of total health expenditures changed in 1974 with impacts that are not known. Fifth-plan expenditures exclude nutrition.

TABLE 17
HEALTH OUTLAYS BY FINANCIAL CATEGORIES

	Third Plan	Plan holiday	Fourth Plan	Fifth Plan	Sixth Plan	Seventh Plan
			Rs millions			
Central	148	168	535	758	4,325	3,396
(%)	(6.6)	(12.0)	(12.3)	(9.5)	(23.8)	(10.0)
Centrally Sponsored	55	111	1,765	1,770	3,638	5,577
(%)	(2.4)	(7.9)	(40.7)	(22.2)	(20.0)	(16.4)
State/Union territory	2,056	1,122	2,035	5,432	10,247	24,955
(%)	(91.0)	(80.1)	(46.9)	(68.2)	(56.3)	(73.5)
Total	2,259	1,401	4,335	7,960	18,210	33,929

SOURCE: GOI 1973, II:232; GOI 1981:382; GOI 1985, II:288
NOTE: This table excludes family planning (100 percent central or centrally sponsored in each Plan), water supply, and sanitation.

1976–1977 Annual Plan, the state share had dropped to 54 percent (Barnett 1977). This pattern of allocations has been repeated in the Sixth Plan, as it was eventually adopted under Congress, but detail on actual expenditures by financial category remains elusive; in the Seventh Plan the states have been allocated a much higher share, apparently reversing the trend from 1975 to 1985.

Three sets of processes are involved in producing government health-sector expenditures. First, the Plan documents are drawn up, and outlays are agreed upon. Second, Plan proposals are turned into actual expenditures. Third, Plan expenditures are integrated with non-Plan expenditures into the overall pattern of health expenditures at the state-government level. The first two of these are usually discussed as the planning process. For each Plan they involve decisions and negotiations between three identifiable events: presentation by working groups of doctors and Health Ministry officials of a proposed Plan for the health sector, publication of the final Plan document, and the end of the Plan period.

Three kinds of information are available on how health planning has taken place within the government apparatus, none of them ideally suited to shed light on these processes. First, are the Plans themselves. They have an advantage in that they represent official statements of policy objectives and some of the rationales for chosen policies. They are readily available and have provided most commentators with much of their material (e.g., Ramasubban 1984). However, they are silent about how competing policies were selected or rejected and how priorities led to the actual distribution of allocations; and they give little information on actual expenditures.

The second source is the minutes of the discussions in the Central Council of Health of the Plan proposals. The information is incomplete but for the Third and Fourth Plans they allow a glimpse into the processes by which proposals from the Ministries of Health are modified in negotiation with the Planning Commission. The third source of material is the background papers prepared for the Planning Commission by working groups. These reports allow more insight into the various arguments, but they say very little about how these competing claims were balanced. Information about state expenditures is provided only by the states themselves. I have collected data on Maharashtra, Gujarat, and Orissa, and these three will form the subjects of the final part of the discussion.

The Planning Process: Creating the Plan

The first step in detailed planning appears to be discussions in which state ministries liaise with central ministries over proposals and projects that are put to the Planning Commission. The Planning Commission collates these proposals and evaluates them in terms of its own assessments of policy in the area and a number of other criteria—such as the implied foreign-exchange requirements, the overall volume of physical and financial resources expected to be available, and priorities between sectors and states. These major decisions are formally the responsibility of the National Development Council, consisting of members of the Planning Commission and chief ministers of the states, and usually chaired by the prime minister. The Planning Commission then translates these essentially political decisions into consistent policies that form the final Plan, and then draws up annual plans that provide justification for state and central ministry budget decision making, and allow state governments to claim back expenditures which fall within Plan allocations.

For health services, the first stage appears to involve the state and central ministries of health providing personnel for working parties and expert groups (dominated by doctors) looking at specific issues, such as medical education or the control of communicable diseases. Each group works independently, and is thus tempted to expand the number of its proposals as far as possible. Similarly, the federal Ministry of Health as a whole is under pressure to submit an exaggerated list of proposals to the Planning Commission, knowing that it is likely to have its total cut whatever is proposed. The eventual plan may lose much of whatever rationality it had because of the need to cut the total to a level acceptable to the Planning Commission, and to divide it into topics and by states in ways that derive from political decisions made in the National Development Council. Looking at these processes, then, gives some idea of the real priorities—what the health officials proposed and what the Planning Commission cut or expanded. Material available for the Third and Fourth Plans allows some insight into how this happened.

During the course of the Second Plan the federal Health Ministry looked at the pattern of expenditures and singled out medical education and family planning as areas where allocations were not being spent fast enough. This kind of information was fed into discussions on the Third Plan allocations. State working groups submitted proposals to a central working group, which reported to the Central Council of Health in 1959. Their proposals form column A in table 18. At the same time the Planning Commission was preparing its own draft outline, that appeared in June 1960 (column B) and allocated only 43 percent of the Central Council of Health proposals. This draft outline was then discussed with the states and the central ministries, and the size of the Plan was increased. Two revised sets of proposals came out of this process before the plan was finalized and appeared in August 1961 (column C). The pattern of actual expenditures is shown in column D.

A similar sequence of events can be identified for the Fourth Plan, summarized in table 19. Matters are complicated by the fact that the original proposals for the Fourth Plan were shelved in 1966 and reviewed only in 1968–1969, because the Fourth Plan period was put back by three years.

These processes created some apparently radical changes in distribution. In the Third Plan, the Planning Commission seems to

TABLE 18

ALLOCATIONS AND EXPENDITURES IN THE THIRD PLAN

	A M of H 1959 Rs. mill.	%	B P Comm 1960 Rs. mill.	%	C Plan 1961 Rs. mill.	%	D Actual 1961-66 Rs. mill.	%
Health:								
Control of communicable diseases	1,200	17	920	30	705	21	971	28
Medical education training and research	750	11	460	15	560	16	668	19
Hospitals and dispensaries	1,370	20	460	15	617	18	495	14
Other health	910	13	300	10	210	6	124	4
Family planning	300	4	250	8	270	8	228	7
Water supply and sanitation:								
urban	2,000	28	630	21	1,053	31	1,045	30
rural	500	7	20	1				
Total	7,030	100	3,040	100	3,415	100	3,531	100

SOURCE: For columns A and B—GOI (CCH) 1961; for column C—GOI 1961:651; for column D—GOI (CCH) 1966:45.

KEY: M of H = Ministry of Health; P Comm = Planning Commission; CCH = Central Council of Health.

TABLE 19
ALLOCATIONS AND EXPENDITURES IN THE FOURTH PLAN

	A P Comm 1965 Rs. mill.	%	B P Comm 1966 Rs. mill.	%	C Plan 1969 Rs. mill.	%	D Actual 1969–74 Rs. mill.	%
Health:								
Control of communicable diseases	1,250	12	870	9	1,270	11	993	9
Education, training and research	2,250	21	1,780	19	980	9	860	8
Hospitals and dispensaries	2,500	23	1,810	19	890	8	827	8
Primary Health centres					760	7	343	3
Other health	550	5	460	5	440	4	437	4
Total health	6,550	60	4,920	51	4,340	38	3,460	32
Family planning	950	9	950	10	3,150	28	2,779	25
Water supply and sanitation:								
urban	1,450	31	3,730	39	3,920	34	4,738	43
rural	1,950							
Total health-related	10,900	100	9,600	100	11,420	100	10,977	100

SOURCES: GOI (CCH) 1965 and 1969; GOI 1964, 1970, and 1973.
NOTE: This table excludes nutrition.
KEY: P Comm = Planning Commission.

have protected the programs to control communicable diseases, family planning, and medical education, and the like, at the cost of hospitals and dispensaries, "other," and water supply. In the Fourth Plan, family planning received a continually growing allocation, and water supply joined the "protected" sectors, while education lost its protected status. It is not clear whether the cuts to hospitals were directed mostly at urban facilities or also at the rural primary health center program.

For the Fifth Plan matters are complicated by several factors. Before the plan could be finalized the rise in oil prices necessitated drastic revisions. Family planning expenditure was raised dramatically during the emergency of 1975–1977; and when the Janata government came to power in 1977 it suspended the planning process, closing the Fifth Plan a year early in 1978. It is difficult to put together information on changes in the pattern of expenditure through the Plan period and in several cases conflicting figures were produced. Comparing the draft plan proposals with steering-group recommendations and with actual expenditures over the five years of the original Plan period, while slightly artificial, gives some idea of the nature of priorities in the mid-1970s. In general, it seems that the Planning Commission protected the rural health program while the plan was being drawn up but this sector was hit hardest by problems of implementation. From 12.5 percent of the draft Plan, its share dropped to 5.4 percent of actual expenditures (GOI 1973; GOI 1981a). In contrast, programs for the control of communicable diseases had a lower priority in the draft Plan (7.2 percent) than the share of actual expenditures (11.9 percent). Finally, while urban water-supply schemes spent over their allocation, rural schemes did not spend their allocation. Other differences were not substantial.

Less information is available about the Sixth Plan, partly because the different sections of health expenditure have not been separately identified. However, it would seem that the return of the Congress government led to a return to an emphasis on rural programs, because the share allocated to (and spent on) rural water-supply schemes rose sharply, and the nutrition programs (largely rural) also rose. However, the rural health program was allocated only about 8 percent, a share of expenditure which it nearly maintained. More significant, perhaps, family planning was allocated 15 percent of health-related funds, but spent 19 percent of actual health-related expenditure.

Part of the explanation for which sectors were "protected," is provided by foreign assistance. This assistance is all channeled through the Planning Commission and tends to be tied to particular sectors. As a result, these sectors may not be threatened when overall cuts have to be allocated to sectors. Foreign aid in the 1960s was heavily focused on preventive programs and, later, on family planning. In the 1970s, water supply and sanitation schemes and some extensions to the primary health structure have also been aid targets (see chap. 8).

The Planning Commission, then, both in its own right and as a channel for foreign pressures, has ensured that the Indian Plans have been fairly consistent in their emphasis on rural, preventive services. It has also presided over a shift of resources, from health to family planning. This shift is exaggerated by these figures, since family planning includes some expenditures directly relevant to the health sector, for example the training of auxiliary nurse-midwives, some of whom worked in health or medical positions. Provision for the training of these personnel originally appeared under the state total for "training," but a reclassification under a centrally sponsored heading such as family planning increased the chances that the scheme would be implemented. Some changes, then, might be little more than cosmetic. Nonetheless, family planning outlays have grown at the expense of "health," as table 20 demonstrates.

Implementing the Plan

The Planning Commission can only restrain expenditures by state governments; it cannot insist on spending targets being met and it is only concerned with Plan expenditures. The actual patterns of total health expenditure may be very different from the priorities laid out in the Plans. Table 21 shows the health-related "outlays" and "actuals" as percentages of total government Plan outlays and of actual expenditures. The percentage allocations to health in each Plan declined steadily, while the other health-related shares rose sufficiently in the Fourth, Fifth, and Sixth Plans to outweigh this decline. The health-related sectors have been less successful at spending their allocations than have either the social services (education being a major component) or the public sector of the Plan as a whole, so actual expenditure shares have been below these levels. Nonetheless, in cash terms the "health-related" sectors have spent over 90 percent of their allocation, except in the First Plan. If inflation is taken into account, this falls to about 80 percent to 85 percent of financial targets.

The extent of central-government control over Plan funds has varied from Plan to Plan and derives mostly from its ability to pay for a particular part of public expenditure. This is a powerful inducement for state governments to follow central policy proposals, and any attempt to reclassify a particular topic from central to state funding is always greeted by protest. But the offer of central funding is not necessarily enough to ensure that a policy is followed. For example, the community health-workers scheme was centrally funded under the Janata government after 1977, but several states (notably Tamil Nadu, Kerala, and Kashmir) refused to introduce it, arguing that they had no need to, because they had alternative ways of meeting the health needs of their rural populations. State governments are also wary of the conditional, time-bound support offered by the central government. When central funding runs out, the states are left with a cadre of workers they do not necessarily want but cannot sack. This limits the ability of state governments to introduce their own pet schemes. For example, as early as 1980 moves were made to transfer some of the costs of the community health-workers scheme onto state budgets, though the central government was not able to enforce its policy on the states in this case. Conversely, the center is unable to prevent some policy initiatives by state governments which contradict central policy if the state is prepared to pay for them. Two examples since 1980 are the opening of short courses for training rural doctors in West Bengal and a new postgraduate teaching hospital outside Lucknow.

Integrating the Plan with Non-Plan Expenditures

So far, I have only considered Plan expenditures. How do Plan and non-Plan spending combine? The main source of information about health expenditures in the states is provided by the Reserve Bank of India, which shows a fairly stable spread of per capita expenditures for the different states, ranging from very high figures in the mountainous northern states (Nagaland, Himachal,

TABLE 20

PLANNED OUTLAYS IN THE HEALTH SECTOR

	First Plan %	Second Plan %	Third Plan %	Fourth Plan %	Fifth Plan %	Sixth Plan %	Seventh Plan %
Health:							
Control of communicable diseases	16.5	28.4	20.6	11.0	6.2	7.5	6.9
Medical Education and Research Training[c]	15.4 {	{ 13.3 } { 2.7 }	16.4	{ 7.4 { 1.1	3.5 0.6	8.3[a]	7.3[a]
Hospitals and dispensaries	17.9	16.0	18.1	14.3	16.3	10.3[b]	8.6[b]
Indigenous systems of medicine	0.3	1.8	2.9	1.4	1.0		
Other programs	14.4	2.7	3.3	2.4	1.5		
Total health	64.5	64.9	61.3	37.5	29.1	26.0	22.8

Family planning	0.5	1.3	7.9	27.3	18.8	14.4	21.8
Nutrition:	—	—	n.a.	n.a.	14.8	3.4	11.7
Water supply and sanitation	35.0	33.8	30.8	35.2	37.3	56.1	43.7
Total health-related (Rs. millions)	(1,400)	(2,250)	(3,415)	(11,555)	(27,376)	(69,910)	(149,180)

Sources: Plan documents.
Notes: Nutrition was not separated from health programs in the Third and Fourth Plans, but was retrospectively identified (in the Fifth Plan draft outline) as having been allocated Rs. 594 million (5 percent of the health-related budget) in the Fourth Plan, of which Rs. 370 millions was spent.

[a] This figure is for Minimum Needs Program for Rural Health.

[b] This figure is for "hospitals and dispensaries, medical education and research, traditional systems of medicine and homoeopathy, and other."

[c] Medical Education is of doctors; Training is of paramedical workers.

TABLE 21

Health-Related Plan Outlays and Expenditures

(as percentage of total public-sector Plan)

	First Plan	Second Plan	Third Plan	Annual Plans	Fourth Plan	Fifth Plan	1979–1980	Sixth Plan	Seventh Plan
Outlay									
Health	3.6	3.3	2.8	–	2.7	1.7	–	1.8	1.9
Family planning	0.03	0.07	0.4	–	2.0	1.3	–	1.0	1.8
Nutrition	–	–	–	–	–	1.0	–	0.2	1.0
Water supply, etc.	2.0	1.7	1.4	–	2.6	2.5	–	4.0	3.6
All health-related	5.6	5.0	4.6	n.a.	7.3	6.5	n.a.	7.1	8.3
Expenditure									
Health	3.3	3.0	2.6	2.1	2.1	1.9	1.8	1.8	n.a.
Family planning	0.01	0.05	0.3	1.1	1.8	1.3	1.0	1.3	n.a.
Nutrition	–	–	–	–	0.03	n.a.	n.a.	0.3	n.a.
Water supply, etc.	1.7	1.6	1.2	1.6	2.9	2.8	3.2	3.6	n.a.
All health-related	5.0	4.6	4.2	4.7	6.9	5.9	6.0	6.8	n.a.

Source: Plan documents; GOI (1983:113), (1983a:66; 1985a:138)

and Jammu and Kashmir) to very low figures in the Ganges plan (Bihar and Uttar Pradesh) (table 22). This pattern reflects differences in the priority given to health and other social-services expenditure (e.g., the relatively high figures for Kerala), as well as the states' financial resources, partly derived from their own tax base and partly from the central government. As George and Gulati (1985) show, "low-income" states like Uttar Pradesh and Bihar have received insufficient central funds to outweigh their poverty, but the "special-category" states (hilly, strategic ones like Himachal Pradesh or Jammu and Kashmir) have received per capita payments many times the national average.

Information on the distribution of these expenditures among different categories is harder to gather, since the states publish budgets and reports that are not centrally collated. Tables 23, 24 and 25 present roughly comparable data from Orissa, Gujarat, and Maharashtra for differing periods since 1971. The Orissa data come from the annual administration reports for the Health Ministry; Barnett (1977) analyzed Maharashtra budget data, and Khan and Prasad analyzed Sixth Plan proposals and accounts for Gujarat and for Maharashtra. Orissa is a relatively poor state, though it has sizable industrial areas that provide it with quite a substantial tax base. Maharashtra and Gujarat are relatively wealthy states.

Table 23 shows that the Plan share varies from less than 20 percent of some categories (e.g., medical relief) to 100 percent of others. However, some distinctions relate to budgetary categories that might be much less distinct on the ground; for example, expenditure on medical college hospitals (in the medical-relief category) is separated from that on medical colleges themselves (under medical education). A further qualification to this table is that other departments in Orissa undertake most public-health engineering works (water supply, sanitation), and so this total is an understatement of Orissa government expenditure on these topics. This makes interstate comparisons very difficult. As table 24 demonstrates, Gujarat and Maharashtra show very different distributions, because their health departments are responsible for most public-health engineering, totaling nearly 30 percent of all health-related state expenditure.

Table 23 also gives some idea of the impact of the state of emergency of 1975–1977 on the health budget. Compensation to clients

TABLE 22

Per Capita Revenue Expenditure on Medical, Family-planning
and Public-health Subjects for Main States

| | Current Prices | | | 1977–78 to |
	1972–73 to 1974–75	1975–76 to 1976–77	1977–78 to 1979–80	1979–80 in 1970–71 prices, 1971 = 100
A: High Income States				
Punjab	11.9	16.8	23.5	143
Haryana	9.7	11.8	22.5	165
Maharashtra	11.5	13.1	21.2	152
Gujarat	9.2	11.6	19.6	148
West Bengal	8.4	12.8	18.1	139
Group A	10.0	13.0	20.2	
B: Middle Income States				
Tamil Nadu	9.4	12.6	15.9	136
Kerala	10.1	14.8	21.9	162
Orissa	6.6	9.0	13.8	134
Assam	7.6	9.4	13.5	135
Karnataka	7.5	11.4	14.2	133
Andhra Pradesh	6.8	9.7	15.6	141
Group B	8.0	11.2	15.8	

C: Low Income States				
Uttar Pradesh	4.7	5.5	9.8	136
Rajasthan	10.9	13.8	20.9	135
Madhya Pradesh	7.3	8.3	13.2	131
Bihar	4.1	4.5	8.5	115
Group C	5.8	6.8	11.5	
D: Special Category States				
Himachal Pradesh	15.8	19.8	47.9	n.a.
Jammu and Kashmir	14.4	17.0[a]	52.9	252
Manipur	13.3	15.1	44.2	n.a.
Meghalaya	19.0	23.9	57.6	n.a.
Nagaland	59.2	76.4	147.6	n.a.
Tripura	10.9	13.7	25.8	n.a.
Group D	16.4	20.2	52.5	
Average of Listed States	7.9	10.2	16.0	

SOURCE: For 1973–74 to 1976–77: GOI (1979:23); for 1972–73, Barnett (1979:16); for 1977–78 to 1979–80, Khan and Prasad (1984).

NOTE: The categorization of states is on the basis of tax-base (George and Gulati 1985); group per capita figures are weighted averages using 1971 and 1981 census weightings. Deflation is by the wholesale-prices index. The system of classifying budget-data changes between 1973–74 and 1974–75, with unknown effect.

[a] Figures for Jammu and Kashmir are unavailable for 1976–77.

TABLE 23

HEALTH-RELATED EXPENDITURES FOR ORISSA STATE: 1972–1979

(Annual Averages in Rs. Millions)

	1972–73 to 1974–75			1975–76 and 1976–77			1977–78 and 1978–79		
	Non-Plan	Plan	Total	Non-Plan	Plan	Total	Non-Plan	Plan	Total
Medical education:									
Undergraduate	8.2	2.0	10.2	12.5	0.4	12.9	12.8	0.6	13.4
Postgraduate	1.2	0.1	1.3	1.9	0.0	1.9	1.9	0.0	1.9
Paramedical training	1.1	0.9	2.0	1.3	0.2	1.5	1.5	0.3	1.8
Medical relief	56.8	9.5	66.3	93.9	9.6	103.5	102.5	19.3	121.8
Prevention/control of disease	5.1	16.9	22.0	9.7	23.7	33.4	11.6	23.0	34.6
Public health, sanitation and water supply[a]	7.0	0.3	7.3	11.0	0.0	11.0	13.0	0.0	13.0
Family planning:									
Compensation	—	3.0	3.0	—	21.1	21.1	—	11.8	11.8
Paramed training	—	0.8	0.8	—	0.7	0.7	—	5.0	5.0
Other	—	17.9	17.9	—	25.8	25.8	—	29.4	29.4
Total	79.5	50.2	129.7	130.3	81.5	211.8	143.3	89.4	232.7
(Column %)	(61.3)	(38.7)	(100)	(61.5)	(38.5)	(100)	(61.6)	(38.4)	(100)

SOURCE: Government of Orissa (Health and Family Welfare Department) for the relevant years.

NOTE: Administration expenses for the medical directorate are incuded in the total for medical relief; for family planning in "other"; and for the public health directorate in public health, sanitation and water supply.

[a] Most expenditure under this subheading is carried out by different departments and so does not appear in these sources.

for sterilization operations rose from 2 percent of the total health-related expenditure in the early 1970s (in both Orissa and Maharashtra) to 10 percent in the two years of the emergency, and remained over 5 percent of the total in 1977–1978 and 1978–1979, poor years for sterilizations. Indeed, of the apparent increase in per capita "real" (1970–1971 prices) health department expenditures in the emergency over the preceding years more than 25 percent can be explained purely as the increase in compensation payments.

Table 24 recategorizes expenditure by whether it is essentially intended to provide primary, secondary, or tertiary care. In brief, primary care is designed to meet the major common health problems of the population, whether curative, promotive, rehabilitative, or preventive in focus; secondary care provides more specialized services, usually after some referral from a primary facility; and tertiary services are the most specialized and the least accessible. There are problems with this analysis; most discussions of the categories are not conceptually clear-cut (see, for example, Cole-King 1977). It is particularly difficult to allocate expenditures on education and training that may produce staff to work in all three sectors. In addition, a facility like a medical college hospital, which is nominally designed to provide highly specialized referral services may actually provide primary care services to the surrounding population. A further problem is that expenditures in one category might really be very different, as in cases where staff are paid from one budget head (say, primary health centers) but are on secondment elsewhere (say, in a medical college). In general, I assume that this will not involve large sums, and that accounting controls are sufficiently tight to ensure that most money is spent in the category for which it is allocated.

The Maharashtra and Gujarat sources also allow some information within these categories about what the money was spent on. During 1980–1984 about 50 percent of medical, public-health, and family-welfare expenditure for each state went for salaries; between 15 percent and 25 percent on drugs, materials, and other supplies, and between 8 percent and 10 percent on family-planning incentives and compensation payments (Khan and Prasad 1985). However, in both states a substantial portion of the total budget was spent by local government authorities that do not provide detailed accounts of what was available centrally, so there is some uncertainty about these figures; Khan and Prasad also exclude water supply and sanitation from their analysis.

TABLE 24

DISTRIBUTION OF HEALTH-RELATED EXPENDITURES BY MAJOR CATEGORIES

	Orissa 1972–73 to 1978–79	Maharashtra 1972–73 to 1974–75	Maharashtra 1980–81 to 1984–85	Gujarat 1980–81 to 1984–85
		Percentages		
Medical education:				
Undergraduate	6.3	} 6	5.1	4.4
Postgraduate	0.9			
Paramedical training	0.9		0.1	0.6
Medical relief	50.7	25	21.1	27.9
Prevention/Control of disease	15.7	14	10.0	12.4
Public health, sanitation, and water supply	5.4	28	39.5	24.5
Family planning:				
Compensation	6.2	5	4.6	5.8
Paramedical training	1.1	} 9	0.4	1.5
Other	12.7		6.0	8.6
Employees state insurance scheme	—	13	9.2	9.3
Indigenous systems of medicine	—	?	1.9	2.8
Other	—	?	1.9	2.3
Total	(100)	(100)	(100)	(100)

SOURCE: For Orissa, as table 23; for Maharashtra, Barnett (1977); Khan and Prasad (1985); for Gujarat, Khan and Prasad (1985).

Table 25 suggests the need for some caution in concluding straightforwardly that public expenditures in health are concentrated on big urban hospitals—though since "large" is undefined, there is room for some dispute on this. The actual total to be regarded as "true" primary care is also disputable; many would argue that family planning is too coercive to be regarded as health care, and even those favorably inclined toward family planning might acknowledge the dubious status of compensation payments. Nevertheless, in an international context these figures seem to show that Indian health expenditures are less heavily biased in the "wrong" directions than might have been predicted.

TABLE 25

DISTRIBUTION OF EXPENDITURES BY LEVEL OF CARE

Category	Orissa 1972–73 to 1978–79	Gujarat 1980–81 to 1984–85	Maharashtra 1980–81 to 1984–85
Administration	8.9	3.3	6.9
Medical	1.9	0.1	} 5.7
Public Health	5.6	1.0	
Family Welfare	1.4	2.2	1.2
Tertiary services			
Medical Education	7.1	4.4	4.3
Secondary services			
Medical Relief	48.6	32.3	20.0
Medical college hospitals	10.9		
Hospitals, dispensaries	20.3	} 20.2	11.6
Primary health centers	17.4		
ESIS	n.a.	9.3	7.8
Indigenous medicine	n.a.	2.8	1.6
Paramedical training	2.1	2.0	0.4
Primary care	33.1	50.7	63.6
Family welfare:			
services	11.4	6.2	3.9
compensation	5.6	5.8	3.9
Disease control:			
malaria	8.2	7.7	5.7
leprosy	3.4	1.0	1.6
other	4.3	3.7	1.2
Health education and			
school health	0.2	0.2	0.1
Water supply and			
sanitation	—	23.8	45.6
Other	—	2.3	1.6
Grand total	100	100	100
(Annual average Rs. millions)	(183)	(1,871)	(3,069)

SOURCES: Orissa, as for table 23; Gujarat and Maharashtra, Khan and Prasad (1985).
NOTE: Nonplan water-supply, and sanitation figures for Maharashtra are not given, and I have assumed the same plan to nonplan ratio as in Gujarat in order to produce a total expenditure figure. Gujarat and Maharashtra figures are for expected expenditures; Orissa figures represent actual expenditures.
KEY: ESIS = Employees' State Insurance Scheme.

Conclusion

First, the Planning Commission has championed preventive, public-health aspects of health expenditures. In both the Third and Fourth Plans, Health Ministry proposals would have given far more weight to urban, curative facilities, but the Planning Commission radically altered the balance of Plan-proposed expenditures toward primary care. Although medical personnel have been dominant in policy proposals within the Health Ministry, they have been less successful in negotiations with more powerful economists and administrators in the Planning Commission. The Planning Commission has also been supported by foreign advice and financial assistance, reinforcing the pressures for preventive, single-disease control programs which were so significant in the 1960s.

Second, the balance between major categories of health expenditure has shifted dramatically toward family planning. This has happened partly because family-planning spending has been a channel under closer control of the Central Ministry of Health than other aspects of health expenditure, and partly because of the ideological commitment to population control. The shift is most marked (somewhat misleadingly so) in Plan expenditures, and some parts of the family-planning budget have a rather ambiguous status (e.g., compensation and paramedical training). Nonetheless, this shift has been a real one.

Finally, the total share of government budget spent on health-related issues seems to have declined steadily over the course of the 1970s. Nonetheless, distribution of health expenditure between functional categories has remained remarkably solid, with at least 40 percent in primary care and, on some definitions, nearer 50 percent. This is surprising given the criticisms that have dominated the literature since 1970. It may be that government expenditures in the 1960s were more inappropriate than these figures suggest for the 1970s and 1980s, but this seems unlikely since the malaria program was very substantial in the 1960s.

The major caveat to this analysis, however, is that it only describes what was spent, not what resulted from the expenditure. Chapters 9 and 10 will look more closely at this issue. The next two chapters, however, attempt to explain how the distribution of Indian government health expenditures might have been arrived at, by considering the internal and external politics of decision making.

CHAPTER SEVEN

The Politics of Medicine in India

I now to turn to Alavi's fourth level of the state—the realm of parties and pressure-group politics. Bureaucrats (in the Planning Commission or in health ministries) frame policy partly in response to their own perceived interests as bureaucrats or as members of particular social classes, and also in response to clients, politicians, and organized pressure groups. These pressures generally reinforce the preferences of those within health ministries— in other words, they share a doctor-oriented, curative-services view. However, conflicts do occur, particularly over medical education and over the role of people practicing Western medicine without a Western medical qualification. Conflicts between supporters of unregistered practitioners and those who regard them as "quacks" have been strenuous and remain basically unresolved. These conflicts provide a useful case study because they illuminate political processes very clearly.

This chapter makes two general points. First, health services are not central to class interests in India, either as benefits to be fought over or as important elements in the reproduction of a class-based social structure. The main protagonists are the various kinds of medical practitioners who fight over shares of the cake, rather than the broader ideological issues. Second, the Indian Medical Association (IMA), the main representative body of doctors, has not been notably successful in attempting to protect its narrow interests or otherwise to influence policy. In other words, health planning has been relatively impervious to party and pressure-group attentions.

The Context of Policy

Political processes have to operate within a framework of institutional forms. Particularly significant for health policy is the division of powers between the center and the states, the structures that link health policy in the center to that in the states, and the internal structure of the health ministries.

The major changes immediately after independence resulted in the end of the IMS as an elite corps of medical clinicians-cum-administrators and the introduction of the Planning Commission. Health ministries, both central and state, were divided (as under the British) into a secretariat, headed by members of the Indian Administrative Service, and a directorate, headed by doctors but including some nurse administrators. Almost all commentators agree that the secretariat is, in the last resort, dominant, for it controls access to the minister, files pass through it, and finance depends on it. This is reinforced by the ability of the generalist administrators to talk as colleagues to the heads of other ministries where they may have recently worked. Doctors, whose careers are restricted within one ministry, can use their technical skills as a political weapon, by claiming that decisions require medical knowledge, or by using their control of medical resources to gain credit directly from politicians. In every state, the Ministry of Health is made up of three categories in potential conflict: the minister, with political advisers and supporters; administrators; and doctors.

State ministries also have to contend with the central ministry, which operates largely through persuasion and its role in dealing with Plan funding. Persuasion is exercised in several ways, the most public being the annual meetings of the Central Council of Health. The role of the CCH was discussed at its second meeting in 1954, when the central minister (Rajkumari Amrit Kaur) complained that the decisions of the first meeting had not been implemented. Several ministers immediately pointed out that health was constitutionally a matter for the states so the CCH could not bind its members at all. Ministers need support from their state cabinets to get finance for any proposals, and a new ministry would be free to change earlier decisions (GOI[CCH] 1954:item 1). This position has rarely been challenged.

The abolition of the IMS meant that the Central Ministry of Health lost its own men in senior positions in state ministries.

Proposals by the center to establish an all-India health service as a replacement for the IMS were discussed periodically after 1950. The states generally argued that they did not want to employ doctors who would look to the central government for promotion, since the states would not have full control over their destiny (GOI[CCH] 1952:item 7). Additional problems are the need to compensate doctors for loss of private-practice facilities and the difficulty of matching staff to the wide variety of clinical and other posts they might fill (GOI [CCH] 1973:366–368). No such service has yet been created. Thus, the central government's medical advisers are all drawn from a small Central Health Service, recruited to fill positions in the health facilities provided by the central government for its own employees and in a few hospitals and medical colleges, mostly in Delhi. The last of the former members of the IMS have now retired, and so recent directors-general of health services have been taken straight from senior clinical positions (often as surgeons) with no experience of medical administrative work in the rural areas or small towns nor of preventive campaigns. This probably weakens the position of the director-general in dealing both with the secretariat in New Delhi and with directorates in the states.

The other agency attempting to coordinate state and central policies has been the Planning Commission. The Central Ministry of Health has operated most effective control when offering financial assistance channeled through the Plan structures and requiring approval of the Planning Commission. State governments routinely threaten not to implement innovations unless they have central-government funding. Consequently, central government is forced to place its priority subjects on either the "centrally funded" or the "jointly funded" list. Since the Planning Commission has not played a neutral role (see chap. 6), the Central Ministry of Health has to look both ways. Central government has also affected state policies by redefining issues that are constitutionally its own. In particular, family planning was expanded to include aspects of maternal and child health when the distinction between the two was regarded as a weakness of the family planning program. This made maternal and child health eligible for direct central funding. Such possibilities have formed the substance of discussions involving central and state ministries and the Planning Commission, not just when a new Plan is being drawn up but also throughout its life.

Changes made in the status of projects during Plan periods form a substantial part of the everyday negotiations between the center and state governments over health policy.

These considerations set the context in which the minister of health or a senior bureaucrat in a state government can maneuver, given certain pressures for action.

Clients and Political Pressure

Clients are not usually well organized to promote a particular point of view about their medical services, and the Indian case is no exception. Patienthood is usually a short-term, undesired state and generating an institutional base on the back of such experience is very difficult. Long-term disabling disorders (blindness, deafness) or those requiring new forms of treatment to solve life-threatening disorders (heart surgery, cancer) may generate client organizations. It is much more difficult to organize client pressure for a particular form of health-service structure or for changing the balance of expenditures or personnel; organizations with such a focus are usually dominated by medical personnel themselves, with their interests as employees uppermost.

In India, in any case, most consumer pressure tends to be weak, sporadic, local, and specific, and to disappear very quickly. Fairly typical is the pressure that can be generated over the siting of a Primary Health Center. Politicians can mobilize local support for a decision that will favor one village over another. Sometimes this support can be sustained to challenge an apparently unfavorable decision, using courts and channels higher in a political party. An unknown number of PHCs have been delayed or built in the "wrong" place in this way. But maintaining pressure to ensure that the PHC is properly funded, staffed, and organized to make best use of its limited resources is often beyond local political resources. An apparent exception is described by Mencher (1980:1782). In Kerala

if a PHC was unmanned for a few days there would be a massive demonstration at the nearest collectorate led by local leftists, who would demand to be given what they knew they were entitled to. This has had the effect of making health care much more readily available for the poor in Kerala.

Zurbrigg (1984:176) quotes a Keralite as saying that if proper care is not given by a PHC doctor, patients write to the district medical officer, local newspapers, or confront the doctor themselves. Such political activism is almost unknown elsewhere in India.

The major medical issues that enter local political debate are strictly limited ones with some general local appeal. First, there are issues over the expenditure of money in one locality rather than another—the building of hospitals, dispensaries, PHCs or sub-centers. Given a higher decision about the sums allocated to health matters under different heads, each state, each district within the state, and each town and village in the district may compete for the money to be spent there rather than elsewhere. Politicians are known for their comparative skill in such battles and voters expect their loyalty to be rewarded by benefits funded from the health budget as much as from the education, industry, and railway budgets. Allocative decisions are not restricted to capital expenditures but may also be found in recurrent decisions. Examples include the filling of vacant posts, staff mobility, the supply of new equipment, funding for drugs, and redistribution of equipment and vehicles. People living in a minister's constituency can expect the major social welfare schemes to be implemented according to plan; those living in the constituency of an opposition member of Parliament can expect a second-rate service at best (though matters are rarely that simple).

Second, there are individual pressures on politicians, which take two forms. Clients want access to medical resources; they may want to be patients or doctors. "Suppliers" and medical and paramedical employees want interventions to further their own careers and incomes.

Medical services are grossly inadequate and no formal mechanism exists to ration access to those services which are provided. At the bottom of the medical hierarchy, in the PHC or subcenter, facilities are often underused. Patients routinely by-pass the PHC using either private practitioners who cluster round about in competition or going directly to district or medical-college hospitals. In these higher services, where demand exceeds supply, "professional" gatekeepers are nonexistent, since there is no referral hierarchy. Financial rationing (charging what the market will bear) can only be done surreptitiously. Would-be patients understand that the decision to admit one patient rather than another is rarely made on technical criteria alone, so they search for intermediaries to bolster their cases for admission, or for cheap or free access to essential treatments. Local politicians write letters of introduction, telephone hospital administrators, or accompany their clients to hospital. Politicians may even use Parliament or the State Assembly to marshal their attacks against doctors who fail to submit to their orders (see, e.g. debates of Lok Sabha, the lower house of central Parliament, in New Delhi, 16 May 1972 and 31 July 1972). Doctors working in the clinics and hospitals for government employees may find themselves criticized during budget debates. A politician may propose a motion to cut the health budget because of the behavior of doctors in a particular clinic or hospital, using the opportunity to try to settle scores in this way. My interviews with government doctors in Delhi in 1976 revealed that they are well aware of their vulnerability, because VIPs not personally known to them are liable to demand favorable treatment for themselves or their clients. As one doctor put it in the Diamond Jubilee Celebration Souvenir of the Delhi Medical Association, "even the senior doctors . . . are often blackmailed and even humiliated by the incompetent bureaucrats and corrupt politicians" (Jain 1974).

Admissions to medical colleges are the other major medical resource controlled by doctors which politicians wish to affect. Paramedical positions have not been particularly popular, largely because there is much less private demand for their skills and less opportunity for emigration. The female categories—nurses, auxiliary nurse-midwives (ANMs) and lady health visitors (LHVs)— have often been short of applicants (see chap. 9). Medical education, by contrast, has always been vastly oversubscribed. Sometimes there has been a collective response; private groups (usually politically well connected) have established medical colleges (notably in Karnataka and Bihar) and concerted pressure by Delhi parents also led to the creation of a fourth medical college in the capital in 1972. The strength of this pressure is indicated by the substantial entrance (or "capitation") fees to private colleges parents are prepared to pay. It is not surprising that allegations of corrupt practice in the admissions to government medical colleges are frequently made though rarely substantiated. Formally, admissions are made on merit, and this probably applies to most entrants. However, many colleges have places reserved for nomination by the governor, and these are subject to considerable pressure quite apart from candidates who improve their chances in other ways. The process does not end with admission, since results in examinations are also vulnerable to political pressure. In 1986 the governor of Maharashtra was forced to resign after admitting that he had pressed to have his daughter's MD marks raised, and the vice-chancellor of Bombay University also resigned over the issue (*Economic and Political Weekly*, XXI, 1986:425–426).

In the case of staff appointments the crude distinction between clients and suppliers breaks down. Medical staff want "desirable" appointments, defined according to criteria such as access to towns (the bigger the better) or to a home area, or near a spouse's appointment, and so on. Politicians use these preferences as part of their political stock-in-trade, offering to help medical staff meet these priorities in exchange for money or political allegiance. Certain lower-level posts may cost a certain amount of money (Wade 1984). At higher levels (posts that can affect admissions to medical colleges or grant other kinds of power) the element to be traded is more likely to include the granting of equivalent favors—a tacit agreement to help the candidates of one political party or faction when requested. The two pressures interact: health personnel want some posts more than others, and politicians want some posts filled more than others, preferably by their own appointees rather than someone else's.

Consequently, staff accede to the desires of some patients more than those of others. Some patients have influence over postings while others do not. In general, the support of the wealthy (or at least, the absence of hostility) may be crucial when the member of staff is engaged in a dispute with another patient or a superior, or is threatened with an unwanted move or denied a wanted one. Following a defensive strategy, staff look over their shoulders to their relationships with their wealthier patients, or potential patrons, even in the absence of financial incentives to engage in private practice, whether legal or illegal. For example, Banerji notes how female paramedical staff tend to visit only the homes of wealthier villagers; he explains this partly in terms of their own comfort (more congenial company, better hospitality), but maintaining good contacts is also necessary for those who want some say over their career possibilities (Banerji 1972).

One exception is if staff members can maintain good relationships with superiors on the basis of their ability. However, in only one field is there any measure of certainty: the meeting of family-planning targets. Staff throughout the health-ministry hierarchy are routinely threatened with transfer or dismissal for failure to meet such targets and are offered support for promotions and desirable transfers for success. This reached its heights during the emergency, but it has been part of everyday practice for much longer (Vicziany 1983).

In general, the higher-paid posts receive much greater prominence. No one is much concerned with the appointments of auxiliary nurse-midwives but the appointment of doctors, especially to higher administrative or teaching medical posts, arouses considerable political dispute. Health personnel themselves expect to spend time negotiating for good posts and avoiding bad ones, while politicians spend a lot of time supporting candidates for posts or (if in power) responding to such pressures. Similar pressures are exerted over purchases of supplies, including pharmaceuticals, and construction contracts. Estimates of the scale or significance of such pressures to engage in corrupt practice are, of course, scarce; occasional cases come to light, usually when more blatant examples are seized on by the press or when allegations are made (and made to stick) as part of factional disputes. Informed opinion is that the medical department generates more staff pressure than most state ministries and that public-health engineering is a lucrative department because of the contracts they have to offer (*India Today*: 1–15 June 1985). Pressures from clients, suppliers, and employees, either directly or mediated through other politicians, tend to dominate the lives of ministers. Dr. Sushila Nayar, central minister of health in the early 1960s, put it to me like this:

Q: As Health Minister, what political pressures were you under?
A: Mostly pressures from my colleagues on appointments. I made some costly mistakes as a result of this, until I realised what was going on. Then they wanted me to open new medical colleges in their areas; they wanted me to get people admission in medical colleges; and there were pressures over the purchase of equipment. I managed to ignore most of these. (Interview:1976)

The prominence of doctors and the absence of ideological debate about medical policy are both enhanced in the process. In addition, staff are under pressure to benefit financially from their appointments in whatever way they can, either to allow them to move where they want to or to fight off attempts to dislodge them from posts they hold. Some of the consequences of this will be discussed in chapter 10. The key point to note, however, is that these pressures are not abnormal or unusual, they are intrinsic to India's political system.

The relative lack of ideological dispute is all the more surprising given the existence of competing medical systems. Conflict is not, of course, totally absent. The proponents of the indigenous systems of medicine have vigorously asserted their claims to larger shares of government expenditure, government employment, and official appointments. These campaigns have had supporters as high as the central cabinet; Nayar had colleagues who wanted equal treatment for indigenous systems of medicine, some for political reasons and some because of their convictions (Interview:1976; see below).

The constitutional divisions described above also limit conventional political pressure through parliamentary activities. In the Lok Sabha, the major opportunity for debate is usually the presentation of the ministry's budget; opponents put down "cut" motions, calling for the budget to be reduced because of the ministry's failure to do certain things. These debates are often dominated by lists of inadequacies in the Central Government Health Service (facilities provided for central government employees, often used by members of Parliament as well). Other topics usually relate to improving facilities in the politician's own regions, or general complaints about shortfalls in facilities. Clear and consistent criticisms of health policies are rarely made; neither are debates sponsored by the opposition on medical topics. Only two exceptions are significant: support for the indigenous systems of medicine, produced on almost every possible opportunity by some members and usually ignored; and requests for more doctors to serve in rural areas (see chap. 9). The absence of informed political debate in the Lok Sabha could be explained by constitutional divisions. However, it also seems to be the case for the state assemblies. Most political activity with respect to health takes place outside the parliamentary forum.

The Indian Medical Association

The main external pressure groups attempting to influence health policy are occupational groups—representative associations of public sector doctors, integrated practitioners,

Western doctors in private practice, indigenous practitioners, pharmacists, medical representatives and so on. The avenues for affecting policy are varied and favor some groups more than others. Allophathic doctors have one great advantage; some of their members are on the inside in positions of influence, though divisions within the occupation (among specialists and generalists, self-employed and employees) mean that they are less able to use this advantage than might be expected.

Almost all medical and paramedical personnel have some association to join, but those for paramedical staff are much weaker than those for doctors, whether Western or indigenous. The most political of the medical associations is the Indian Medical Association, but other notable associations of Western doctors are those of specialists (surgeons, physicians, etc.) and of doctors in specified employment (by the Employees' State Insurance Scheme, coal mines, etc.). Groupings for "integrated" doctors (with joint training) and for Ayurvedic and Unani practitioners are less stable. There is even an association for those who practice Western medicine without formal qualifications (the Private Medical Practitioners Association of India). By far the best documented is the IMA, and I shall concentrate on its history, organizational form, and mode of operation.

Early organizations of doctors in India either admitted only European doctors, or were dominated by them; they were often affiliated with the British Medical Association (BMA). A Bengal branch of the British Medical Association, established in 1863, broke up in 1867 over the reading of a homoeopathic paper. Several other Indian branches were short-lived until separate membership for officers in the IMS became popular in the 1890s (Johnson and Caygill 1973:198–209). But there were also more academic medical societies. In Bombay in the 1880s a Grant Medical College Society (open to Indian and European doctors) and a Bombay Medical and Physical Society (apparently restricted to members of the IMS and Royal Army Medical Corps) predated the Bombay branch of the BMA in 1889. (Cursetji 1934:255–262).

Indian doctors began to establish alternative societies (e.g., the Bombay Medical Union, dating from 1883), which also received fluctuating support. These societies were often active on political issues, presenting memorials and sending witnesses to appear before royal commissions that considered medical matters in London or in India. They lacked a stable all-Indian organization until regular All-India Medical Conferences were held in the mid-1920s and the IMA was founded in 1928 as a coalition of local medical associations. Its original membership of 200 doctors grew steadily to over 3,000 ten years later.

The IMA was closely linked to the nationalist movement (Jeffery 1987). M. A. Ansari, on the founding executive committee, had been president of the Congress Session of 1921. In his address to the 1928 All-India Medical Conference, Dr. Sir Nil Rattan Sircar made no secret of his view of medical backwardness in India.

> The secret of this unfortunate situation is not hard to discover. An alien trusteeship of a people's life and fortune is almost a contradiction in terms. For among the governing factors in all sanitary reforms and movements are the social and economic conditions of life, the environment, material as well as moral, and above all the psychology of the people— and an alien administration, out of touch with these living realities, will either run counter to them and be brought up against a dead wall of irremovable and irremediable social facts or, wearying of fighting half-understood obstacles in the path, grow timid and fight shy of all social legislation even in the best interests of the people's lives and health. (Ray 1929:5)

Such sentiments were frequently repeated at this conference. The most hostile comments were reserved for the Indian Medical Service, seen as dominated by racist sentiment. B. C. Roy, also prominent in the Congress party, used similar terms in his presidential address in 1929 when he spoke of the "determined and systematic efforts (that) have been made in the past to keep us in a perpetual state of inaction and stagnation" (Roy 1964:276): the British had not developed medicine in India far enough. However, because of the link between cultural renaissance and Indian nationalism, the leaders of the IMA also had to offer cooperation to indigenous practitioners. Sircar's address included an assertion that "we must put ourselves *en rapport* with the genuine living representatives of the ancient medical art" (Ray 1929:9). Roy wanted to open membership of the IMA to those who "honestly believe in their own system of medicine and practice it with real sincerity" (Roy, 1964:275–276). But these views had little support and they were pushed aside during the disputes over the international recognition of Indian medical degrees.

The proximate cause of the establishment of an all-Indian medical association was the claim by the General Medical Council in London that Indian medical degrees were no longer adequate as sufficient evidence of a doctor's ability to practice in the United Kingdom and, by implication, to be a member of the IMS (Jeffery 1979). The General Medical Council promised to withdraw from this position if an Indian Medical Council was established. Such a council would be respectable in British eyes only if its membership was largely nominated and official. This led to the medical cause célèbre of the 1920s and 1930s. The IMA accepted the desirability of a national medical council to coordinate the work of the provincial councils, established since 1912. However, it argued for the inclusion of licentiate doctors on the all-India register, and for a larger elected, nonofficial element, in line with nationalist arguments. The early sessions of the IMA, and the editorials of its journal are dominated by this issue until 1933, when the new Indian Medical Council was established.

In 1936, when Congress policy changed from opposition to the reforms of the 1935 Government of India Act to willingness to contest elections and enter assemblies, the IMA also became involved with the work of the Indian Medical Council. B. C. Roy was a member of the council and was later its chair. By 1945 he argued against maintaining licentiate qualifications, though he still held the view that licentiate doctors should be registered on the all-India Register with graduate doctors (Roy 1964:290–291). But it was always clear that close association with indigenous practitioners would be incompatible with international recognition, and this ensured that barriers between Western and indigenous doctors would be reinforced.

Medical politics are not the IMA's sole activity. Since 1931 it has published a journal containing mostly academic articles, and branch meetings also have academic sessions. But the unavoidable impression is that the political activities of the IMA have been dominant. That was certainly how the British government saw it. Prior to 1933 the government tried to prevent its own employees from joining, arguing that the IMA would recommend its members to vote for certain candidates (presumably Congress) and was thus a political body, out of bounds to government servants (NAI File 18–6/237–H). This bar was dropped when IMA rules were changed to delete those clauses urging support for candidates sponsored by the IMA. But the image of official disapproval has remained, and some doctors have claimed that their IMA activities have caused problems in their careers.

This record of nationalistic opposition to British rule, and the links between the Congress party and prominent members of the IMA might suggest that the IMA was well-placed to influence policy after 1947. Dr. B. C. Roy, after all, became chief minister in Bengal in the 1950s. However, the IMA has not been very influential, and its leaders claim that they have had little importance.

First, the IMA has attracted a membership of no more than about 35 percent of Western doctors in the country. Membership at independence was about 10,000, reaching 18,000 in the mid-1950s, 26,000 in 1965, and 41,000 in 1975 (IMA [Annual Reports] various years). In the 1960s the IMA attempted to draw the associations of specialists into a closer relationship, preferably under its own specialty wing, but this was largely unsuccessful. Doctors in employees' associations have occasionally sought the IMA's assistance. Some campaigns (such as the agitation against "quackery" and for improvements in service conditions in 1969) have been jointly organized. But longer-term relationships have been resisted.

Second, the medical association is identified with the interests of private practitioners. Early government hostility left a residual bias against membership on the part of doctors in the public sector. Also, the benefits offered by the association tend to be directed toward private practitioners. Most local branch activities are organized at the convenience of private practitioners, taking place in the afternoons when most private clinics are closed but when employed doctors probably have to attend to their duties. Membership in the IMA has sometimes meant preference in the allocation of telephone connections, cars, and motor-scooters, with government doctors having separate access to these scarce resources. Government and doctors concur in seeing the association as representing only the general, private-practice fraction of Western doctors.

Nonetheless, the IMA is the largest association of doctors and has attempted to present its views on medical policies as widely as possible. Its headquarters were moved from Calcutta to Delhi in 1948 to be nearer the center of power, and the IMA has worked constantly to be "taken into confidence" by politicians and medical civil servants. Its representatives attend a wide range of committees—the Annual Report for 1973–1974 lists 18, all with some governmental involvement. The most prestigious are the meetings of the Central Councils of Health and Family Welfare. The IMA president is usually invited to attend, though not as a full member.

Association officials, however, generally complain that they are not taken into official confidence in medical decision making. During the 1960s the IMA made a concerted attempt to enhance its influence. A public relations standing committee was established in 1963; its rationale was the progress of modern medicine and the enlightenment of laymen. The IMA was to study proposed legislation and publicize its views in the press and "through personal approach to the legislators or health department officials, administrators and others directly concerned" (IMA [Annual Report]:1963/1964). The committee's main objectives included communicating medical news and information and generating a positive image of the profession by preventing internal conflicts and "presenting a true, realistic picture of the medical men of today" (ibid.). In the late 1960s and early 1970s the government was planning to regularize the practice of medicine by unqualified personnel, and the IMA tried to generate public support to oppose its action, using protest days, marches, and more concerted approaches to the press (see chap. 9). However, this strategy was largely abandoned by 1975 (when the emergency made public protest illegal) and the IMA reverted to its former methods. Its officeholders visit ministers with memoranda about policy proposals; they hold conferences on topics such as rural medical relief, and invite politicians to open or close the proceedings and medical civil servants to give papers or chair scientific sessions; and they use contacts (such as doctors who are members of Parliament) to improve relationships with government. Perhaps it is surprising that the IMA has not followed a clear-cut policy of promoting private medicine; for a period during the 1970s it favored a complete nationalization of medical services as a way of dealing with the problems of overcrowding in medicine. Nevertheless, IMA officeholders still believe that their access and relationships do not result in policy influence.

The political weakness of the IMA is partly due to its dependence on the very government it wishes to influence. The IMA is not wealthy; it does not employ any doctors full-time and depends upon the commitment of working private practitioners to do office work in the Delhi headquarters, or attend meetings and conferences during working hours. Many of its proposals (such as the involvement of the IMA in school health and family planning activities) are only viable if they are underwritten by government funds. The IMA could expand its headquarters staff and employ doctors or other professionals in an executive capacity only with government support. Its major sources of patronage—access to priority allocations of scarce goods—are provided by the government. Its prestige activities—conferences, buildings, overseas tours—also depend on government funds and permission.

Its political weakness also arises from internal disputes. Litigation connected with elections of the president and vice-president has in some years taken over 5 percent of IMA income. For example, the medical association president for 1970–1971 could not take office because of a legal dispute over whether Bombay was entitled to branch status separate from that of Maharashtra State. By contrast, the posts of secretary and assistant secretaries are rarely contested and have stayed in the hands of a small group of Delhi GPs. Only six people have held the post of general secretary since 1948, several with only licentiate qualifications. Factional political disputes have sometimes surfaced when office-bearers attempt to discipline IMA staff, whose cause, in turn, is championed by some IMA members. Such divisions have weakened its ability to act decisively.

A third reason for political weakness is the limited spread of doctors into rural areas. This may cause some doctors embarrassment at being unwilling to go where they are most needed. When political policy was largely the preserve of the urban intelligentsia this may not have mattered much, but the changing structure of political life, described as a "ruralization of politics" (Rosenthal 1970), leaves doctors less well placed than unregistered practitioners to arouse rural public support or factional followings. Political success has increasingly depended on such resources, except during the emergency of 1975–1977.

The IMA has demonstrated several features typical of professional associations in postcolonial states. Johnson (1973) argues that these associations have a limited range of activities, their membership is low, and advancement and prestige within them is mostly sought by marginal practitioners. Two other criteria in his model fit the IMA less clearly—that ambitious young doctors would use an organization such as the IMA to advance their public careers and that international networks would be of crucial significance. The first was true around independence; several men were active in the IMA and then moved onto a wider political base, most notably Dr. B. C. Roy and Dr. Jivraj Mehta. Mehta was the first secretary of health and director-general of health services in independent India before becoming an ambassador. By the 1960s such links had waned. In 1970 ten doctor-M.P.s, were invited to attend a meeting of a committee concerned with monitoring legislative proposals, but only one turned up.

The role of international networks is also difficult to substantiate. The IMA is certainly proud of its membership in the World Medical Association and the Commonwealth Federation and of hosting international conferences. Further, since foreign exchange is difficult to obtain, attendance at conferences abroad can be a prized right. However, doctors attending such conferences have often had to pay all their own expenses and there has been little competition to go. Rather, doctors who happened to be in the relevant country at the right time have represented the IMA, without playing any further part in its activities.

Other medical associations in India share these characteristics. On the one hand, associations of specialists have not actively attempted to affect medical policies except for relatively technical issues, such as conditions for the import of medical equipment. They also depend on the government for financial support. On the other hand, they are generally dominated by doctors in the public sector, with official posts usually held by professors from senior medical colleges, and factional disputes rarely erupt into public or legal arenas. The associations of employees, such as those in state governments, and the diploma-granting bodies have a wider significance. The employees' associations tend, not surprisingly, to be concerned mainly with the terms and conditions of employment. In the Employees' State Insurance Scheme the main debate has been over its basic form of organization. Initially, especially in Maharashtra, there was a panel system where private practitioners could apply to be included. Panel members were paid according to the numbers of insured people registered with them. But this fell out of favor with the Employees' State Insurance Corporation which increasingly offered care provided by salaried doctors, often seconded from the state health services. The Association of Employees' State Insurance Scheme doctors still favors the panel system, but it has had to acquiesce in a scheme where panel doctors are a small minority, and capitation allowances have not kept pace with inflation.

Professional associations of employed doctors have acted essentially like other Indian trade unions. The associations, proving grounds for budding politicians, protect the interests of their members only insofar as this is compatible with the wider political interests of the leadership. Nonetheless, their strikes for higher pay, for improved status for junior hospital doctors, for reinstatement of sacked or suspended colleagues, and for protection of rights to private practice have sometimes brought medical politics into the forefront of general politics. In the late 1960s and early 1970s they often collaborated with the IMA in actions resisting the "legalizing of quackery"; and some issues (such as the right to private practice) are potentially very significant for medical policy. Nonetheless, most such associations have generally had an episodic life and have not shown a sustained ability to raise the status or the conditions of their membership. Doctors in employment still complain about their subordination to administrative staff, their failure all to be awarded class-one status (or senior class-one), and discrimination among doctors on administrative grounds (such as the distinction between those allowed to prescribe a full range of drugs and those restricted to a basic list).

The British royal colleges have no real equivalent in Indian medical life. The Colleges of Physicians and Surgeons in Bombay and Calcutta were involved in establishing undergraduate medical colleges, but traditions of higher or specialist qualifications did not develop partly because of the dominance of the British royal colleges. Associations of Indian specialists have attempted to give recognition to excellence, but most post graduates have continued to seek Indian university qualifications (an M.D. or M.S.), or British or American diplomas. This has begun to change since the mid-1970s. In 1975 Indian medical qualifications were again "derecognized" by the General Medical Council in London. In retaliation, the government of India insisted that British qualifications would no longer be recognized in India. At about this time, too, it became much more difficult to enter the United States for higher training. The government turned to the Indian Academy of Medical Sciences (IAMS) to resolve these problems. The academy was formally established in the 1960s, to play a role somewhere between the British royal colleges and the Soviet academies of science. It was entirely dependent on government sponsorship and did little more than award honorific titles until, in 1975, the government chose to use it as a vehicle for providing medical qualifications in India, separate from the university sector. The IAMS sprang to life, established specialist subcommittees, and began to offer curricula and regular times for examination. However, it does not have the prestige of foreign qualifications because it cannot insist on the same minimum requirements of work in prestige hospitals. Although it claims to offer training requirements and examination standards which are relevant to Indian conditions, it remains but a pale shadow of its overseas parallels.

Control Over "Quackery": A Case Study

Medical politics, the tactics of the various participants and the values they are trying to establish, can be further understood by looking at a case study. The primary issue that has exercised the IMA since 1947 has been policy toward practitioners unqualified in western medicine. Before independence, the expressed attitudes of doctor-politicians were not very hostile. In the 1930s, indeed, several presidents of the IMA called for a rapprochement between allopathic and indigenous practitioners. Even so, the hand of friendship was only offered to "sincere, genuine" practitioners who maintained a "pure" practice of the ancient arts. But since 1947 the IMA has consistently drawn a clear line between allopathic graduates and licentiates, on the one hand, and all other practitioners, usually called "quacks," on the other. It has reluctantly admitted that trained vaids and hakims should be permitted to practice in their own line but has protested vehemently against integrated practice (training and treatment from more than one system) and the use of allopathic treatment by untrained personnel. In 1963 the public relations subcommittee commented: "Quackery is rampant in our country. It would be the duty of the Association to acquaint the public and educate the illiterate masses about the same with a view to elicit their cooperation in rooting out this menace."

Unfortunately for the IMA, the public and many politicians and civil servants do not see the matter this way. Propaganda against traveling sellers of cures has been undertaken by the government, but neither the government nor most patients view established practitioners with dubious qualifications and the prescription of allopathic medicines by vaids and hakims as the same kind of issue.

In many areas trained doctors are few and far between. The government has therefore argued that the unqualified practitioner is entitled to earn a living as long as he is not an actual threat to his patients, at least until there are enough trained doctors to replace him. This view is held despite legislation designed to:

1. Restrict unqualified practice by registering existing practitioners and then outlawing any future additions to the register (following a Bombay Act of 1938 as a model).
2. Prevent any medical practice by those unqualified in modern medicine (enshrined in a clause of the Act which amended the constitution of the Medical Council of India in 1956).
3. Prevent prescribing of drugs contained on a list of dangerous drugs (enshrined in the Drugs Act of 1940).

The IMAs frequent assertions that this legislation be enforced have usually been ignored, maybe because, at the local level, the relevant agencies (district medical officers, or the police) prefer to maintain illegal practices for considerations, or as part of the favors and obligations which are the everyday currency of political life. However, when government proposed to change that policy to overrule aspects of this legislation, the Medical Association has prevented most of these changes from being implemented. The "barefoot" doctor scheme of 1972–1973, and the proposal by the Kerala government in 1974–1976 to establish a common register for qualified and unqualified personnel, were two cases where sustained action succeeded, in combination with other factors, in preventing change. But IMA opposition to the schemes developed since 1975, again based on a "barefoot doctor" scheme, has not prevented the establishment of community health volunteers. The rural populism of the Janata Government led it to overrule medical opinion, and the 1980 Congress Government eventually decided to implement the scheme (Jobert 1985).

The associations of indigenous practitioners have also been concerned with this issue. These associations have divided into two opposing camps—those insisting on a "pure" Ayurveda and those in favor of some integration of Western and indigenous practice (Brass 1972). Before the 1960s, most Ayurvedic and Unani colleges integrated modern subjects, such as anatomy and physiology, into their curricula. The political case for indigenous medicine rested on its suitability for Indian culture, diet, and climate, and on its claim to be providing services in rural areas that western medicine was unwilling and unlikely to supply. However, students generally wanted more Western medicine, since they were often studying indigenous medicine as a second-best option, having failed to get into Western medical colleges. Then, after training, they claimed that they were entitled to employment at the same rate of pay and on the same conditions as Western graduates. These contradictions were resolved in the early 1960s. Most indigenous colleges removed "modern" science from their curricula and followed the "pure" line. This position was also preferred by Western doctors, because it might lead to a sharper delineation of the distinctions between the systems of medicine and a greater capacity to stop outsiders from encroaching on Western medical territory (GOI 1961b).

But this dispute continues. Deep contradictions remain between representatives of "pure" Ayurveda and the actual practices of most graduates of indigenous colleges. The practitioners routinely use aspects of Western medicine and usually insist on their right to prescribe any legal drugs. The logical problems of producing an integrated system of medicine are usually regarded as insurmountable; but in everyday practice, many practitioners and clients move without embarrassment between these apparently incompatible systems. In addition, indigenous graduates have been almost as unwilling to work in rural areas as their Western counterparts. The debates over policy have thus taken place at considerable remove from everyday reality.

Indigenous practitioners continue to exist, with a measure of state patronage for their colleges and some public employment for their graduates. In the early 1980s, graduates of indigenous medical colleges were supposed to be employed as the third medical officer at Primary Health Centers. In private practice they prescribe Western medicines with varying degrees of impunity and run successful clinics in urban as well as in some rural settings. Since 1977 Western doctors have also had to accept the creation of a vast number of community health volunteers, also with state patronage. The IMA has been powerless to prevent what it sees as state sponsorship of "quackery." The result is a weak form of medical oligopoly.

Conclusion

The IMA campaigns have generally been unsuccessful. Its officeholders feel excluded from the informal policy-making process, and formal attempts to influence policy have been of limited success. Other organizations of practitioners have been even less influential, whether they have been paramedical practitioners or from other systems of medicine. The main strength of Western doctors comes from their representatives within the official hierarchy, where they have traded on their control over scarce, desirable resources—access to hospitals and medical colleges. Health policy has thus been made in the absence of sustained ideological debate, whether over the system of medicine to be supported, the role of private medicine, or the distribution of resources between uses.

Key doctors involved in health policy seem to be medical administrators, especially those who control major national medical institutions or are at the apex of the medical hierarchy in the Ministry of Health in New Delhi. Indicators for this are few. Some directors-general of health services appear to have effected some policy changes. For example, P. K. Duraiswami was identified with the introduction of mobile hospitals in the late 1960s. But perhaps the most significant policy changes followed the report of the Group on Medical Education and Support Manpower, established in 1974, and chaired by J. B. Srivastava, then director-general of health services (see chap. 9). Its membership included directors of the Indian Council for Medical Research, the Post-Graduate Institute in Chandigarh, the All-India Institute in New Delhi, as well as the member-secretary of the Indian Council of Social Science Research, an administrator from the Central Ministry, and a deputy director-general of health services as member-secretary. Notably absent are members from state governments.

These medical influentials operate on an international stage. For specific purposes they might include the heads of more specialized research institutes, such as those for nutrition, mental health, and population studies. Their careers are almost entirely within a research-cum-higher-education framework (which excludes most academic doctors, who do very little research), and generally within the Central Health Service. Very few of them have worked in a State Health Service, or as district medical officers (the normal route to the directorship of State Health Services). Within the Central Health Service accelerated promotion is possible for clinical specialists, who may vault over competitors who have worked for years as medical administrators in junior positions in the New Delhi directorate. After serving in top jobs in New Delhi, they may move into the international bureaucracies of the United Nations.

Thus, elite doctors tend to be open to ideas and proposals of foreign agencies. They may make apparently radical proposals often poorly related to everyday medical bureaucratic realities. Their networks usually do not include the leadership of the IMA or employees' associations for which they have no need. They are probably members of the general intellectual elite by virtue of birth, marriage, school education, or overseas research careers. Jobert (1985) implies that this elite acts almost like a Mafia, but he exaggerates its cohesion and exclusiveness and its power to affect wider policy. But if any doctors' voices are heeded in India, these are their owners.

CHAPTER EIGHT

India in the World Health Economy

The Indian economy is affected by world technology and markets. Culturally, this promises a desirable future especially for people who are influential in government decision making or who have skills that can be sold on world markets. Economically, multinational corporations operate in India, affecting production and investment. Politically, foreign governments and international institutions have brought resources and advice. While these forces have not been as powerful or substantial in India as in many other peripheral capitalist economies, they set a context which cannot be ignored.

Indian health policy is similarly influenced not solely by internal forces. The influence of the world economy on the health sector has not attracted as much attention as has its impact on other policy areas. Nevertheless, a growing number of critics since the mid-1970s have influenced key decision makers in donor agencies and health ministries. They have advanced aspects of three distinguishable arguments about the impact of international relationships—they increase dependency, support inappropriate health service patterns, and are Malthusian in intent. These critics focus on three aspects of the international context: health aid, medical migration, and the operations of pharmaceuticals companies.

Arguments that focus on dependency point to the ways in which aid, migration, and international investment benefit donors, recipients of migrants, and "home bases" of multinational corporations and, furthermore, how such processes may thwart developmental potentials within dependent countries by overwhelming local sources of capital and knowledge. Measuring the benefits to the capitalist "center" and the costs to the "periphery" (and vice versa) is difficult. Medical dependency is reproduced by doctors who have trained in another country and who use and demand medical equipment and pharmaceuticals from that country. Health "aid" in the form of scholarships or training encourages medical migration which more than repays original costs, either directly, through the work of overseas doctors and nurses within the country, or indirectly, through expanded exports of medical supplies (Doyal 1979; Cleaver 1977). Multinational companies that establish production within peripheral countries also, critics argue, siphon out in profits more than the original investment. This argument applies to companies supplying medical markets at least as much as to others.

A major weakness of this kind of analysis is that it gives the impression that "metropolitan" countries are almost totally dominant. But class formations and state apparatuses within the "periphery" may well affect the kind of health aid, the nature of migration, and the terms under which multinational companies can invest and operate. In particular, the Indian government uses India's size, its geopolitical position, and its links with the Soviet bloc to improve its bargaining position vis-à-vis donor agencies, and international companies. On occasion it has resisted political pressures and accepted the reduction in aid or withdrawals of foreign companies that followed, though when its position has been weak, it has had to accept much less favorable terms, as in 1965. Overall, however, a dependency analysis of India's position must be a qualified one.

Dependency analysts sometimes verge on conspiracy theories when they assert that material benefits (such as a better environment for multinational investment) determine health-aid policy. While such arguments may be used by supporters of health aid, these supposed benefits may not materialize nor affect the decisions taken after the assistance has been sanctioned. Debunking the claims that health aid is purely philanthropic is useful, but the relative insignificance of health aid in the overall picture must not be forgotten.

The part played by health aid, medical migration, and multinational pharmaceuticals firms in maintaining and reproducing the mode (or modes) of production in underdeveloped countries has been neglected. Most health aid is channeled through the state and thus helps to expand the resources available to the state and those who control it. Health-sector aid thus tends to strengthen the position of ruling groups in general as well as the position of public-sector doctors over those in the private sector, and modern bureaucratic cosmopolitan medicine over informal, indigenous, and traditional systems. Similarly, the access of Western-style medical personnel to a world market reinforces their claims for preferential treatment by the state and benefits the social classes they come from. Finally, the role of the state as defender of the interests of indigenous manufacturers and the source of access to the Indian market, also reinforces its general position.

Furthermore, medicine is an ideological form—one of the ways in which poverty and exploitation can be explained away, or at least one way those responsible for it can deny responsibility (see Frankenberg 1981). The provision of individualized medical (and other) services by the state helps to defuse pressures for change in the underlying social structures ultimately causing the patterns of morbidity and mortality (Jeffery 1978). Health-sector aid channeled through the government tends to support these processes; medical migrants return with more fully developed ideas of how such individualized health systems might be run; and pharmaceuticals companies operate with a perspective in which health care tends to be identified with the supply of their products, making health into a commodity.

Funding health services from outside the community also tends to weaken its capacity to provide for itself, which can be seen as an important aspect of development. However, if the alternative is that the poorest groups are left with the job of managing their own poverty, then external assistance may not worsen the situation (Briscoe 1980). Banerji (1978) has argued that medical services can also have liberative effects—and some of the projects supported by international agencies could well fall within this category—by threatening established powerful groups. Perhaps this is possible because health is rarely perceived as central to a pattern of domination; but attempts to make significant changes in the health status of the poor can easily lead to confrontation (Chowdhury 1978).

The most familiar criticism of the way the world market has warped health services in the Third World is that it has supported inappropriate patterns of health-service delivery. The inappropriate model involves large hospitals, expensive equipment, and high-level personnel. The costs of maintaining such large projects can swallow up a considerable proportion of the budgets of poor countries and usually benefit only a small proportion of the population (elite, urban groups); they have been designed to cope, in an expensive way, with diseases that are relatively insignificant in the morbidity pattern of the country as a whole (Bryant 1969). Health aid has often supported new investment in such projects. Migrant personnel learn this way of delivering health services and multinational companies can profit most from these trends. International pressures have tended to move resources out of primary care into secondary and tertiary care; away from rural areas into urban ones; away from preventive, community health and into hospital-based curative facilities; and away from female healers and toward male healers (Doyal 1979). The legacy of inappropriate institutions—for training, and hospitals, and in the skills of available staff—makes change very difficult to achieve.

Large aid projects may fail if no attempt is made to adapt to local economic, social, and cultural conditions (Newell 1975). For example, the malaria eradication program was based on experience from other parts of the world, but it was inadequately adapted to local conditions, notably the weakness of Indian basic health services (Sinha 1976; Aggarwal 1978; Harrison 1978). Another example is the early clinic-based approach to supplying family-planning services, inappropriate to a large rural country (Banerji 1972; Demerath 1976). Some critics go further and argue that Western solutions can never serve underdeveloped countries, because they are not effective even in the West; while others take the more radical view that these services are counterproductive in health terms, because they generate dependencies which are antithetical to people's ability to manage their own lives (Illich 1976).

Criticism of inappropriateness is rarely located in a political economy of decision making, but assumes that errors are a result of ignorance (and so knowledge alone will bring changes) or the particularly narrow form of medical education. Introducing community elements into decision making is expected to correct this imbalance. Perhaps this very willingness to propose technical solutions has made such criticism acceptable to decision makers and given this critique more influence on the policies of donor agencies than the more political dependency perspective. In addition, it offers the possibility of gathering support on populist grounds—keeping "our" doctors to serve "our" people, supporting "our" drug companies, and producing "our" solutions to "our" problems.

The third set of criticisms focuses on the explanations of poverty that underlie much health aid—the Malthusian assumption that the cause of a country's poverty can be found in the size and rate of growth of its population. The idea that world affluence was threatened by population growth in poor countries provided a clear justification for assistance to family planning programs from the mid-1960s onward (Piotrow 1973). The Ford Foundation and USAID led this process and continue to support these programs on a substantial scale, but other donors also became involved at different levels. Critics argue that such programs can become another way to ensure that the poor are blamed for their poverty and are designed to prevent social revolutions. Resources that could be used to assist the poor are instead put into programs the poor do not want and which meet few of their perceived needs. Concern for preventing births is not matched by concern for those already born, and some critics interpret this as essentially racist and antifeminist (Doyal 1979).

Many writers, however, are also aware of the ambiguities involved and of the fine line between providing services that allow men and women to control the number of children they have, and forcing them to have fewer than they want (Balasubrahmanyan 1986).

Although I shall not discuss the overall character of family-planning programs in India, I shall examine whether or not family planning has taken an undue share of health-sector aid to India.

Health-Sector Aid To India: 1947–1977

Critics of health sector aid argue that any health policy must be understood in the context of an international political economy. Health policies supported by the World Bank or other capitalist institutions must be seen in the light of the interests which they serve; and capitalist institutions have no interests which would be served by reductions in infant and child mortality for India's rural population (Banerji 1981). Health aid must therefore meet different interests—to support medical exports, improve the image of the donor, and help safeguard social systems within which capitalism can flourish. My concern here is to outline the pattern of aid to the health sector in India in order to assess the extent to which this pattern has been distorted by the interests of the donors. A substantial project on health-sector aid was carried out in the Institute of Development Studies in Sussex (Cole-King 1977; White 1977), but it concentrated on assessing patterns of activity by donors. By contrast, I am concerned with one recipient country. More detailed information is available in Jeffery (1986).

Several general points need to be made about health-sector aid. (Aid and assistance are of course contested terms, but I shall use them for simplicity.) Health-sector aid may or may not affect health: aid to other, apparently unrelated areas, such as female education, may have much more impact. Aid is fungible: funds nominally given for one project (say, a new hospital) releases money for other projects (say, a new hotel). Since we cannot know what would have happened in the absence of the aid, we cannot know how far the aid really funded the hospital (Singer 1965). Health aid also poses problems of classification, since any particular project may have several features, some inappropriate or Malthusian features as well as appropriate ones. I shall ignore the fungibility problem, and spell out how I have classified the data when necessary.

Table 26 summarizes the main sources of foreign assistance to Indian public-sector health activities. The major donor has been the United States, providing $107 million in assistance between about 1950 and 1973 (see table 27). After the U.S. government's "tilt to Pakistan" in the Indo-Pakistani War of 1971, it stopped all new assistance to India for several years. However, a new loan to malaria control was negotiated in 1978, and since 1980 new grants have been made to area development programs in five states. Before 1971 most U.S. health aid was on a grant basis, and health took about 37 percent of technical assistance to India in this period. In addition, a 1969 grant of $20 million was not tied to specific imports or advisers, but 50 percent of the extra resources were to be

TABLE 26

Major Sources of Health Aid 1947–1979

	1947–49	1950–54	1955–59	1960–64	1965–69	1970–74	1975–79	Total
U.S. Government								
Technical Aid		21	46	25	12	2		107
PL–480			70	136	160			366
Other						10	15	25
UNICEF	0.3	8	10	20	26	40	50	154
WHO	0.2	2	5	6	6	11	23	53
UNFPA						5	37	42
World Bank:								
Population						6	15	21
Water supply, etc.						1	69	70
Ford Foundation				3	4	3	1	10
Rockefeller Fndtn.	0.1	0.2	2	1	2	0	–	5
Swedish IDA						2	9	11
Norwegian IDA						4	24	28
U.K. (ODA)							6	6
Total	0.6	31	133	191	210	84	249	898
(excl. PL–480)	0.6	31	63	55	50	84	249	532

Sources: For US aid, see table 27; UNICEF Financial Report and Accounts, UN General Assembly Official Records New York 1950–1976. (Because of changes in classification and the expansion of activities to include education, the 1970–1974 and 1975–1979 figures are estimates); India: Report of Mission on Needs Assessment for Population Assistance, UNFPA, New York 1979; "Twenty Years in South East Asia, 1948–1967," WHO, New Delhi 1968; "Twenty-five Years in South East Asia, 1948–1973," New Delhi 1973; Financial Reports, WHO, Geneva, 1973–1977; Annual Reports, Rockefeller Foundation, relevant years; Ford Foundation Annual Report, Ford Foundation, New York, relevant years. (Details provided change from year to year and the absence of payments information from seven years means that there may be some double counting); Norwegian aid: personal letter, June 1985.
Key: PL–480, Public Law–480; UNFPA—United Nations Fund for Population Activities; ODA—Overseas Development Administration

TABLE 27

U.S. PUBLIC-SECTOR ASSISTANCE IN HEALTH AND SANITATION

	Technical assistance (U.S. $ million)	PL-480 Grants (Rs. million)	Loans (Rs. million)
Malaria control/eradication	83.3	852	210
Filaria control	2.4	*	*
Smallpox control/eradication	*	103	27
Other communicable disease-control programs	0.4	*	*
Water supply	6.4	*	587
Medical education	2.8	*	*
Nursing education	1.2	*	*
Family planning	6.2	*	*
Miscellaneous	3.9	*	*
Total	106.7	1249	999

SOURCES: Technical assistance completed projects and activities, Office of Controller, USAID, 1976:259; Shenoy 1974:243.

* Categories are not recorded separately.

NOTE: *The Times of India Directory and Yearbook* reprints press releases from the United States embassy in several editions from the mid-1950s onward until 1969–1970. This incomplete listing gives some evidence on the timing of this assistance, and notes Rs. 29 million to All-India Institute of Medical Sciences, Rs. 134 million to primary health centers, and Rs. 74 million to the training of medical educators before 31 March 1966.

Report on Currency and Finance, Reserve Bank of India, lists loans from 1969/1970 onwards. A loan from USAID for malaria control was agreed in 1978, and Rs. 120 millions ($15.4 million) was spent in 1979/1980 under this head.

spent on improving the delivery of rural health and family-planning services.

The final category of U.S. assistance is Public Law-480 rupee counterpart funds. Some of the grain supplied as "aid" by the United States under the provisions of PL-480 was paid for in rupees; the Indian government could only spend these with the agreement of the U.S. government. Nearly Rs. 1,000 million from this source (approximately $166 million) went in loans to the health sector, and Rs. 1,250 million (about $200 million) went in grants. The major share of technical assistance and PL-480 funding was to malaria control and eradication (78 percent of technical assistance and 47 percent of PL-480 funds), water supply and sanitation took another 6 percent of technical assistance and 26 percent of PL-480 funds. Indians also have been trained abroad on U.S. government funds; for example, between 1952 and 1960, 249 were trained in health subjects, roughly 10 percent of the total (Shenoy 1974; Times of India 1951–1967).

The next largest sources of aid have been the UN agencies, especially WHO and UNICEF. India is a contributor to both so figures for these agencies are not net assistance, though they do reflect the extent to which Indian government spending is tied by foreign advice. WHO has operated a tacit division of labor; while material supplies have come from U.S. aid, technical advisers (many of them American) have been provided under WHO's auspices (Mayer 1967). WHO aid, which totaled over $40 million between 1948 and 1976, was spread over most parts of the Indian government health program. Substantial proportions went to malaria control and eradication (13%), smallpox eradication (24%), and tuberculosis control (8%). Communicable disease control programs (including technical advisers and fellowships for Indians to study abroad) have taken roughly half of total assistance, while education and training have taken 8 percent. Although other countries in the region are increasingly encouraged to send their medical personnel on WHO fellowships to India for training, 90 percent of Indian fellows study outside the region. WHO provided 1,184 fellowships between 1948 and 1972, mostly in public health (570), malaria eradication (83), and control of other communicable diseases (161), but 208 were for medical education and 162 for clinical subjects.

WHO's "non-political" status has probably meant that its advice has had more weight than that of other donors. WHO has continued to send advisers to meetings of the Central Council of Health. It has assessed plans and projects; its support was crucial in the establishment of malaria-control and eradication programs in the 1950s, and the smallpox eradication program of the 1970s; and it continues to play a large part with, for example, its Expanded Program on Immunization.

WHO has collaborated with UNICEF, particularly in aid to maternal and child-health services, tuberculosis, and leprosy-control programs, the production of vaccines, and the applied nutrition program. From 1947 to 1970, UNICEF provided over $64 million, mostly in the health sector, though in recent years it has diversified its assistance into education. This excludes emergency relief.

A detailed breakdown of UNICEF assistance to India by purpose is not available, but the largest share was in supplies and equipment—antimalarial and antitubercular materials, milk for child feeding, jeeps for primary health services, and so on. In the 1980s, UNICEF assistance has been increasingly targeted on child survival, in a program known as GOBI-FF which concentrates on growth monitoring, oral rehydration, breast feeding, immunization, and pregnant women.

Since 1971 the UN Fund for Population Activities (UNFPA) has provided substantial assistance, with $43 million allocated up to 1979. Smaller grants have been handled by WHO or the International Labor Organization (ILO); large awards have been managed direct by the UN Fund for Population Activities or by the UN Development Program. Some of this assistance has been firmly within the family-planning program of the government of India, such as $14 million for the expansion of the sterilization program. Other grants have been concerned to strengthen training for paramedical workers who do more than just family planning work, as in the grants of $20.5 million for training indigenous midwives and paramedical workers, and for the employment of nurse-midwives and female health-workers.

The United Kingdom government has usually been the largest bilateral donor to India, but its health program has been small. First, it has offered "maintenance aid," in which the government of India imports what it wishes from the U.K., funded by a sterling credit. Some of the goods imported in this way have been medical in nature—about $720,000 a year in the 1970s (White 1977). Second, aid for specific health projects amounted to very small sums, for example $120,000 in 1974, nothing in 1975, and $250,000 in 1976 (Overseas Development Administration [ODA], 1971; Overseas Development Ministry, [ODM] 1978). The third area is technical cooperation—fellowships in the UK and the provision of technical advisers, partly handled through the Colombo Plan. Over 100 medical fellowships were offered in Britain in the 1960s (Colombo Plan 1969). In addition, the Post-Graduate Institute of Medicine in Chandigarh was linked to the Postgraduate Medical Federation at the Hammersmith Hospital in London. Fourth, a grant of $6 million, available for spending in rupees, was made in 1977 to equip operating theaters at Primary Health Centers and subdivisional hospitals, largely for sterilization operations; at the same time each medical college was given three mobile clinics.

Other bilateral donors have given aid for specific projects and for training abroad. For example, New Zealand provided $2 million for the All-India Institute of Medical Sciences (AIIMS) in New Delhi in the mid-1950s; in the 1970s and the early 1980s the Norwegian government provided assistance to a postpartum family-planning program; the Swedish government provided $10 million to WHO for smallpox eradication in India in the early 1970s and cofinanced a major project with the World Bank; and Danida (Danish International Development Agency) has also provided assistance to maternal and child-health programs and nutrition programs since 1975.

Except for Rockefeller and Ford, most private-sector agencies have not supported government programs in India. The Rockefeller Foundation began assistance in India in 1920, with aid to health programs in Mysore state, and provided $675,000 to the All-India Institute of Hygiene and Public Health in Calcutta before independence. Since 1950 major grants have gone to the Virus Research Center in Poona (over $1.2 million by 1973); to the All-India Institute for Medical Sciences (over $1.2 million) and its rural training center at Ballabgarh (over $250,000), and to selected medical colleges—Christian Medical College at Vellore, Trivandrum Medical College, and King George's Medical College, Lucknow, in particular. Rockefeller has also provided overseas fellowships; one report lists over 250 fellows in medical subjects who completed their study program between 1917 and the end of 1968—a list that includes most of the prominent nurses and doctors in India in this period (Rockefeller Foundation 1972). Rockefeller assistance tailed off from 1967.

Ford Foundation aid dates from 1959 and reached a peak in 1970. To begin with, rural sanitation took a large share, but then population programs run by the government of India ($3.7 million) or by the research/action center at Gandhigram (nearly $1 million) took an increasing proportion. An early and continuing interest was research in reproductive biology (nearly $2 million, with one-third going to AIIMS). Ford also supported research fellowships of the Indian Council for Medical Research (ICMR) as well as offering research fellowships abroad.

The many other private-sector agencies provide so little documentation of their activities that their involvement cannot be easily summarized; only general indicators of their scale and form can be provided. For example, the Federal Republic of Germany has provided assistance, through charitable agencies, to voluntary hospitals and other health facilities amounting to DM 66.4 million (roughly $23 million) between 1950 and 1980. In the United States, CARE and Catholic Relief Services have both been heavy users of U.S. surplus food. The Catholic program handled around $30 million of PL-480 food in India in 1978–1979, while CARE has supplied over $830 million worth of food in India from its inception up to mid-1979 (Catholic Relief Services 1979; CARE 1980). Some critics argue that like PL-480 "donations," this should not be seen as nutritional aid or even as aid at all, on the grounds that major beneficiaries have been U.S. farmers and the import of food has tended to have adverse effects on local food production. Food aid has been handled by the Department of Social Welfare, and not the health ministry. The Catholic program also provided nearly $2 million in medical supplies. In 1973/1974 roughly a quarter of all British voluntary agencies' health-sector aid went to India—about $2 million (Cole-King 1977).

In quantitative terms voluntary aid, apart from food aid, has not been very substantial, but it has supported the employment of foreign doctors and nurses, provided basic supplies, and, on occasion, funded sizable medical investments, such as much of the advanced equipment at the Christian medical colleges in Ludhiana and Vellore. A number of rural hospitals have been supported; the voluntary sector (mostly church-related) in India accounts for a substantial share of hospital beds in the country, and many of these depend on funds from outside. Finally, some of the main innovative health schemes in India (see chap. 11) have had considerable support from overseas agencies to help them get started.

A number of points can be made about the significance of this pattern of aid. To begin with, while it has formed a small part of total aid to India, aid funds in three Plan periods contributed more than 15 percent of public sector expenditures on health (see table 28). The malaria programs were heavily dependent on outside assistance after 1952 when, in the following six years, the United States contributed over half the cost of the control program, and nearly 40 percent of the cost of the eradication program in 1959–1961 (Meyer 1967). When this aid ceased (around 1965), Indian expenditure on malaria control dropped substantially. Similarly, the family planning program has received substantial aid, permitting a much larger program than would otherwise have been possible, even though population assistance has not been the largest item of health-sector aid.

TABLE 28
HEALTH AID TO INDIA

	1947–49	1950–54	1955–59	1960–64	1965–69	1970–74	1975–79
				($ millions)			
1. Health aid	1	31	133	191	210	84	229
2. ,, exc. PL-480	1	31	63	55	50	84	229
3. Total aid utilized	{ 443 }		2,954	5,973	3,956	4,763	7,682
4. Line 1/Line 3	{ 7.0% }		4.5%	3.2%	5.3%	1.8%	3.3%
5. Line 2/Line 3	{ 7.0% }		2.1%	0.9%	1.3%	1.8%	3.3%
6. Health expenditure	108	353	668	1,230	1,280	2,767	6,092
7. Line 1/Line 6	1%	8.8%	19.9%	15.5%	16.4%	3.0%	4.0%
8. Line 2/Line 6	1%	8.8%	9.4%	4.5%	3.9%	3.0%	4.0%

SOURCES: Lines 1 and 2: as table 26; Line 3: *Report on Currency and Finance*, Reserve Bank of India, various years: "Utilizations of external assistance." Line 6: Reddy 1972; Barnett 1977; and RBI (op. cit.) for figures after 1975.

Prior to 1965–1966 an exchange rate of Rs. 4.76 = $1 has been used; afterwards the rate assumed is Rs. 7.8 = $1.

KEY: PL = Public Law

Exc = excluding

TABLE 29

DISTRIBUTION OF HEALTH AID TO INDIA: 1947–1979

Category	General health aid	Population health aid	Total health aid
		U.S. $ millions	
Primary care	575	85	660
	(63%)	(10%)	(73%)
Secondary/Tertiary care	35	24	59
	(4%)	(3%)	(7%)
Medical education/research	30	5	35
	(3%)	(1%)	(4%)
Paramedical training	15	20	35
	(2%)	(2%)	(4%)
Administrative support	5	10	15
	(1%)	(1%)	(2%)
Unallocated	–	–	94
			(11%)
Total	660	144	898
	(73%)	(16%)	(100%)

SOURCE: as in table 26, above.

Table 29 uses crude indicators to show that aid has favored primary care (rural health services, water supply and sanitation, communicable diseases programs, etc.), appropriating some 75 percent of total health aid. Aid to medical education has not been substantial, but because it has been concentrated on elite colleges (notably the All-India Institute for Medical Sciences) and their hospitals, its impact has probably been much greater than the figures would suggest. These institutions have trained a considerable proportion of leading Indian doctors, both educators and practitioners, and the concentration of funding has probably meant that these institutions have been markedly different from the other Indian medical colleges. Nevertheless, it seems reasonable to conclude that the pattern is by no means the straightforward disaster story the critical perspective would suggest. In particular, hospitals, family planning, and medical education have not taken a dominant role.

The second general point is that only family planning and smallpox and malaria control and eradication owe their origins or natures to the impact of foreign aid. Population policies supported by external agencies were clearly very important in expanding the size of the family-planning program and affecting its nature (Banerji, 1972). Their impact should not be exaggerated. Local bureaucrats were able to minimize the significance of many innovations that foreign advisers attempted to introduce (Minkler 1977). But in the rest of the health sector, very little before 1975 was not foreshadowed in the plans and structures established under the British (Hanson 1966).

A third general point is that the pattern of assistance to India has probably been affected by the constitutional distribution of functions between the central government and the states. The central government has generally restricted aid to areas for which it is responsible—control of communicable diseases, family planning, maintenance of standards of medical education, and medical provisions in the Union Territories. Most aid has been distributed through the Plan, under the control of the Planning Commission. Aid has gone to new areas after 1977, partly because the Janata Government decided to include maternal and child health in the tasks of the Family-Planning section of the Union Ministry, then renamed Family Welfare. This recognized that much of the basic rural health service was being funded under this head by the central rather than the state governments, and also reflected the ambivalence about family planning in the immediate postemergency period. It also, perhaps, opened the way of the new aided projects which have dominated the period since 1980.

Finally, the scale of health-sector aid to India has been totally inadequate to cope with the scale of Indian health problems. Of course, health aid is not necessarily the most effective way for donors to improve health but, even so, India has not been treated very favorably in terms of assistance to match its needs. Donor agencies appear to have shared the views of Indian planners (see Cassen 1978) and regarded health expenditures as a social rather than economic area, and health has never been seen as a core part of donor-agency discussions. However, the growth of the basic-needs approach to development led to India's minimum-needs program in the Fifth Plan, which gave more prominence to health programs. At the same time, aid to health took on increasing importance in the eyes of donors like the World Bank. I shall deal with the new pattern of aid which characterized the period of 1975 to 1985 in chapter 11.

THE ROLE OF HEALTH AID

Health aid must be seen in the context of overall aid policies, which are undoubtedly perceived by donors as extensions of foreign, industrial, and trading policies designed to benefit the donors themselves. This sets limits on the aid donors will offer and provides a lever that can be used to prevent other policies of which the donors might disapprove. But it does not thereby mean that health aid is precisely attuned to the interests of capital, broadly defined. In some cases, professional judgments might only be permitted because the appearance of autonomy is useful to "global capital" (Johnson 1978). Nevertheless, some autonomy is usually allowed and aid is given and used in an institutionalized form that permits some freedom for the exercise of professional judgment. This judgment, in turn, is not restricted to the imposition of received technical solutions derived from European and American experience, but responds to the major problems and considers alternative ways of dealing with them. These analyses and proposed solutions are of course limited by the scientific and administrative paradigms which are part of the learned environments of the experts involved; how could it be otherwise? But the experts do learn from past mistakes. Their limitations, of course, do have political consequences; medical experts may rule out some solutions because of a narrow definition of the medical, and these may be the solutions that imply radical changes in the organization of society.

But even with all these caveats, the pattern of health-sector aid to India after 1947 suggests, on the one hand, that major threats to health *were* given priority, that "appropriateness" *did* enter into decisions about the training needed, and that the proposed solutions *were* plausibly connected to the problems identified. On the other hand, because of political concerns, assistance to malaria control tailed off just when it was most needed and the resources put into smallpox eradication did not match its importance as an Indian health threat. Finally, an indicator of the limits of donor-agency influence is the donors' inability to redirect Indian priorities sufficiently to ensure that government will take over when assistance ceases. This is perhaps an inevitable feature of the aid relationship, though it also reflects tensions in Indian center-state relationships.

Migration of Health Personnel

Data on the migration of health personnel from India are highly unreliable. The emigration of trained personnel costs a substantial amount, but the loss is almost impossible to quantify, or to see when it occurs or whether it continues. Furthermore, the microeconomic models used to estimate the costs of migration are misleading; the very inappropriateness of medical education that enables doctors to migrate, also reduces the value to India of their contributions to health care had they stayed. Their migration is a symptom of failure to relate job content and training to local needs; this failure imposes much broader costs than the specific loss of personnel through migration. Nonetheless, I will start by considering what is known of the extent, direction, and trends in emigration.

THE NUMBERS OF MEDICAL EMIGRANTS

The historical roots of medical migration from India were set almost from the beginning of medical education in India, when a group of graduates from the Calcutta Medical College accompanied one of their teachers to London for further training (Johnson and Caygill 1973). The staff at the Indian medical colleges probably fostered the idea that local education was incomplete, rather than different. Teachers measured their teaching against standards derived from their own education. Until the First World War candidates for the IMS had to travel to London to take the admission examination, and many took additional qualifications while they were preparing for this. Before 1914 few doctors traveled to Britain, and most of them returned to India after relatively short stays—but this has to be conjecture since the address of a doctor in the Medical Register is a poor guide to where he actually lived. Other sources give some partial idea of the numbers involved; for example, 177 doctors with Indian names and coming from India received the Triple qualification from Scottish colleges in 1900–1909, another 83 in 1910–1919, 73 in 1922–1929, and 43 in 1930–1936 (ibid:115).

After 1918 travel to Britain was quicker and cheaper, and more doctors with Indian qualifications registered with the General Medical Council in London. By 1939, for example, some 10 percent of

1921–1923 Indian medical-college graduates had registered with the Medical Council through their Indian qualifications. Some registered with the expectation of traveling (but did not) and others registered on the basis of additional qualifications gathered in Britain. Indian doctors did not travel only to Britain, but relatively few followed the same routes as other Indian emigrants—to Burma, Malaysia, the Pacific Islands, and the Caribbean, or to other parts of the Commonwealth.

This situation changed with independence, when major international institutions began to introduce schemes to take doctors to Britain and America for higher training. No formal count seems to have been made of who went where and when nor whether they returned. Evidence from analyses of passport applications (which assumes that doctors gave their occupation) first became available in 1960, when 1,000 doctors were issued passports; this figure rose to 2,000 in 1970 (Indian Academy for Medical Research 1974). Once again we do not know how many used these passports to travel abroad nor for how long they did so.

THE DESTINATIONS OF EMIGRANTS

Estimates of the stock of Indian doctors in different foreign countries become more frequent and more reliable from about the middle 1960s. For example, the law on immigration to the United Kingdom changed in 1962 so that doctors wishing to enter the United Kingdom to work had to apply for vouchers; in the next six years nearly 6,400 Indian doctors applied for vouchers and roughly half of these were probably taken up (Johnson and Caygill 1973:69–70). The total receiving vouchers is equivalent to roughly 20 percent of the output of Indian medical colleges in this period. In 1968 a United Nations survey estimated 9,000 Indian medical personnel were abroad, two-thirds of them with higher qualifications. In the six years between 1963 and 1969 under the scheme run by the Indian Council for Scientific and Industrial Research to provide temporary posts for returning migrants almost 70 percent of the applicants were at the time in the United Kingdom, with another 25 percent in the United States. The U.S. share was much larger toward the end of the period, but we know very little about migration rates between the two countries (Mejia et al. 1979:293; see also *Technical Manpower* Vol. XV, no. 3, March 1973). The earliest U.S. data come from a survey carried out by the American Medical Association in 1970 which reported 3,957 Indian doctors, followed by a survey two years later which reported 6,303 (Mejia et al. 1979:291). Data on doctors in U.S. training schemes in the 1970s showed that India was the largest supplier of foreign medical graduates (see table 30).

Combining different sources gives an estimate of 12,000 Indian doctors abroad in 1970 and 15,000 in 1975 (Mejia et al. 1979:277; 291–292). The numbers abroad probably grew most rapidly in the late 1960s and early 1970s, when the numbers of Indian doctors entering the United Kingdom and the United States were about 1,000 a year in each case. About 40 percent of Indian doctors entering the United States in 1970 had not come directly from India, but we do not know whether 1970 was typical or not because the data on these movements are so poor. Similarly, the data on return flows to India are restricted to the information from the Council for Scientific and Industrial Research plan (CSIR), and then only for the late 1960s when an average of 220 a year entered the scheme. These figures suggest that, if anything, the 1975 estimate of 15,000 abroad is an underestimate.

Since 1975 the situation has probably changed considerably. The United Kingdom and the United States have both made entry by Indian doctors much more difficult. The General Medical Council in London withdrew recognition of the degrees from Indian medical colleges granted after May 1975, so that all Indian doctors qualifying after that date have to pass tests of "linguistic and professional competence" if they want to work in the United Kingdom. This

TABLE 30

MEDICAL GRADUATES IN TRAINING IN THE UNITED STATES

	31.12.72	*31.12.74*	*31.12.76*	*31.12.77*
India	2,988	3,900	4,009	2,782
Bombay	336	397	n.s.	248
Baroda	n.s.	269	n.s.	179
Total FMGs	17,712	22,301	15,097	10,108
(% India)	(16.9)	(17.5)	(26.6)	(27.5)

SOURCE: *Journal of the American Medical Association* vol. 226, 8:939; vol. 234, 13:1,356; vol. 240, 26:2,837.
KEY: FMG = foreign medical graduate.

had a phased effect on emigration of doctors from India. In the early tests only about 40 percent of Indian candidates passed (Mejia et al. 1979:278). In the United States new legislation introduced in January 1977 designed to restrict the inflow of doctors probably took effect more rapidly than the U.K. restrictions. As table 30, above, shows, the numbers of foreign medical graduates in training schemes dropped sharply between 1976 and 1977. Emigration of Indian doctors in the mid-1980s was below that of the mid-1970s, and involved different destinations—in particular the oil-rich nations of the Middle East and Nigeria. The predominant form of such flows is limited; most doctors enter on fixed-term contracts, which may or may not be renewed but which do not imply longer-term rights of residence or citizenship, as was the case for migrants to the United Kingdom and the United States.

Not all medical colleges contribute to the emigration of doctors. In part this probably reflects both the social origins of the student body and the closeness with which the medical faculty is able to tailor the education they provide to standards current in the West. As table 30 shows, Bombay and Baroda graduates contribute disproportionately to the numbers in the United States. The Baroda case is interesting, and illustrates the closest link between health aid and medical migration. Baroda Medical College was linked to the Edinburgh Medical School under a WHO program in the late 1960s and early 1970s. A study in 1976 suggested that half of all Baroda graduates were abroad at the time (Bhatt et al. 1976).

THE IMPACT OF EMIGRATION

The costs of this emigration have been variously assessed. In percentage terms, in both 1970 and 1975, about 10 percent of the stock of Indian doctors was abroad. In each year, this represented about 1.2–1.3 years output from the medical colleges; had these doctors remained, they would have raised the doctor population ratio from about 2 per 10,000 population to about 2.3 (Mejia 1979:166). India is the largest contributor of emigrant doctors, but these indicators suggest that the impact of this emigration on India is less than that on many other "exporting" countries. India is ranked twenty-second in terms of the impact of emigration on the domestic stock of doctors, and twenty-ninth in terms of the time it would take to replace the emigrant doctors at current level of output (ibid.). If the outflow in 1975–1980 was reduced because the main importing markets contracted, as suggested above, then the impact will have declined. The total stock of Indian doctors by 1980 was probably more than 210,000, of whom perhaps 17,000 were abroad.

If the impact is measured in terms of the loss of return on the investment in each of these doctors, the calculations produce rather different results. One estimate of $9,600 (Rs. 75,000) to educate a doctor generates a cost to India of $144 million to educate its doctors abroad in 1975 (Mejia 1979:288). Estimating the benefit lost to India by a neoclassical economic analysis based on earnings figures, generated an estimate of $44,000 per emigrant doctor to the United States for 1970 (Conference on Trade and Development 1975:8).

Any strictly financial calculation, however, has to take into account the remittances of these doctors back to India (figures for which are unknown, though remittances in general have been very significant to the Indian economy since 1975) and the employment the doctors would have had if they had not emigrated. India probably has a surplus of doctors, relative to its ability to pay them at the levels currently accepted by employers and doctors, so it makes little sense to attempt to value the contribution the doctors might have made had they stayed. In addition, the skills of these particular doctors were probably even less appropriate to the tasks needing to be done in India than the skills of those who stayed, so one might argue that Indians benefited more from their absence than their presence. Clearly, it would have been better if other forms of personnel had been trained, or if the individuals emigrating had paid a higher proportion of the costs of their training. But these are all interrelated factors. The demand for medical education (which led to the rapid expansion of medical colleges in the 1960s and early 1970s) was in part fueled directly by parents who saw the chances of emigration for their children. Emigration has also helped reduce medical unemployment and to keep medical salary levels higher than they might otherwise have been.

In general, then, the emigration of doctors and other medical personnel from India has had contradictory effects on medical policy making. On the one hand, emigration has probably tended to reduce medical unemployment, rather than create shortages of valuable skills; unintended benefits have been remittances and a reduction in political pressures to increase employment prospects in "high-technology" medicine. On the other hand, the demand for medical education has increased, contributing to the neglect of other forms of personnel, medical salary levels have been higher than they might otherwise have been, and the pressure for medical education to be organized so that doctors can continue to be acceptable abroad has been reinforced. The barriers to migration which have developed in the past ten years have probably quite dramatically altered the balance on this issue, but it may be too late; systemic inertia may now ensure that the costs continue to be felt, while the benefits are of declining significance.

Pharmaceuticals Companies

Multinational drug companies are obviously powerful. Sixty large pharmaceuticals companies dominate the supply of drugs, with about 60 percent of non-socialist-country production in the early 1970s. These companies are almost all based in either France, Germany, Italy, Japan, Switzerland, the United Kingdom, or the United States (Lall 1977:22). They are often diversified companies, with interests in a variety of chemical-based industries, and they vary considerably in the range of products they produce, in their major markets, and in the kinds of strategies they follow with respect to the Third World (Stoker 1984:115–118). Three factors, it is said, give these companies considerable influence: the size of the major companies; their apparent dominance over different sectors of the market for pharmaceutical products; and the significance of drugs bills in health budgets. This influence affects the supply of drugs, the type of drugs available and promoted, and the health policies of all countries, but especially those of underdeveloped countries (Khaliq 1976:5; Muller 1982; Melrose 1982; Medawar 1982).

The first major criticism of the activities of these companies in underdeveloped countries is that the cost of drugs has been much higher than need be. Companies are able to maintain high prices through patent protection, which reduces competition, through aggressive marketing and brand names, through control over the supply of raw materials, and by policies which are designed to maximize profits, such as transfer pricing (shifting profits to low-tax countries). Second, the drugs supplied have usually been designed with the disease patterns, socioeconomic conditions, and drugs markets of advanced capitalist economies in mind, leading to a concentration on the drugs suitable for sale to the relatively wealthy in urban areas, with far less emphasis on providing low-cost basic drugs for common diseases. Third, some companies appear to be less concerned about the interests of patients in the Third World than they are forced to be in some developed countries, failing to show the same concern with accurate prescriptions and warnings of possible side effects and contraindications. Fourth, some companies have attempted to stop governments who have tried to alter this situation, as well as making it very difficult for local companies to be established (Lall 1977; United Nations Conference on Transnational Corporations [UNCTC] 1983).

Several UN agencies (WHO, UNCTCS, and UNIDO [Industrial Development Organization]) have attempted to influence the pattern of drug development, production, and marketing and to limit what they regard as undesirable patterns (UNCTC 1979). In particular, WHO has led efforts to encourage countries to draw up lists of essential drugs, to use generic names, and to follow purchasing policies that will cut costs and lead to drug purchases more closely related to dominant-disease patterns (WHO 1977). Several agencies have supported Third World production of pharmaceuticals to reduce costs and to match health needs and drug supplies (UN Industrial Development Organization 1980). WHO also started to control the quality of drugs entering international trade to prevent the possibility that companies might export outdated drugs or drugs that have been banned because of adverse reactions, and to standardize marketing information (WHO 1978). Finally, the agencies have encouraged research, development, and the training of staff to produce more drugs to help in the control and treatment of six major diseases found mostly in tropical countries—such as malaria and leprosy (WHO 1976).

However, different Third World countries are not all in the same position with respect to pharmaceuticals production and marketing. UNIDO (1978) and UNCTC (1983) have produced classifications of production capabilities, placing countries in one of five or three categories respectively. In each case India is one of the very few underdeveloped countries in the highest category—and it is by far the poorest in this category. Indian companies can manufacture most of the intermediate products used in the country from bulk drugs, and the local chemical industry can make some bulk drugs from simple chemicals. Indian pharmaceuticals companies also carry out research and development activities of their own. As a result, they import relatively small amounts of raw materials, and export intermediate products, raw materials, and production plants, to several other countries (UNCTC 1983:88–92).

India nonetheless shares many of the problems of other poor countries. Here I shall describe how government policy has contributed to the development of the Indian industry, the current state of production and ownership, some of the problems that remain, and how far the pattern of drug production and its ownership, drug marketing, and consumption have affected health policy and health in India since 1947.

THE PHARMACEUTICALS INDUSTRY IN INDIA

The history of the modern pharmaceuticals industry really starts in the nineteenth century. India contributed to its development by supplying Britain with raw materials. The first substantial local production was in government factories in Madras and Bombay of quinine and later of a wider range of drugs (Stoker 1984:295). Production by Indian capitalists is usually dated from 1901, when P. C. Ray established Bengal Chemical and Pharmaceuticals in Calcutta. The Alembic Company was established in Baroda soon afterward (Hathi 1975:16). Few foreign companies had production facilities in India before World War II. In 1939 only about 13 percent of total consumption was produced in India (Khaliq 1976:131; Rangarao 1975:3–4).

The disruption to trade caused by the war made a dramatic difference. The decline in imports and the growth of government demand stimulated a large growth in local production drawing on the basic knowledge and capital available in India. By 1943 this met almost 70 percent of consumption, and the country was nearly self-sufficient in some areas, such as sera and vaccines (Stoker 1984:296). Production was largely in the hands of a few big British and Indian companies that were already established before 1939, but many small-scale firms also contributed to total production.

Pharmaceuticals production has changed rapidly since independence. Three major processes have been at work: technical changes associated with massive expenditures in the West on research and development; support for public-sector production; and public policy with respect to the private sector (in affecting the balance between public and private production, the ownership of companies, and attempts to promote production of certain drugs and to control their prices). I will describe each of these briefly in turn.

Most of the drugs currently in use throughout the world were not discovered or fabricated until after 1930. The first major discovery was the group of sulfa drugs, followed by antibiotics (penicillin and then others), discovered and produced in the 1940s. Estimates in the early 1970s suggested that some 30,000 drugs were then available, some of them little more than variants on others, about 8,000 of which were regularly prescribed (Stoker 1984:88). Most of these are new and were discovered in laboratories run by the larger firms that patented their discoveries not only in the country of origin but elsewhere as well. Research and development expenditures for these drugs are often considerable, and companies point to these costs to justify their control of production and prices through patents in order to gain sufficient profits to recoup their investments and pay for new research. However, critics suggest that many "new" drugs are merely minor variations on existing patented drugs and that the process of technical change is artificially managed in the interests of maintaining higher profits (Lall 1977:25). One particular feature of the medical market in many parts of the world reinforces the pharmaceuticals companies' ability to do this. Most drugs are purchased on the advice of or through prescription from a doctor, and pharmaceuticals advertising and marketing is thus focused on the doctor, not on the final consumer. In general, the cost of a drug is not a very salient point for doctors, other considerations (including the perception of "quality") possibly being more significant. Attempts by governments to affect prescribing patterns are also hindered by the desire of doctors to maintain clinical freedom of choice, based on their own assessment of which drugs will suit individual patients.

The figures on the numbers of drugs and clinical prescribing patterns thus probably exaggerate the extent of technical change. Nonetheless, these changes favor large producers over small and help to create a market divided into a very large number of small submarkets, where competition is artificially restricted and production runs are small. All these make it difficult for many countries to organize local production in order to replace foreign imports and to support local producers against the competition of foreign multinationals.

In India several factors have combined to make the impact of technical change in production of pharmaceuticals different from that in other Third World countries. An existing production capacity had already been developed during World War II by Indian and by foreign companies. The absolute numbers of consumers makes India a profitable market, even if only 5 percent or so of the total Indian population are wealthy enough to be included. In addition, the public-sector drug companies and an active government policy toward foreign-owned companies in general, and pharmaceuticals companies in particular, have tended to reduce the effect of these technical changes.

After independence India expanded its public-sector drug production. In 1951 the establishment of a Penicillin Enquiry Committee "marked the beginning of government entry in modern drug manufacture" (Rangarao 1975:4). A Pharmaceuticals Enquiry Committee reported in 1954 in favor of the creation of large-scale public-sector manufacturing of penicillin and other drugs in order to reduce prices and conserve foreign exchange (Hathi 1975:54). The Indian government then started negotiations with Western firms and the Soviet Union (Kidron 1965). Western commercial interests used diplomatic and other pressures to ensure that they supplied technical advice to Hindustan Antibiotics Limited at higher prices and with less control over technical data than the offer from the Soviet Union. The reason announced publicly was "technical superiority," but the extent of diplomatic pressure exerted suggests that technical considerations were not the only ones involved. However, the second public-sector company, Indian Drugs and Pharmaceuticals Limited, was based on Soviet advice. Completion of its major plant in Hyderabad was delayed until 1968 (Stoker 1984:320–326).

Public-sector production of pharmaceuticals has not been impressive. The two main companies involved have had considerable production difficulties and have been unable to produce up to their licenced capacity. Profitability has been lower than for most foreign and many private-sector Indian companies, with Hindustan Antibiotics Limited, taking a loss for much of the 1970s, whereas foreign-owned companies routinely make a higher profit than the averages for Indian industry (Stoker 1984:304). Nonetheless, by

1980 the public-sector companies were producing about 26 percent of bulk drug production, and 6.5 percent of formulations (UNCTC 1983:88). But government production may have had more political significance in demonstrating that the Indian government is prepared to reduce its dependence on imports and on foreign-owned companies. In addition, Indian Drugs and Pharmaceuticals is now in a position to export technology on a wide range of drugs, mostly to Middle Eastern countries, as are several private companies, suggesting that a significant technical barrier has been overcome (ibid.:89).

The government has also attempted to control the private sector through the terms they impose on foreign multinationals wanting to work in India. In the 1950s high tariff barriers and other restrictions on imports of finished goods led most companies to establish manufacturing plants within the country. However, this affected formulations mostly, with bulk drugs being imported. After 1970 the government restricted new production licenses to firms committed to some production of basic drugs. As a result, the foreign sector share of the bulk market rose from about 11 percent in 1972 to about 40 percent in 1980, but, because of a reduction in the number of companies defined as foreign, the 1983–1984 figure was only 22 percent (Stoker 1984:308; UNCTC 1983:88; Scrip 1985: 194).

In 1970 the period of patent protection was reduced to seven years and companies had to allow production of their products by competitors under license after three years. The government also systematized control of drug prices, introduced in 1962 at the time of the war with China. A Drug Price-Control Order was issued, setting maximum prices for seventeen bulk drugs and attempting to control the prices of formulations by limiting markups. In addition, the 1973 Foreign Exchange Regulation Act (FERA) stipulated that foreign equity must be reduced. Drug companies were originally placed in the core sector and excluded from these controls (Stoker 1984:309), but by 1978 policy had hardened and most companies had to dilute their shareholdings, with only two (Roche and Parke-Davis) being allowed as much as 74 percent, the rest being restricted to smaller shares (ibid.:310–311). The expansion of shareholding does not seem to have influenced policy or made these companies more accountable to Indian pressures, but companies regarded in this way as "Indian" find it easier to get licenses for new production (ibid.).

Pressures on drug companies in general, and foreign ones in particular, were strengthened by the 1975 Hathi Committee Report. It proposed some unexpectedly radical measures, including nationalizing all foreign drug companies, establishing a National Drug Authority, a phased abolition of brand names, and a change in the form of drug-price control (Hathi 1975:84–85, 96, 104, 180–188, 257). It provoked a heated debate over the next few years, complicated by the change in government in 1977. The most radical proposals were watered down under strong lobbying from the drug companies and the medical profession; there was no similarly well-organized support for the proposals (Hasan 1980). The one partial exception is that the organization representing the larger Indian firms (Indian Drugs Manufacturers Association [IDMA]) supported the nationalization of foreign firms, believing that this would improve their market position. The new drug policy, which emerged in 1978, took a markedly less forceful line on foreign ownership (allowing the maintenance of equity holdings above 40 percent) on the removal of brand names (making the process more gradual) and on a National Drug Agency (not created but replaced by a number of smaller statutory bodies with fewer powers) (Stoker 1984:366). Some of the price control, research and development, and production policies were, however, more far-reaching than Hathi had proposed (ibid.).

Political debate continued after the policy document was issued and the new Drug Price Control Order was passed in 1979. The introduction and implementation of several elements of the proposals were delayed or seem to have failed to have the desired impact. Legal moves by companies delayed the abolition of brand names and, in 1984, the Bombay High Court permitted a new drug to be marketed under a brand name, pending the settlement of cases in the Supreme Court challenging the new regulations. Foreign companies have claimed that the New Drug Policy has reduced the growth of drug output because of uncertainty and poor profitability, as companies have lost some elements of market protection (UNCTC 1983:50, 91). But these policies have been designed to limit foreign domination, make Indian drug production more appropriate, and limit drug company interventions in health policy. I shall now assess their success on each front.

FOREIGN DOMINATION

A simple indicator of foreign domination (but one which is nonetheless difficult to construct) is the share of production. Estimates of total output are not very reliable because many small companies rarely report their output accurately. However, the United Nations Center for Transnational Corporations' estimates, by major producing category, for the production of allopathic drugs and their distribution are given in table 31.

This indicator, however, takes no account of the sizes of companies in each sector nor how far drug production in all sectors was influenced during an earlier period when foreign companies were more dominant. Thus the foreign-owned sector (in this case defined as companies with more than 40 percent of equity owned by one foreign company) includes only 26 firms, five of which are among the ten largest pharmaceuticals firms in India. Their retail sales in 1980 were Rs. 1271 millions ($163 million), about 10 percent of the total. The five largest Indian-owned companies had sales of about Rs. 1,004 millions ($129 million), about 8 percent of the total (UNCTC 1983:152). The 3,000 or so small Indian producers are not all active (Stoker 1984:317). In addition, foreign companies concentrate more of their activities in formulations, where market conditions are more favorable. Thus the market power exercised by the average foreign company is much greater than that of the average Indian company. One further indicator of

TABLE 31

PRODUCTION OF DRUGS IN INDIA BY COMPANY OWNERSHIP:
1979–1981

| | *(Annual averages, U.S. $ million)* | | | | | |
	Bulk	drugs	Formulations		Total	
Companies:		%		%		%
Foreign-owned	71	(22)	568	(43)	639	(39)
Local private	163	(52)	669	(50)	832	(51)
Local state	82	(26)	87	(7)	169	(10)
Total	316	(100)	1324	(100)	1640	(100)

SOURCE: UNCTC 1983:88, 154.

this (again, not perfect) is profitability; in the mid-1970s, 30 foreign companies reported gross profits of 14.3 percent of sales, whereas a sample of 12 Indian companies reported gross profits about half that level (Stoker 1984:304). Finally, some companies are defined on these criteria as Indian, but a controlling-share interest (say 25 percent or more) is held by one foreign company. Others share in production arrangements with foreign companies: at least 26 Indian companies received foreign know-how between 1962 and 1972, for example, through technical collaboration agreements (ibid.: 341).

Overall, despite nearly thirty years of attempts by the Indian government to control the operations of foreign pharmaceuticals companies, they remain the most substantial element in the pharmaceuticals market. They set the framework for the industry in the period when they were far more influential still. As the UNCTC report puts it, "the product mix of both kinds of firms [local and foreign] tends not to reflect social priorities" (1983:89). Both kinds also have fought to protect the competitive advantages provided by brand names (ibid.:91); they spread product information to doctors by an active network of company representatives and by company advertising, rather than by a more "arms-length" method. All these are typical of pharmaceutical company organization in advanced capitalist countries and seem likely to outlast any future decline of direct influence of multinational corporations in India.

THE PATTERN OF DRUG PRODUCTION

Controlling the price of drugs has formed a growing part of government policies since 1962, but it is not easy to assess its success. Certainly, informed opinion before 1970 was that Indian drug prices were high but probably not as high as in some other parts of the world. In part, this resulted from the system of import licenses, which reduced the possibility of transfer pricing. Companies were forced to make at least a pretense of justifying the prices they paid for raw materials—with Hoffman-La Roche's ability to overcharge for Librium and Valium a notable exception (Stoker 1984:378–379). Insisting on production in India as far as possible, however, may have increased general price levels above those of the world market. The position is complicated by the very large number of formulations, often very similar and probably more expensive than if they were all sold by generic names.

The Hathi Commission claimed that prices had declined, relative to world levels and their previous Indian levels, after the introduction of the 1970 Drug-Price-Control Order (1975:174), and the industry says that prices have continued to fall since the strengthening of these controls in 1979 (Stoker 1984:372). Unfortunately, the only drug-prices index in India is probably a poor guide to general price levels, being constructed from common drugs that are out of patent protection. This shows very stable drug prices, well below the general price level, but it may be misleading. Indian drug prices are probably not notably high, and may well be relatively low, and this can be attributed to direct government policy, to the existence of an indigenous manufacturing capability in both the public and the private sector, and probably to the size of the Indian market which permits economies of scale and competition which are not always possible elsewhere.

The picture for the product mix of drugs is less satisfactory. The UNCTC argues that remedies for diseases that afflict the mass of the population are not produced in the same quantity or variety as those that suit the purchasing preferences of the relatively wealthy (1983:89): vitamin preparations, cough and cold preparations, tonics, and "health restorers" made up some 25 percent of all sales covered in one survey in 1978 (Stoker 1984:399). Furthermore, most of the "essential" drugs listed either by WHO or by Indian writers on the subject are produced in India, but production is well below both installed capacity and consumption (ibid.:404). In addition, because the drugs rules (introduced in 1945 on the basis of the 1940 Drugs Act) have not been enforced, many drugs remain on the market despite little evidence of their efficacy. Furthermore, the products of many small Indian producers are of dubious quality (UNCTC 1983:89). None of the legislation has made any comment about the efficacy of the drugs, only the methods by which they are produced, standards of hygiene, and so forth. In general, drug policy has had economic and political goals—the harboring of scarce foreign exchange, control over the prices that affect the middle-class market, and the nationalistic desire to foster local industries. Policy has been the concern of the ministry which has included chemicals, with the Ministries of Commerce, Finance, and Industry more closely involved than the Health Ministry. Drug policies have been relatively uninfluenced by health policy concerns (Stoker and Jeffery 1987).

In sum, drug production has hindered health-policy development by failing to provide basic, crucial drugs in large quantities and at low prices. This is due as much to the structure of the Indian market and the location of Indian purchasing power as to conscious decisions by individual companies or the industry as a whole. A glaring exception to this generalization is the behavior of some American companies when the public-sector companies were being established in 1956. Several American companies attempted to prevent the establishment of sizable companies to produce basic drugs outside their control. A more appropriate structure of production might have been developed if this had not occurred. However, the record of the Indian public sector is not good compared with the private sector. It may not have made much difference if governmental companies had started earlier or on a larger scale, since the dominant ethos of the industry would have remained the same.

THE IMPACT OF DRUG PRODUCERS ON HEALTH POLICY

Attempts by drug companies to affect health policy per se are not well documented. Evidence abounds of their attempts to influence the narrower sphere of drugs policy itself—to restrict government intervention, to limit the more radical proposals, with the most obvious examples being their opposition to controls on equity shares (and the extreme nationalization) during the 1970s (Stoker 1984:356–371). Despite the importance of government purchasing in total drug sales, most companies have worked on their market shares (through advertising and intensive marketing) rather than to increase the total market size by pressing for larger health budgets or a larger share of drug purchasing within them. Government drug budgets are totally inadequate to meet the demands of most patients, so companies may reckon that the best contribution to overall sales is by affecting the prescriptions written by government doctors and purchased by patients from commercial pharmacists. Alternatively, companies have focused on influencing the distribution of government drug purchases by bribing those who control the drug-purchase committees (Shepperdson 1986).

The major criticism of the operations of pharmaceutical companies in India is probably the least tangible: the creation of, or at least support for, a perspective on health policy in which technical interventions in the bodies of individuals (using drugs or surgery) are regarded as crucial contributions to the health of the nation. In looking after their own interests, they draw attention away from environmental, social, political, and economic contributions to improved health. In this way, they have probably helped Ayurvedic and Unani preparations acquire a similar meaning, helping to generate the growth of indigenous pharmaceutical companies along similar lines. Their liaison with doctors is close, but they also spread their products through networks of practitioners without formal qualifications in Western medicine, by competing to offer these people profitable opportunities. Some benefits have undoubtedly been produced by these means, but they may not have outweighed the costs.

Conclusion: The International Context

The Indian experience in health policy does not neatly fit the models derived from dependency analyses. Health-sector aid has been concentrated on primary care, particularly the prevention and control of diseases, medical migration has not constrained health policy-making, and local production of pharmaceuticals has permitted controls over the operations of multinational corporations so that excesses reported for other countries have been curbed. In less substantial ways, the international context has supported a view of health services that has limited their effectiveness by reinforcing the dominance of doctors, reinforcing the symbolic value of individual rather than environmental improvement, and by orienting medical education and provision to international standards rather than to Indian needs.

CHAPTER NINE

Medical and Paramedical Personnel

Over the past thirty-five years, India has seen a dramatic expansion in the number of medical and health-related personnel and in the variety of specialized positions they occupy. But some categories have grown faster than others, and a discussion of how this occurred must consider the government's ability to control whoever has been trained. Some categories cover health workers who have not been trained at all, or not before the late 1970s.

For some health workers a private as well as a public market exists; others are virtually dependent on public-sector employment. The categories are not clear-cut and unchanging, but doctors would fall into the first, and ANMs into the second. The government has responded largely to pressure from potential applicants for the first category, whereas for the second category, it has adjusted training to meet its own recruitment demands. Nonetheless, although the numbers of doctors trained has routinely exceeded the planned expansion, the numbers of paramedical personnel have grown much more quickly, though in a more discontinuous fashion.

Official plans assume that only trained personnel are of relevance and that those trained actually practice what they have been taught. But substantial numbers of people have acquired some form of training unofficially (e.g., as assistants to doctors or by correspondence course) or have received one form of training (e.g., as an army medical orderly or as a pharmacist) but practice in a different capacity (usually as an independent practitioner). There are no worthwhile estimates of the numbers involved here. The inclusion of the training of personnel outside the Western system introduces yet further complications. Training in indigenous medicine has been solely for the equivalent of doctors—there are now several degree and diploma courses for Ayurvedic and Unani practitioners—but not for supporting personnel. This reflects the absence of government demand for such workers. However, many of these graduates attended courses with substantial Western components, and even those from pure indigenous courses may actually use the Western pharmacopeia.

The major health-policy documents since 1947 have all stressed the need to expand the numbers of Western personnel rather than practitioners of the indigenous systems of medicine (including homoeopathy); and within the Western sector, to increase the numbers of auxiliary personnel more rapidly than doctors. No attempt has been made to define an overall desirable number of indigenous practitioners nor to set targets for achievement in individual plan periods, and the discussions of Western personnel make no reference to any form of integration with indigenous practitioners until the late 1970s. I shall therefore deal with the indigenous sector separately, and here focus on Western personnel.

The formal commitment to expanding the number of "nonmedical" health workers dates from the Bhore Committee, which called for four times as many doctors in 1971 as in 1941, but one hundred times as many nurses and health visitors, and twenty times as many midwives. (GOI[CPHB] 1948:102). The rationale was spelled out in the meeting of health ministers and secretaries in 1948. Paramedical workers can carry out a variety of tasks "under the direction and supervision of doctors," such as inoculations, antimalarial work, and sanitation; they are cheaper to train and employ and they are more suited to work in rural areas (ibid.). This emphasis was repeated in the Five-Year Plan documents. The First Plan specified nurses, midwives, and dais (traditional birth attendants) as categories of health workers that could be trained more rapidly in existing institutions (GOI 1951:203), while the Second Plan noted that "shortages in personnel other than doctors have been more marked and are likely to persist longer than in the case of doctors" (GOI 1956:538). Similar sentiments are expressed in the succeeding Plans.

The outcome was slightly different. To begin with, the problems of training more doctors have always been discussed first. This symbolic precedence is matched by a financial precedence: policymakers allocate much more money per head to the education of doctors in order to maintain standards (see further below), and therefore financial allocations favor medical colleges over paramedical training. The financial distribution is difficult to establish very precisely. The Planning Commission has usually included the two together (along with research), distinguishing the outlays under the two heads only in the Second, Fourth and Fifth Plans, and the Draft Plan for 1978–1983. In these Plans, medical education and research was allocated between four and seven times as much as paramedical training. Actual Plan expenditures are only available for the Fourth Plan, when an allocation imbalance of 6.5:1 in favor of the doctors (Rs. 853 million to Rs. 129 million) was translated into an expenditure imbalance of nearly 11:1—Rs. 790 million to Rs. 73 million (GOI 1969; GOI 1975:22). Non-Plan expenditures may reinforce this imbalance. Table 32 shows that in Orissa, for most of the 1970s, Plan expenditures on paramedical training exceeded those on medical education, but over 90 percent of non-Plan expenditures were for medical colleges.

While expenditure figures are probably fairly reliable, the data for physical targets and achievements, expressed as numbers in practice or in service and summarized in table 33, are much more uncertain. Considerable problems are involved in estimating total numbers of doctors, nurses, and others, in the workforce: I deal with some of them in more detail later in this chapter. But in addition, many of these targets appear to have been precisely met and, in some cases, planners have used "likely" or "estimated" figures for "achievements" when they had virtually no data to go on. Thus, as late as 1972, the Directorate of Manpower declared that "there are no stock estimates of health visitors worked out on a systematic basis" (p. 46). Other inconsistencies exist between the figures produced by different agencies, and the Planning Commission itself has provided contradictory figures for 1950 and 1955. Therefore, table 33 should be regarded as only a guide to rough magnitudes and proportions.

It is possible, through rather heroic assumptions, to summarize table 33 in terms of the proportions between different personnel as in table 34. What this suggests is that the balance of personnel around 1980 was probably far more "appropriate" (less heavily dependent on doctors) than it was around 1950.

In dealing with the evolution of proposals and patterns of health

TABLE 32

ANNUAL AVERAGE EXPENDITURES ON MEDICAL AND PARAMEDICAL
EDUCTION AND TRAINING, ORISSA: 1972–73 TO 1978–79

| Category | Rs. Millions | | | | |
	Non-Plan	State Plan	Central Plan	Total	(%age)
Undergraduate	10.8	1.1	—	11.9	(73)
Postgraduate	1.6	0.1	—	1.7	(10)
Paramedical	1.3	0.2	1.3	2.8	(17)
Total	13.7	1.3	1.3	16.3	(100)
(percentage)	(84)	(8)	(8)	(100)	

SOURCE: *Annual Administration Reports*, Orissa Department of Health and Family Welfare, Bhubaneswar.
NOTE: Medical figures exclude expenditures on Medical-college Hospitals. Paramedical figures include expenditures on Regional Family-Welfare Training Centers, which also train doctors.

personnel I shall reverse the normal order and deal first with community health workers, then with health assistants and paramedical workers (mainly male) under the heading of Health Auxiliaries, then with nurses of various categories, and finally with doctors, first allopathic and then indigenous.

Community Health Workers

As early as the National Planning and Bhore Committee reports, it had been argued that the existing categories of personnel might not suit the kinds of tasks that were regarded as the most essential, and that some new categories of health workers should be trained. Two kinds of proposals were made: for what we would now call community health workers and for a medical auxiliary category.

The NPC provided as good a description and justification of the potential and role of a community health worker as any to be found in the international policy documents of the 1970s. Because of the dearth of trained medical personnel, the health needs of India could "only be met by training specially a very large body of men

TABLE 33
Plan Targets and Achievements in Numbers of Health Personnel
(thousands)

	Base-Line 1951 Ach.	First Plan 1956 Ach.	Second Plan 1961 Tgt.	Second Plan 1961 Ach.	Third Plan 1966 Tgt.	Third Plan 1966 Ach.	Annual Plan 1969 Ach.	Fourth Plan 1974 Tgt.	Fourth Plan 1974 Ach.	Fifth Plan 1979 Tgt.	Fifth Plan 1979 Ach.
Doctors	56	65	77	70	81	86	102	138	138	176	178
Nurses	17	19	24	27	45	45	61	88	88	123	113
ANMs	—	—	—	3	4	22	34	54	54	n.a.	58
LHVs	0.5	1	3	2	4	4	4	7	n.a.	n.a.	8
Nurse-dais	—	6	41	12	40	25	(no further figures)				
SIs	—	4	7	6	19	18	20	32	33	n.a.	
Pharmacists	—	4	n.a.	42	48	48	51	66	66	n.a.	

SOURCES: Columns 2, 4, 5—GOI 1961:653; column 3: GOI 1956:61, 538; columns 6, 9, 10—GOI 1975:23, except for column 6 for LHVs, which is from GOI 1964, and for ANMs, midwives, and nurse-dais, which come from GOI (CCH) 1973:24; column 8—GOI, 1969:291, except for midwives, which comes from *Directorate of Manpower* 1972; column 11—*World Health Statistics Annual* 1983.

NOTES: In each case these are figures for those estimated to be in practice or in service in the country. In some plan periods, no physical targets seem to have been set for some categories.

KEY: ANM = Auxiliary Nurse-Midwife, now Health Worker (female).
     LHV = Lady Health Visitor, now Health Assistant (female).
     SI = Sanitary Inspector, including Health Assistants (male).

TABLE 34

PROPORTIONS OF MEDICAL AND PARAMEDICAL PERSONNEL

	1950	1960	1970	1980
Doctors	100	100	100	100
Nurses	25	39	60	60
Auxiliary Nurse-Midwives	—	4	35	—
Sanitary Inspectors	6	9	20	—
Multipurpose personnel (male and female)	not applicable			100

SOURCE: table 33.
NOTE: For more detail on multipurpose personnel, see further below in the section on health auxiliaries. This total includes male and female health assistants and health workers.

[sic] to perform some of the simpler tasks,'' and "thus the corner-stone of the scheme we recommend is a Health Worker." (NPC 1946: 43) The health worker was to be an intelligent young man or woman selected from the village itself, sent for nine months training in community and personal hygiene, first aid, common ailments, and simple remedies and then returned to his or her village to "spread the gospel" (ibid.: 44).

> The health worker will be one of the villagers themselves, only somewhat better trained than themselves. He will not appear to the villagers as a strange imposition of a strange system, but their kith and kin who desires to help them.

The proposal involved retraining after five years, with the prospect that in twenty years some of these workers would be of degree standard.

There were several problems with this proposal: no thought was given to the problem of finding trainers; selecting candidates in villages divided along caste, gender, class, and religious lines; of supervising his or her activities; and finding suitably educated women who met the age requirements and could attend a long training course away from their homes or marital villages. Further, the financial implications of the proposal were enormous, involving more than double the current total levels of health expenditure just to pay the salaries of health workers.

The main reason no attempt was made to implement the proposal was the perspective used later in the more official and "authoritative" Bhore report, which focused on top-down planning based on health centers staffed by doctors and ancillary staff. In addition, the issue of rural medical relief was sidetracked away from the idea of a new category of worker at the village level. Several states were running schemes to encourage doctors to settle in rural areas, using subsidies for the establishment of dispensaries, and offering honoraria. There were also arguments about whether to continue the training of licentiate doctors on the grounds that they were more willing to settle in rural areas, though there was no evidence for this. Supporters of indigenous systems of medicine also argued their case in part on the same lines. The concept of the health worker also fell because it was argued that villagers should not be offered an inferior standard of care from that of towndwellers, and that medical standards in India should be modeled on those of Britain and America (GOI[CCH] 1951:item #4).

For whatever reason, no new proposals for village-level health workers were made before the early 1970s. International thinking on development in general was then critical of the previous belief that the benefits of economic growth would trickle down to the poor. Increasing evidence suggested that the efforts of the preceding twenty years still left most villagers with little access to state medical services; it was argued that one reason for this was the slavish adherence to models derived from the colonial period and based on structures copied from the West. In this period the Chinese use of "barefoot doctors" after 1966 received a great deal of positive comment and analysis. The critique of the "professional" model of health services found a crusading voice in Ivan Illich, who counted in his circle of supporters several well-placed Indians, particularly V. Ramalingaswami, the director of the All-India Institute of Medical Sciences (AIIMS) and J. P. Naik, the member-secretary of the Indian Council for Social Science Research (ICSSR).

The critics could also point to the evidence from some of the voluntary-sector health projects in India, described in more detail in chapter 11. A common feature of these projects is the use of auxiliary personnel. In Narangwal, in Punjab, most of the experimental programs were run with auxiliary nurse-midwives and lady health visitors or their equivalents as the lowest levels of auxiliary personnel, recruiting village women only for child care (crèches). At the other extreme is Jamkhed, in Maharashtra, whose village health workers have usually been illiterate, middle-aged women. Hardiman (1984:132) points out that this was not part of the original planning for Jamkhed. The project founders had intended to use ANMs until they discovered problems in recruiting and placing such women in the project villages. Pyle (1979:20–21) reports that several of the Maharashtrian projects discovered that village workers with less education were performing better than those who were educated, and almost all report better experiences with women than with men. This is partly because the focus of many of these projects has been on maternal and child health.

These projects were very influential in reasserting the idea that community health workers were not only good in principle, but that they could be trained successfully and used under Indian conditions. Jamkhed was widely publicized by WHO and UNICEF, and its example was behind some of the proposals of the 1975 report of the committee chaired by J. B. Srivastava (GOI 1975a) on the future of medical education. This committee was originally established by Health Minister Dr. Karan Singh as a result of a bruising strike of Delhi junior hospital doctors in 1974. The report came at a very inauspicious time—the emergency had just been declared and grassroots political initiatives in general were unwelcome. Furthermore, within a year the whole of the health sector was to be dominated by an attempt to make a dramatic breakthrough in the sterilization program. While the report was accepted, no moves were made to implement it until the Janata government was elected in 1977. The Janata Manifesto mentioned community health workers and the new health minister, Raj Narain, adopted the proposal as a personal commitment (Leslie 1981; Jobert 1985). Unlike the 1938 National Planning Committee proposals, the community health worker (CHW) was to be offered training in the indigenous systems of medicine as well as Western medicine; and for training purposes an additional doctor was to be appointed at each Primary Health Center. The course was reduced in length to three months, and the stipend offered was based on the assumption that the health worker would only work part-time.

Much to the surprise of many commentators, the community Health-worker scheme was indeed implemented, beginning in late 1977. Progress was slower than planned and was delayed further when Mrs. Gandhi was reelected in 1980. It took several months before the Congress government was prepared to continue a scheme that was so clearly identified with the opposition, particularly with Raj Narain. Eventually just a change in title, from worker to volunteer, or village health guide, a new emphasis on appointing women where possible, and a few other small changes were sufficient to permit the scheme to continue; efforts were made to complete the training of community health volunteers for all villages by the end of March 1984.

The chequered history of the community health worker has posed some problems for orthodox Marxist interpretations of health policy in India. It is relatively easy to explain the failure to use this means of providing health care prior to 1977: it fits a model of health-service provision that is dominated by the interests of urban, propertied classes allied to the medical profession's desire for dominance over the medical division of labor and protection from competition. How, then, can we explain the change in policy? It certainly does not fit easily into a "labor's demands/capital's needs" view of reform. It is not clear that "improving villagers' health" would safeguard capitalism, and villagers themselves have never articulated a demand for this kind of service. Attempts to dismiss the significance of the scheme as merely a smokescreen, or designed to buy off demands for a doctor in every village, seem equally unacceptable (though a realistic assessment of the outcomes, if not the intentions, of the change). Jobert (1985) argues that this policy is populism par excellence, and it seems that a confluence of forces support the move, of which the emerging "agrarian populism" and clientelism of the Indian state, the potential for using these workers for population control, and a changing international climate are the most important. I will return to these points at the end of this chapter.

Health Auxiliaries

Proposals for auxiliaries emerged in the 1950s and 1960s. The first meeting of the Central Council of Health, in January 1953, considered whether to reintroduce licentiate training as a way of solving the shortage of medical personnel in rural areas. The meeting resolved against licentiates but in favor of medical auxiliaries, and the central government proposed a scheme in 1954 to produce a cadre similar to the Russian feldshers, living "in the midst of the villagers," trained in environmental sanitation, and also able to attend to minor ailments (GOI[CCH] 1954). The discussion was heated, with the major objection being that these people would set themselves up as doctors if they had any curative training. While under the proposal, it was insisted, medical auxiliaries would be under the supervision of a doctor, it was argued that in practice this was highly unlikely: the auxiliary would thus become a quack. Nonetheless, there was majority support, and the Planning Commission promised money. But the following year a revised scheme was announced, apparently as a result of pressure applied through the Planning Commission, to reduce the curative training to the level of first aid only. At this point, the representatives of several states reiterated their belief that the new category would overlap with the sanitary inspectors (GOI[CCH] 1955).

Although the scheme did appear in the Second Plan, very few states seem to have followed up the proposal. Health assistants were apparently trained in Nagpur, and in Andhra Pradesh, Bihar, and Rajasthan (GOI[CCH] 1963:191) and possibly in Uttar Pradesh (GOI[CCH] 1964:286), and some of them were given jobs as medical officers in Primary Health Centers. The idea was reintroduced in the ninth meeting of the Central Council of Health, in 1961, as a three-year course. Once again, reference was made to experience in Russia and other countries and again it was suggested that the new health assistants should work under the supervision of doctors and should not be able to set themselves up as independent practitioners—and the same criticisms were made as before. A subcommittee reported favorably on the proposal the following year and the matter was discussed again in 1963, when some opposition was reported from the international agencies which were then more in favor of sanitary inspectors (GOI[CCH] 1964:284–318). By 1965, WHO and UNICEF were in favor of the scheme for training health assistants (GOI[CCH] 1966a:70–72), but by 1967 a new version of the scheme was being mooted—for B.Sc. courses in public health and in maternal and child health. Finally, in the early 1970s, the attempts to integrate the different specialist cadres—sanitary inspectors, family planning, malaria and smallpox workers—began to bear fruit with new proposals that called for multipurpose health workers (MPHWs) (GOI[CCHC] 1973:368–369). Only after 1975, when the multipurpose-health-worker schemes were joined by the resurrected community health worker and backed by international agencies, was there finally a completely new look to health personnel training in India.

The exact course of these fluctuating proposals and the reasons for their almost total nonimplementation prior to 1975, are not clear. However, what seems to have happened is that the problem of rural medical relief was seen as the absence of doctors. Discussion and effort thus went into schemes to persuade graduate doctors to work in rural areas. Proposals to use different personnel never received the same support—no existing cadre's training could be expanded. No political benefit was to be gained by promising villages an unknown, incomprehensible, health assistant, but if a doctor could be offered, a strong response could be evoked. The final proposals evolved through two routes, both of which addressed themselves to existing groups of health personnel—indigenous practitioners and existing cadres of "unipurpose" health workers (for smallpox, tuberculosis, family planning, etc.).

The most notable attempt to involve indigenous healers as health auxiliaries was made in 1972, during the first flush of the Congress government's election in 1971 on the "abolish poverty" slogan. The 1972 proposals emerged and disappeared very rapidly. As late as the 1971 meeting of the Central Council of Health the master plan to provide health services to rural areas followed previous patterns in being based on improving facilities and incentives to encourage staff to serve in rural areas (GOI[CCH] 1972:41–71). After the 1971 elections a completely new set of proposals was introduced, to give substance to Mrs. Gandhi's election promises. In 1972 the new minister of state for health, D. P. Chattopadhyaya, proposed a "national health scheme for rural areas," first announced in the Lok Sabha in May and passed at a conference (not a full meeting) of the Central Council of Health in July. The government apparently gave this scheme a very high priority, considering the rapidity with which further meetings were held: in July the Planning Commission approved pilot projects, and the subcommittee set up in July reported in time for modifications to be made in November and a public discussion in December.

Pilot projects were to start in 1972–1973 and the scheme itself in 1973–1974. Press comment suggested that the prime minister had put her own weight behind this scheme as "an earnest of [the central government's] desire for social services to reach to the rural communities" (*Statesman* 27 July 1972). The scheme envisaged using the estimated 300,000 registered medical practitioners from indigenous systems of medicine, training them for four months in simple treatments from "Ayurveda/Unani, Homoeopathy, and Allopathy including first aid" (*Journal of the Indian Medical Association* 1973, 2:77) and then employing them at Rs. 150/- per month, providing them with a medical kit with simple Western, homoeopathic, and Indian medicines. In this way, it was argued, medical relief and care could be provided to rural areas rather in the way Russia and China had solved similar problems (ibid.:76).

But it soon became clear that powerful forces were ranged against the proposals. The Indian Medical Association predictably called it a "cocktail" of systems that would legitimize quackery and discriminate against doctors at a time when increasing numbers were unemployed. The president of the IMA used his position on Planning Commission subcommittees to argue for amendments to the proposal (IMA [Annual Report], 1971–1972). The Planning Commission itself began to suggest problems, such as the difficulty of integrating different medical systems after a short course of training when there were no trainers who understood all three; and once again it was argued that it would be politically unacceptable to offer the rural population a level of practitioner below that to be found in urban areas (*Hindustan Times* October 1972). In addition, some states opposed the scheme: Punjab, for example, argued that it had enough Western doctors, and Rajasthan sponsored a discussion of its "problem of increasing numbers of unemployed doctors."

This coalition was sufficient to prevent the scheme from being implemented, even as a pilot, although Mrs. Gandhi addressed gatherings of vaids and hakims in 1973 and talked of the need to use all available medical resources (JIMA 1973, 6:211). But Chattopadhyaya left the ministry, and without his personal support the proposal died. The IMA was able to call off its proposed Black Day of action, April 16, 1973. But this was not the last attempt to introduce auxiliaries, for an alternative approach was introduced at about the same time.

This alternative route was through the retraining of the existing paramedical staff. The previous twenty years had seen the expansion of paramedical categories linked to the so-called vertical campaigns against specific diseases or for family planning. In the mid-1960s hopes were high that malaria would soon be conquered;

this gave rise to some discussion about what to do with the malaria workers. The "problem" disappeared with the resurgence of malaria, but the approaching elimination of smallpox reintroduced the issue in the early 1970s. In addition, some argued that the separate campaigns were hindered by their isolation from one another. They were unable to call upon workers from other campaigns at moments of urgency—in epidemics, or at seasonal peaks of activity such as spraying against mosquitoes. In addition, there was—if work schedules were conscientiously followed—a great duplication of visiting, and time spent in travel was a major source of unproductive time. Thus, it was argued, the full potential of the existing staff was not being realized. The proposed solution was to integrate the different cadres to provide the full range of preventive and public health services, and, after 1977, to include basic curative training as well.

Finally, two research projects were used to provide evidence in favor of health auxiliaries. The Narangwal project was designed to test the benefits of different combinations of services—nutrition, family planning, maternal health, and general women's programs. Its conclusions were weakened by its unplanned ending before the research design was complete. The Narangwal team was led by a group from Johns Hopkins University, and its members became personae non grata in the wake of President Nixon's tilt toward Pakistan during the Bangladesh war of 1971. Nonetheless, the team made strenuous efforts to ensure that the Narangwal results were passed on to Indian decision makers, through special conferences. However, for political reasons, the Narangwal experiment is never referred to as a pilot for the new health auxiliaries; credit is given instead to some research carried out by the Ministry of Health's own project in Haryana, managed by a group from the National Institute of Health Administration and Education (NIHAE).

The institute's action research in 1971–1972 was a more direct guide for government to follow, since it employed government personnel in approximately the same numbers as were available in the rest of the country. It apparently showed the benefits of the integration of single-purpose workers into multipurpose ones, and the implementation of the revised system, though the results came from only a short experiment in a relatively well-run state. Nonetheless, the government responded enthusiastically and initiated training programs, though it took some time before these were properly established (Jeffery 1976b). The proposal was part of the Fifth Plan, but that Plan was set back by the inflation of 1973–1974, when the social services sectors were cut back to allow core sectors, such as heavy industry, to go ahead. In addition, within health, the malaria control program ate up more than its budgeted share of funds.

By the time retraining was under way, more problems surfaced. First, the family-planning drive of the emergency took precedence. Then there were difficulties in resolving differences in pay scales: the workers involved were not educated to the same levels, and the state governments were not prepared to bring all workers onto the highest pay scales. It is not surprising that this generated conflicts that took ten or more years to resolve in some states.

Further problems arose because of the different numbers of the different categories. Thus, the Plan calls for one male supervisor for every four male workers, but in Orissa, if sanitary inspectors were included there would be one supervisor for every two workers (Indian Institute of Management 1980:39). Finally, not all workers were involved in multipurpose work; the national campaigns against leprosy, filaria, and tuberculosis retained an independent organization in some states. Some levels of the administration re- mained unintegrated: District-level medical officers in Orissa are still organized according to specific diseases, and report to state and central disease-specific officers (David and Narayana 1983). As a result they place divergent pressures on their subordinates. In- tegration within the health sector has thus only been halfhearted; wider integration, with the work of nonhealth staff, has yet to be seriously considered.

The Supply of Nurses

A detailed consideration of the expansion of nursing education complements the preceding section in part, since the junior nursing cadres—lady health visitors and auxiliary nurse- midwives—provided the female multipurpose workers. Compared to doctors, nurses have been systematically relegated to a minor po- sition in the organization and funding not only of training but also of employment. This is, of course, common to many countries, but the problem is probably more extreme in India. Nurses have a low status in the community. They are mostly women. They are drawn either from marginal or disadvantaged social classes, because of the "polluting" connotations of their work, or from the one group that clearly rejects this conception of nursing activities—Christians, mostly from Kerala. They have failed to exert forceful pressure to raise their standing. As a result, key aspects of national health policies (in particular, for maternal and child health) have remained understaffed and inadequate, despite frequent formal commitments to increase the number of nurses and improve their education and employment conditions.

Nurse training was not well developed under the British. Most nursing for the armed forces was done by male dressers, with the first nursing sisters arriving in Bombay only in 1888. In 1914 female nurses were recruited in India for the first time for military purposes and were formed into an Indian Military Nursing Service in 1927 (Wilkinson 1958:11). Nursing schools in government civil hospitals were established in the 1870s (in Madras) and the 1880s (in Bombay and Calcutta). In Bombay, Poona, and Calcutta early nurse training was done by Anglican sisters, and mission hospitals trained more nurses than government hospitals did, using European or American nurses as trainers.

Nursing students in government and mission hospitals were originally Anglo-Indian and, later, mostly Indian Christian. Nursing education was increasingly standardized after 1909, when mission hospitals in north India established a common examining board (ibid.:32). In the 1920s the first steps were taken to establish a category of Lady Health Visitors, whose focus was to be in public-health work (Seal 1975:433). A Trained Nurses Association of India was established in 1922, bringing together two regional associations, and acts to register qualified nurses were passed, first in Madras in 1926 and by 1939, such acts had been passed in most provinces (ibid.; Nandi 1981:158).

At independence, the two categories of registered nursing personnel included about 15,000 general nurses who might also have midwifery qualifications, and 500 Lady Health Visitors. In addition, some traditional birth attendants—dais—had received training and might be employed as subordinate nursing staff and an unknown number of others carried out duties that could be defined as nursing.

The Bhore Committee recognized that the nursing situation in India was totally unsatisfactory. It pointed out that conditions for nurses were "deplorable" (GOI 1946, II:386) and went on to list the main problems: no professional status (by which it meant no gazetted rank [official standing] in government service); low pay for senior nurses; understaffed hospitals leading to overworked nurses; deplorable living conditions, diet, and leisure facilities; and no pension rights. The Bhore report argued that all these were within the power of government to remedy, but it did not believe, in any case, that enough women would come forward for training to meet its long-term goal of one nurse for every 500 in the population. In marked contrast to its view on doctors, the committee proposed two grades of nurse—junior and senior—with the addition of nursing degrees as soon as possible. The report specified the proposed curriculum, standards of training centers, and so on. Almost as an afterthought, the committee referred to male nurses, noted their role, and the difficulty of recruiting men to nursing while pay rates were so low, and suggested that an expansion of the number of male nurses for male wards would release female nurses for other work—presumably with women and children.

One indicator of the low priority given to nursing is the very poor quality of information about how many nurses there were and what kind of work they were doing. This makes it very difficult to assess the significance of the changes since 1947. The study carried out by the major organization of voluntary hospitals in India, the Coordinating Agency for Health Planning (CAHP), notes that the Indian Nursing Council registered only 87 percent of the general nurses trained between 1951 and 1971, 69 percent of LHVs, and 62 percent of ANMs but the census errs in the other direction by including "untrained and unqualified self-styled nurses" (CAHP 1975:9). In addition, double counting is a serious possibility, since recruitment to higher grades has often been from lower ranks. Using the results of a 2 percent sample of registered nurses, figures for graduation from nurse-training institutions and estimates of mortality, migration, and "preretirement resignations" the study estimated a nurse population in 1971 as shown in Table 35.

The Coordinating Agency study also provides an estimate of how marriage interrupts nurses' work careers. Based on an admittedly small sample, it suggests that about 11 percent of all nursing personnel were not currently working for "temporary" reasons, while another 2.5 percent regarded themselves as "permanently" out of the nursing work force (ibid.:12–13). Medical administrators resist the appointment of married nurses jointly with their husbands when both are employed by the health department, because administrators like to use job transfers as the principal means of disciplining staff. It is also not clear how many nurses might return to government employment if service rules were amended to make their jobs more compatible with their domestic obligations. In general, little reliable information exists about the numbers of trained nurses of different grades who are in employment or who might be available for employment. The survey found most of its employed LHV and ANM respondents working for the government (97 percent and 85 percent respectively), but far more general nurses working in church-related (31 percent) or private (13 percent) employment. The report also suggested that estimates of unemployed nurses, provided by the Ministry of Labor, were probably highly unreliable. These estimates included large numbers of male ANMs and LHVs (!), and many employed staff members who nonetheless register as unemployed in the hope of bettering their positions (CAHP 1975:19–21).

The basic level of nursing worker has remained the dai, the nursing orderly, and the ayah. Virtually nothing is known about who they are, how many there are, what tasks they carry out, what education they have, and so on. As we shall see, there are relatively few trained nurses for hospital and health-center work, so much of it is carried out by these untrained personnel. Only in the case of the dai has there been any attempt to provide training. The Bhore Committee accepted that this category, however undesirable, would inevitably remain necessary for a period and described a successful training scheme from the North-West Frontier as a model (II:398–402). It did not propose replacing indigenous midwives by trained birth attendants from outside. Instead, it suggested improving the methods used by dais by offering help and advice, particularly to the "younger women of the dai community (ibid:402)." Such women were indeed employed in primary health centers as "trained dais" during the 1950s, and many are still at their posts today—though once again no national estimates exist. Trained dais' courses were stopped when ANM training was introduced in the 1960s, but more dais have been brought into government service since 1977 as assistants to nurse-midwives working in subcenters.

This recent move is part of the shift in the orientation of health

TABLE 35
STOCK OF NURSES AT THE END OF 1971

Category	After estimating loss from mortality	After estimating loss from mortality, migration retirement, and resignation
General nurses		
male	4,231	3,977
female	68,377	64,275
ANMs	44,172	41,522
LHVs	6,414	5,914

SOURCE: CAHP 1975:10, 14.

services described above. In the case of the dais, the shift has involved attempts to train at least one dai from each village for each 500 villagers over a three-week training course held at a local subcenter. This target has been achieved, though the longer-term goals of maintaining contacts and supervision are less likely to be reached. The dais are not employed after training (except for perhaps one to help the nurse-midwife), but they are offered a small inducement to report pregnant women to the auxiliary nurse-midwife to allow for prenatal visits. Assessments of the dai training program have been published for some states. The program for Uttar Pradesh suggests that very few dais there, trained or untrained, have any regular contact with any health personnel (NIHAE 1980; Jeffery, Jeffery and Lyon 1985), probably because the dais fear that they will become involved in family-planning activities. Furthermore, they rarely receive the payments due them for reporting pregnant women.

Two main changes since independence affected the more established grades of nurses. One substantial new category was introduced—the auxiliary nurse-midwife—and nursing colleges have trained staff for a number of positions, such as nurse-tutors and public-health nurse. Table 36 summarizes the available data on the numbers in each of the larger categories.

Auxiliary nurse-midwives' training was introduced in 1952 as a way of expanding the number of junior nurses, mainly for public-health work. The two-year course accepted women with eight years of schooling. In contrast, the general nursing course takes three

TABLE 36
STOCK AND SUPPLY OF NURSING PERSONNEL

	1951	1961	1971	1981
Graduates	100	385	1,100	
(annual outturn)	(21)	(43)	(108)	
General nurses	17,000	35,000	72,600	115,000
(annual outturn)	(1,105)	(2,663)	(5,778)	(5,000)
Health visitors (LHV)	500	2,475	6,400	
(annual outturn)	(55)	(369)	(377)	
Nurse-midwives (ANMs)	—	6,550	44,000	
(annual outturn)	—	(2,085)	(5,036)	

SOURCE: For 1951, 1961, and 1971 figures, CAHP 1975:10–16. For 1951 and 1961
I have taken the outturn figures quoted there, added to the estimates of stock in 1950,
and adjusted downward by 2.5 percent to allow for mortality (probably an overes-
timate, especially for ANMs, a young group especially in the early years), and
rounded. GOI 1972 estimated the stock of general nurses in 1971 at about 70,000,
of lady health visitors at 6,000, and ANMs at about 45,500.
NOTE: Stock here refers to outturn figures adjusted only for estimated mortality.

years, with a minimum entry requirement of ten years of schooling. ANMs are also not as well trained as the Bhore-proposed junior
certificate nurses would have been. The numbers of ANMs that
qualified rose steadily until 1970, but since then they have varied
from year to year, according to estimates by state governments of
the number of new recruits they want. Thus, in 1968 there were
about 10,000 admissions, but in 1970 this figure dropped to about
7,750 because some states closed down training institutions believing they had a surplus, and only about 500 new posts were filled
in the two years from 1969 to 1971 (GOI 1972:49–52). The original
target, to provide one ANM for every 10,000 people, was achieved
in most states by the mid-1970s. Since 1977, with the move toward
multipurpose health workers, the ANM has provided the bulk of
the new category health worker (female). Current attempts to meet
targets of 1:5,000 population (with 1:8,000 as an interim measure)
have led to a reopening of training schools.

Matters have been complicated still further by the role of the central government through the family-planning program. The ANM
has family planning as well as health responsibilities, and therefore some of the training schools were established and funded by
the central government, and some by state governments. Some

nurse-midwives (not necessarily those trained in central-government institutions) were then employed under the family-planning program, with funds from the central government, on slightly better terms than those in the maternal and child-health program on state government funds. Under the multipurpose scheme, terms and conditions should have been equalized; even though the variation in background and training of the ANMs is small, this equalization process has been slow.

Public-health nurses are organized in two cadres: the first, established in the early 1920s in Delhi on the model of health visiting in the United Kingdom, is the Lady Health Visitor (LHV). The second is the Public Health Nurse (PHN), an additional one-year qualification available to nurses or to LHVs, introduced in the 1950s. The Bhore Committee report was scathing about LHVs, claiming that none of them was ''rendering that type of service to the individual, family, and community which is considered necessary in health programs today'' (GOI 1946, II:394). It called for the establishment of PHN training, but the category has not been popular. PHN posts were scarce until the late 1970s and a staff nurse had little incentive to take the training. For example, before 1975 there were only two sanctioned posts for PHNs in the Orissa government service, though nearly 50 qualified women were available (IIM 1980:34). The main category of public-health nurses has thus been the LHV, now retitled Health Assistant (female) under the multipurpose scheme. Their position has been very unclear, with two states' nursing councils (in Madras and Kerala) apparently having no such category. The Planning Commission has argued that the estimates of ''stock'' are so unreliable that it has not given any (GOI 1972:46–47).

The first courses for senior nurses, and for degrees in nursing, began in the 1940s. A nursing college was formally established in Delhi in 1946, the inheritor of intensive training programs created during World War II to meet the demand for administrative nursing staff in military hospitals. Courses for nurse-tutors and nursing administrators were also held in Madras and Vellore before independence, and after 1947 such courses have been expanded. Graduates have gone on to take up most of the senior nursing positions, with holders of degrees most likely to progress within the administrative hierarchy. However, their chances of wielding any significant power are strictly limited. Very few high positions are open to nurses and in all cases they remain subordinate to doctors.

Policy toward the nursing categories has thus been contradictory. On the one hand, with support from Western and international agencies, attempts have been made to professionalize nursing by lengthening training courses, establishing nursing colleges, and providing new posts for career nurses. On the other hand, nurses have remained divided into separate cadres (unlike doctors) and have failed to gain any substantial support in their everyday attempts to raise their position and to overcome the "polluting" legacy attached to their work. As women, most nurses remain very vulnerable to sexual harassment if they are unmarried or separated from their husbands. Nursing education has remained unequal to the task of providing women with the self-confidence that marks women doctors, probably because recruits have not come from high enough social backgrounds. Elite women have not adopted nursing. Some changes have followed the improvement of female education and changes in the evaluation of female employment. This is, perhaps, the feature which most sharply distinguishes nursing from medicine: nurses are predominantly in employment, whereas doctors can earn a living in their own clinics as well as in government or private employment. I will now consider the difference this has made to policies on medical education.

The Training of Doctors

Medical education has been affected by three kinds of pressures. To begin with, the Indian elite has attempted to ensure that its doctors would be the equal of those elsewhere in the world, and able to supply them with medical services similar to those available to the elites of other countries. Second, the elite has demanded access to medical colleges for its sons and daughters, and has therefore pressed for a steady expansion in the numbers of colleges and their intakes. Third, the medical establishment has attempted to relate the numbers and kinds of doctors being produced to its perception of India's needs. Pressure to expand numbers obviously generates conflicts with pressure to maintain standards, and their resolution underlies the patterns that have emerged.

The insistence on keeping up standards was carried over from colonial-policy proposals before World War II. The major medical-political issue of the interwar period was precisely concerned with ensuring that the General Medical Council in London would continue to recognize Indian medical degrees. In order to achieve this, the government of India established a Medical Council of India in 1933 which excluded from its registers the holders of "inferior" qualifications (i.e., those not recognized in London as adequate for British registration). In this way, the all-India council differed from its provincial counterparts, which registered all those with Western medical qualifications. Even the political doctors of the Indian Medical Association who opposed the founding of the Medical Council (MCI) were prepared to work within it and to follow policies designed to maintain international recognition. This had two consequences: accepting the long-term desirability of raising the standards of licentiate qualifications to degree standard and opposing any involvement of indigenous practitioners in Indian medical colleges.

The government of India's leading medical advisers—British and Indian—won general acceptance of the phasing out of the medical schools in 1938. Medical administrators used the existence of large-scale medical underemployment to counter the arguments of those who opposed reducing the numbers of doctors trained every year. Over the following eight years several medical schools were closed or upgraded to medical colleges, but the process was not complete when the Bhore committee submitted its report.

The Bhore Report endorsed this policy, though not without some dispute among its members. The report argued that the country should focus its limited resources on the training of only one kind of doctor "the highly trained type of physician whom we have termed the 'basic doctor' " (GOI 1946, IV:60). However, a minority of six members of the committee argued that, because of "the overall shortage of doctors" this policy should not be implemented immediately, but that the training of all types of medical personnel should be expanded as fast as possible (ibid.). The majority view won the day and the policy of unifying medical education was implemented during the first ten years after independence. Nonetheless, prominent nonmedical policymakers have continued to argue for a lower level of medical personnel to meet rural needs—and in the early 1980s the West Bengal government introduced three-year medical education for this reason.

Pressures for raising standards were not lessened by the abolition of licentiate training but were then channeled into attempts to ensure the second basis of international recognition—freedom for Indian medical colleges from any taint of Ayurveda. The 1948 meeting of the Central Provincial Health Board had a note from the government of India to the effect that they should consider whether "the establishment of higher and more desirable standards in existing colleges" was not more urgent than expanding the output of doctors (GOI[CPHB] 1948:98). This was part of the response to the Chopra committee report, which was submitted in 1948 and had proposed that all students of medicine should be taught both Western and Indian systems. However, the "modernizers" in government—including Prime Minister Nehru and Health Minister Rajkumari Amrit Kaur—followed the advice of Western doctors in the ministry, especially K.C.K.E. Raja and A. L. Mudaliar (GOI[THMC] 1950:31–33).

Raja, then director-general of Health Services, reported to the Third Health Ministers' Conference in 1950 that there was a real danger of confusion, since the various systems were not reconcilable. He brought in the country's obligations to WHO to support his argument that all medical practitioners should have Western medical degrees first, and should then be free to specialize or practice in an Indian system if they wished (ibid.:15–30). This was a line also promoted by Nehru in his speech to the conference, pointing to the British system as a model (ibid.:6–7).

A. L. Mudaliar, later to chair the major review of the development of medical services in India in 1959, was prominent in his support of the abolition of licentiate training before the war. As a member of the Bhore committee, and chair of its Professional Education Advisory Committee, he embodied a major link between medical policymaking before and after independence. He was appointed chair of two committees in 1948, one to draw up plans for an All-India Medical Institute (eventually the All-India Institute of Medical Sciences, or AIIMS) and the other, to strengthen existing teaching departments. He argued at the first meeting of the Central Council of Health in 1953 that undergraduate education at AIIMS should be "along the most modern lines that are accepted in international circles"; and that

It is very important for us to realise that we must look to international standards. . . . When it comes to a question of helping in the cure of the sick and the general welfare of the community you cannot afford to forget international standards or lower your standards below the international level. If you do that, you will be the worse for it. (GOI[CCH], 1954)

The major issue that dominated policy in the 1950s was how to produce more doctors without compromising on this minimum level defined as basic by the Bhore committee—that is, an internationally acceptable MB, BS degree.

The Bhore committee also established a tradition of defining medical need by a doctor-population ratio. This procedure has a number of well-recognized weaknesses, which do not apply just in India. It neglects the uneven distribution of doctors; the national average may be reached, yet many areas may have very few doctors while others may have surplus. It ignores differences among doctors, for example by specialization, and language, so that shortages or surpluses become hidden. It also ignores the role of other medical personnel. In this way it draws attention away from alternative providers of care and from nurses, pharmacists, and so on, who are needed by doctors to enhance their productivity. Finally, reliance on doctor to population ratios ignores issues of the employability of the doctors who have been produced. All these problems have characterized the history of policy with respect to medical training in India since 1947.

Table 37 summarizes the available data on the numbers of doctors trained and the expansion of medical colleges. The sources for these data are fairly straightforward. The main problems are posed

TABLE 37
SUPPLY OF DOCTORS

	1947	1951	1961	1971	1981
Medical colleges	22	30	57	95	106
Annual admissions	1,983	2,489	6,446	12,500	12,500
Annual outturn	959	1,696	3,900	10,449	11,500
(% female)			(22)	(24)	

SOURCE: Row 1—Institute of Applied Manpower Research 1967; rows 2 and 3—from *Technical Manpower* XVI:9–10, 1974 with 1981 figures from *World Health Statistics Annual 1983*; row 4 from IAMR 1967, using 1965 intake figures to estimate female outturn percentage in 1971.

by the establishment of medical colleges by private associations in the 1960s and 1970s, which gave rise to disputes about their standards and thus conflicts over whether they "really" existed. The further complication posed by the existence of medical colleges offering integrated degrees—in Ayurvedic or Unani medicine but with substantial components of Western medicine—is sidestepped; these colleges and their graduates are always excluded from the calculations.

The expansion of medical education took place in two main phases. Once the initial confusion of partition had been overcome, a dozen new medical colleges were established by upgrading medical schools, the last being those in Madhya Pradesh in 1955. New medical colleges were also opened in a steady trickle of three or four a year up to 1962. Then, during the war with China, the armed forces found great difficulty in recruiting doctors on short-term contracts to supplement their own medical services. They called for a dramatic expansion in the number of medical students, and forty-six medical colleges received Rs. 40 million in emergency central-government funding to admit 2,000 more students in 1963 than in 1962 (GOI[CCH] 1964:560). The Medical Council of India was persuaded to consider reducing the length of an M.B. B.S. course (it did not agree), and was forced to waive its norms on staff-student and bed-student ratios so that existing colleges could admit more students. In addition, twenty-two new medical colleges were opened in the four years between 1962 and 1965.

For all the formal insistence on international standards, this rate of expansion was much faster than should have been permitted if the available number of medical educators had been a prime consideration. The government was aware of likely shortages immediately after World War II, and had established a scheme to send doctors abroad for higher training. In the four years from 1945 to 1948, 183 were sent at government expense, and traveling fellowships were also provided for senior teachers (GOI[CPHB], 1948:100–101). In the 1950s and 1960s, international agencies provided fellowships, some specifically for medical-education purposes.

By 1953 official policy was to discourage overseas training, and Mudaliar stated that it was time India was self-sufficient, with AIIMS to play a major role in achieving this (GOI[CCH] 1954). But, as the secretary to the MCI pointed out in 1958, the expansion of medical colleges called for 320 new teachers every year (GOI[CCH] 1959:41). Most medical colleges still depended on part-time teaching by local specialists, except in preclinical posts. They found great difficulty in recruiting staff, especially where there were no private practice opportunities, as in the nonclinical departments. Thus, in 1956, only one medical college was fully staffed in its pathology department, and there was a total shortfall of over 1,900 teaching staff (GOI[CCH] 1961:96). The Mudaliar committee estimated a shortage of 4,400 teachers in 1960. In 1964 roughly 22 percent of all teaching posts were vacant, with 28 percent of preclinical posts empty (GOI 1972:14–15). These shortages did not inhibit plans in the late 1960s to open new medical colleges, using the Mudaliar committee's proposed norm of one college for every 5 million persons in the population as justification (GOI[CCH], 1969:119). Of all medical teaching posts in 1970, 18 percent were vacant, but the vacancies were not evenly distributed: the Madhya Pradesh colleges were short 363 teachers (out of an unknown total), and it is difficult to understand quite how medical education was carried on in these circumstances.

The main solution to these shortages was to increase the pool of potential teachers by expanding postgraduate medical education. Some departments in existing medical colleges were given extra funding to open courses at a master's level, and several of these received substantial amounts from the Rockefeller Foundation to train staff and to provide equipment. In addition, new postgraduate institutes were opened in Punjab (Chandigarh) and in Pondicherry as prestige institutes by politicians jealous of the preeminence of Delhi's All-India Institute of Medical Sciences. Those in favor of the expansion of specialist training pointed to the shortages of medical teachers and argued that medical education in India should be available at all levels at the standards of Britain or America. Thus, a subcommittee on postgraduate education preparing a perspective plan for health in 1962–1963 managed to get the lion's share of the funds for education and training earmarked for postgraduate education (Rs. 750 million out of a total for all health workers of Rs. 1,830 million) and to propose a medical-education grants committee. This committee would have had access to foreign exchange, clearly stated by the subcommittee as essential but inaccessible (GOI[CCH], 1964:570–574).

These recommendations were not implemented (partly because

of the collapse of the planning system between 1965 and 1968), but the number of places and scholarships for postgraduate students expanded steadily. By 1969 there were 6,000 places a year (as against 11,000 undergraduate places), but only about 3,500 of them were taken up. This did not inhibit the expansion of postgraduate places by another 1,600 or so during the Fourth Plan (GOI 1972:14). The apparent surplus of specialists in medicine and surgery, noted during the discussions preceding the Fifth Plan (GOI 1971a: 25) finally led to a curb on the expansion of postgraduate education.

The issue of foreign standards was highlighted by the dilemmas posed by Indian doctors who traveled abroad to receive higher training (see chap. 8). Here it is worth pointing out the attempt to encourage such doctors to return to India to fill empty teaching posts. From 1958 a "pool" scheme had been in operation, by which doctors who returned received an honorary post and a salary while they looked for more permanent positions. This had very little appeal to doctors; those who came back to the pool often returned abroad again on the grounds that they were not being offered posts at the right level. Those who had received Indian training were often better placed to get higher posts (because of their contacts and sponsorship by professors and politicians) and resented attempts by those returned from abroad to leap over them (GOI[CCH], 1967:40–41). In the mid-1970s, the journal Technical Manpower reported that around ten doctors a month were being offered places in this pool, of which only half took up the offer, so the contribution to the return of Indian doctors was insignificant.

Control by the Medical Council of India over the standards of medical education was made more difficult by the establishment of new private medical colleges. Most medical colleges in India were founded by the state, with staffing and hospital provision all part of the normal state health budget. In a few cases (especially in Uttar Pradesh) medical colleges are part of the university, and thus funded by the state education budget. Private medical colleges also exist, some Christian foundations (Ludhiana, Vellore), some established as part of medical nationalism before independence and based on colleges of physicians and surgeons, and some municipal colleges in Maharashtra and Gujarat.

After independence, however, a new form of private medical college was established, with funds subscribed to committees dominated by politicians who expected to control admissions to the college as both financial and political rewards. Here admission was based largely on ability to pay, rather than on merit, and there was strong pressure to cut costs and standards in the interests of profitability. Minister of Health Karmakar, who served from 1959 to 1962, argued in favor of these colleges, saying that they would save government funds. He also argued that such colleges should be permitted to start in a modest fashion and then be given time to improve, and that prominent medical men could be used as teachers even if they were not qualified up to the level required by the Medical Council. During his time as minister more than Rs. 6 million was given to five private medical colleges in Andhra Pradesh, Karnataka, Bihar, and Kerala (GOI[CCH] 1964:155). A committee set up by the new health minister, Sushila Nayar (who had been a physician to Mahatma Gandhi), reflected a shift of power toward the medical establishment. It reported in 1964 that no new colleges should be established and existing colleges should be taken over by the state, with central government assistance, to root out corruption and low standards. Dr. Nayar seems to have resisted pressures from her cabinet colleagues to open medical colleges in their areas, but under her successors four more private medical colleges were opened in Bihar and three in Uttar Pradesh, from 1969 to 1972. In fact, the government decided it would be too expensive to take all of them over, but official disapproval was reiterated in 1971 (GOI[CCH], 1965:125–128 and 1972:4).

The MCI is essentially unable to control this kind of college and its standards. It can inspect a college after it has been running for two years and make recommendations, but it makes a final decision only when the first group of students are graduated. At that stage the university degree undergoes scrutiny, not the individual college. If the college has gained affiliation to a university, MCI has to threaten students from other affiliated colleges with nonrecognition of their qualification as well. But by then it is too late, in practical political terms, to act; students may organize to ensure that their degrees will be recognized, and they have strong support from the political heavyweights on the college managing committees. In any case, the MCI cannot act but can merely advise the government of India, which is free to ignore its advice. This position was established under the 1933 Act, and thus Rajkumari Amrit Kaur, as health minister in the early 1950s, was able to overrule the Medical Council in its attempt to delay recognition of the degrees of five medical colleges. She retained this power when the Medical Council of India Act was amended in 1956 (Lok Sabha Debates 10 December 1956). When the MCI attempted to withhold recognition from nine medical colleges in 1974, the government of India again did not support it (*Hindustan Times* 19 and 21 March, 1974).

The Guru Gobind Singh college, established in Faridabad (just south of Delhi) in 1971, was the most blatant example of political profiteering. Its sponsors were responding to unmet demands for medical-college places among the Delhi middle classes. The government itself had broken its own resolve to open no new medical colleges, capitulating to student and parent pressure in 1971 by forcing Delhi University to open a university medical college and then attaching it to one of the central government hospitals in New Delhi, Safdarjang. But the Faridabad college had no hospital facilities at all. The managing committee were all relatives of the Congress party's chief whip in the Punjab State Assembly, and the students went on a hunger strike when the promised facilities did not materialize. The issue was resolved by the college moving to Faridkot, in Punjab, with all its paid-up students, and being allowed to continue in existence (Lok Sabha Debates 19 December 1972; *Hindustan Times* 28 April 1973). After 1973 no new medical colleges were opened in this way for ten years, but proposals were made in 1984 to do so in Maharashtra.

Policy on medical education has thus not been entirely in the hands of doctors, despite the nominal power of the MCI. The subordination of the authority of the MCI by politicians was probably going on in the 1960s but did not surface into public debate. The effects of this subordination on the quality of medical education also provided the manifest grounds for the General Medical Council in London to refuse to recognize degrees from most of the medical colleges established in India after 1947, and for the final break in 1975, when the General Medical Council decided that it would admit no Indian medical degree as sufficient evidence of competence for practice in Great Britain. Keeping the lid on the expansion of medical education has only had partial success in maintaining quality and the incomes of doctors. But that success has fueled the demand for medical education, a demand politicians find impossible to ignore for long.

Patterns of Employment of Doctors

Little reliable information is available on where doctors go, how they practice, and what typical careers are like. One frequently cited source is the 1971 Special Census of qualified personnel, but it provides information on fewer than half the doctors estimated to be in practice in India at the time. We cannot tell how this sample relates to the whole population, or whether it includes some marginal practitioners, for example with integrated degrees. In table 38, I have therefore relied on more indirect estimates of the total stock of doctors and their distribution by employment category; this represents the result of a complex set of assumptions.

To begin with, different authorities provide estimates of total "stock" which varies quite considerably, ranging from 51,000 to 56,000 in 1951, from 70,000 to 81,000 in 1961, and from 115,725 to 141,000 in 1971. In part, these variations result from different methods and sources. For example, the MCI estimates are based on the numbers of doctors registered with it, but since no annual fee is payable, doctors who have died or retired tend to remain on the list and council estimates are high. Attempting to estimate the effects of death, retirement, and emigration does not produce clear agreement among the other sources (the Planning Commission, the Council for Scientific and Industrial Research, and the Institute for Applied Manpower Research). The figures in table 38 thus represent an approximate average of the estimates which include doctors who may be abroad, but attempts to exclude doctors who have retired or died.

These estimates suggest that despite some fluctuations, about 25 percent to 30 percent of doctors have been in public employment of one kind or another—central, state, or local government, Employees State Insurance scheme, defense, railways, coal mines, and so on. In some places (such as Delhi) the proportion in public employment is much higher (Jeffery 1976) and I have assumed that most of those in genuinely rural areas have also been in public employment. The most dramatic feature of table 38 is the rise in numbers of the residual category. I would not place great reliance on this figure, since the margins of error in the other categories are considerable (there seem to be no national figures even of employment in the public sector). Public-sector employment, private-sector employment, and emigration are unlikely together to have

TABLE 38
DISTRIBUTION OF STOCK OF DOCTORS

	1944	1961	1968	1971	1974	1978
Public sector	13,000	29,000	39,000	43,000	45,000	50,000
Self-employment	*	43,000	57,000	67,000	73,000	82,000
Private employment	*	*	6,000	7,000	8,000	9,000
Abroad	*	*	8,000	9,500	13,650	21,000
Rest	*	3,000	3,000	3,500	10,350	38,000
Total	47,400	75,000	113,000	130,000	160,000	200,000

SOURCES: 1944 figures from GOI 1946:12, referring to British India; 1961 figures from Mathur 1971; 1968 figures from IAMR 1970; 1974 figures from IAMR 1974; 1978 figures from IAMR 1974; and Ramaiah and Bhandari 1975.
NOTE: "Rest" (row 5) is a residual, including doctors who are attempting to establish private self-employment, practicing part-time, in employment with pharmaceutical companies, in postgraduate training, temporarily out of the labor force, etc.

risen fast enough to cope with the level of output of doctors since 1971. Most of the "residual" doctors are probably self-employed, at varying levels of income. Since demand for medical education remains unabated and there have been few accounts of serious unrest among the unemployed or underemployed doctors, the market for medical services has probably grown faster than the growth in national income. But little evidence suggests how this might have been happening, beyond isolated examples of expansion of private qualified medical services in rural areas in some states.

INDIGENOUS PRACTITIONERS

Policy with respect to indigenous practitioners has been restricted to issues concerning the formal education of practitioners, including attempts to produce social closure of the category by making all new practitioners undergo training. The battles between advocates of "pure" and "integrated" courses of training have probably slowed down the growth in the number of indigenous medical colleges and their intakes. Table 39 presents some indicators of the trends.

TABLE 39
Supply of Indigenous Medical Practitioners

	1962–1963	1972–1974	1977 ISM	1977 Homoeo-pathy
Practitioners:				
Qualified	30,000	50,000	130,000	20,000
Registered	87,000	150,000	142,000	74,000
Enlisted	?	?	?	51,000
In practice	?	200,000	?	?
Total	?	400,000	?	?
Colleges:	95	115	108	116
Annual admissions:	1,375		4,199	?

Sources: 1962–1963 figures from Brass 1972:348; 1972–1974 figures from Gwat-kin 1974:90, and Djukanovic and Mach 1975:85; 1977 figures from GOI, 1979a: 47, 53.
Key: ISM = *Indian Systems of Medicine*

These numbers are not mutually compatible, since more seem to be added to the "qualified" category than are trained every year. Some people probably are counted two or three times, because they are registered in more than one state (each of which has different rules); others are able to be registered on the basis of "postal" education, usually in homoeopathic colleges, not listed here; and still others may have found different ways of gaining access to the "qualified" registers. The estimates of the total numbers in practice also vary according to the principle used. For example, the UNICEF/WHO joint study quotes figures which are said to include dais (among the 200,000 personnel who were untrained and un-registered)—but at 1 dai for every 1,000 people (the government es-timate in 1977) there would be 650,000 dais. Gwatkin grosses up the 1961 census estimate in order to produce his figure of 250,000–300,000 who would report themselves as practitioners, but notes that the Narangwal-based estimates would expand that figure mul-tifold. Finally, estimates of the proportion of the total who are qualified vary from about 25 percent to 33 percent (Gwatkin 1974:90; Chuttani et al. 1973:996). All these estimates depend crit-ically on assumptions about whom to include as healers: those who are registered, qualified, financially dependent on practice, those engaged in practice full- or part-time, or someone known locally as having particular expertise. If all these categories are included, the number of healers would be not less than 1.5 to 2 million.

Very little is known about the whereabouts or employment of indigenous practitioners from these different categories. Gwatkin (1974:90) reports one estimate for 1972 of 25 percent of "certified" (qualified?) practitioners in government employment. This seems to be unduly high, generating a figure of about 20 percent of all government doctors being "integrated" or "pure" indigenous graduates. Beyond government employment, jobs seem to be scarce: other reports are concerned solely with those with their own clinics or working from their own homes (e.g., Alexander and Shivaswamy 1971; Neumann et al. 1971).

Conclusion

The introduction in the late 1970s of grades similar to feldshers and of community-health workers was not the result of new ideas, but of social forces that finally allowed old ones to be implemented. The social forces were rural populism, personified by the Janata Health Minister Raj Narain; the programs of international agencies; and the pressures for job improvements by employees of the erstwhile "vertical" disease programs. Men have generally taken advantage of the new opportunities, and are establishing themselves as new kinds of healers, formal and informal, but women have been much less affected, either as nurses or as dais, and have been largely excluded from the community health worker scheme. The other major changes since 1947 have been the loss of international recognition for Indian medical degrees and the growing significance of practitioners outside the control of the Western medical profession. Doctors have failed to "close" the occupation of medicine.

On paper, India now has an infrastructure of personnel capable of implementing health policies in every village. Its peripheral workers should have supervision and support through a graded hierarchy of male and female workers who have received an integrated training, able to deal effectively with some of the major health problems—environmental hygiene, infectious-disease control, nutritional advice, and support. However, the reality is significantly different.

CHAPTER TEN

Structure and Process in Health Services

Examining how health services in India developed and how they work in light of the most common criticisms made of them, must include a closer look at the medical colleges and hospitals, the primary health centers and their peripheral workers, and the ways that "clients" perceive what they are offered.

Medical Colleges

The major criticism of medical colleges is that they are unable to relate to the main health problems of most Indians. Because the dominant ethos of college teaching staff is said to mimic that of British and American medical colleges—which are often accused of concentrating on hospital medicine and within that, on unusual conditions—the Indian medical student is not prepared for the everyday work of the general practitioner. Indian medical colleges are said to compound these problems of "irrelevance" by focusing on hospital medicine of Britain and America, thus doubly distancing themselves from the common problems of the mass of the Indian population.

These issues have not escaped the attention of higher medical policymakers nor of the Medical Council of India. However, the concern with "maintaining international standards" has usually overcome "ensuring that doctors fit local conditions," as central health minister, Rajkumari Amrit Kaur, described the twin goals in

1954 (GOI[CCH] 1955). She presumed that these two goals were compatible. She stated in 1956:

> We must take full note of these developments [in the rest of the world] as well as our own special needs and then attempt to solve our problems in respect of medical education to suit the conditions prevailing in the country. (GOI[CCH] 1957)

The Medical Council of India has frequently revised medical curricula to stress the significance of social and preventive medicine (SPM), and to insist on periods of rural residence for interns (graduates who have completed their medical training but have to complete a year's experience for full registration) and, latterly, of medical students as well. Notably absent has been any sustained effort to ensure that these changes are implemented in the actual practice of medical colleges or to monitor their impact. Similarly, few attempts have been made to change the views of medical educators, or in other ways to raise the status of staff in departments of social and preventive medicine or working in rural posts.

Social and Preventive Medicine

One of the earliest attempts to change the social orientation of medicine in India came through the establishment of departments of social and preventive medicine. For example, in the central provincial health-committee meeting of 1948 there was a report on a survey of medical education which revealed that "the emphasis laid on the teaching of preventive medicine and public health is quite inadequate" (GOI [CPHC] 1949:97). Similar sentiments were repeated in speeches and resolutions from the Central Council of Health. A special medical-education conference held in Delhi in 1955 called for the strengthening of social and preventive medicine departments as a way of raising the prestige of preventive medicine in health services generally, and these recommendations became regulations of the Medical Council of India in 1961 (Taylor et al. 1976:7).

The main fallacy in the discussions was the belief that the cause of the low status of preventive work could be traced solely to India's colonial heritage and that its status could be raised by changes of a minor kind within medical curricula, but without changes in career opportunities and rewards for medical practitioners.

Throughout the world, the prestige rankings of medical specializations seem to show a common pattern. General surgery and other surgical specialties are almost always near the top, while public health, social and community medicine, and preclinical specializations are usually at the bottom (Taylor et al 1976). General practice and family medicine have never gained a foothold in Indian medical colleges. Indian medical students surveyed in the 1970s consistently ranked social and preventive medicine at the bottom of a prestige hierarchy, and showed little interest or knowledge in, for example, primary health care (Nichter 1981:226; Ramalinga-swami and Shyam 1980). Madan (1980:93) describes "the received image of preventive and social medicine as a 'soft choice,' something that only the second-rate medical students specialise in," as the view held by most of the doctors he interviewed at the All-India Institute of Medical Sciences. Banerji (1974:2) argues that this is not merely a matter of image; when the new social and preventive medicine departments were created after independence, the teaching positions were taken by discards, those who fell off the ladder to senior positions in more prestigious specialties. One indicator of their low status is that in many medical colleges the posts are held by women, who often find access to medical and surgical specialties more difficult (Bhargava 1983).

An exaggerated concern for curative specialties, in particular those with the masculine glamor of the "activist" model of surgery (passive patients in a life-or-death situation, rescued by dramatic knife work) is not restricted to India. However, it takes on an additional pathos in a context where policy statements by politicians and senior medical bureaucrats repeatedly argue that generalist skills are the most pressing needs. Most doctors at the All-India Institute took the view that national concerns might require social and community medicine, but not all doctors should follow that model and that they, in an elite institution, should be the first to be exempted (Madan 1980:94).

Rural Orientation

The 1955 medical education conference also called for the establishment of rural field-practice areas attached to medical colleges, in order that undergraduates and interns would be exposed to rural conditions and health problems. It took the Medical Council of India nine years to respond by making three months of such experience mandatory for interns; revised recommendations were drawn up in 1971 (Aggarwal et al. 1975:277–278). In 1961 only half the medical colleges had active rural internship programs, and of the seven colleges in one study (drawn from those with "better" programs) only two had full three-month programs (Taylor et al. 1976:43). When studying the situation in 1974 (Aggarwal et al. 1975:282–285) 60 percent of the forty-seven medical colleges that replied to their inquiry reported that rural internship lasted less than two months, with one-third reporting less than one month. Only three colleges claimed they were following the objectives of the rural internship program as defined by the Medical Council of India.

Following the Srivastava committee report of 1975, proposals were again made to "Re-Orient Medical Education (ROME)." In 1978 medical colleges were each given responsibility for health care services provided by three primary health centers. Money was provided under this scheme to build hostels for medical students to use while receiving rural orientation as part of their training. In most cases, responsibility for the primary health center and for rural training has been vested in the social and preventive medicine departments. No consistent attempts have been made to evaluate the progress of this scheme. In Orissa, at least, the primary health centers controlled by the medical college are organized differently from the rest, since they have a resident associate professor from the medical college, and occasional visits by the professor of social and preventive medicine. But in no case does the work of the primary health center figure largely in the training of undergraduates or of interns, most of whom never spend a night in the ROME hostels.

Two assumptions have underpinned these efforts. The first is that exposure to rural conditions will lead to an awareness of rural problems and a desire to help solve them. The second is that having more doctors working in rural areas is the best way to solve rural health problems, and that persuasion is a desirable way to achieve this, at almost any cost.

Some attempts to evaluate the effect of rural exposure on orientation to rural work have been made. The most sustained attempt, by C. E. Taylor and his colleagues (1976), was based on their experience and research linked to the Narangwal Project in Punjab, but drawing material also from Mysore (Karnataka) and other states. They argued that doctors were, if anything, given a negative orientation toward rural work from their medical college training. There was some evidence to suggest that views before rural exposure were more favorable toward rural work than afterward, when the full extent of the isolation and working conditions were made manifest. In general, since the dominant ethos of the medical college was centered on urban hospital work, two or three months spent in a primary health center could not redress that imbalance.

The assumption that the medical problems of rural areas can be solved by increasing the numbers of doctors prepared to work there predates 1947. The discussion is limited by an almost unchallenged further assumption that doctors cannot be sent to rural areas. No such direction exists, nor has it been tried, for other trained personnel—engineers or scientists. The 1972 National Service Act provided that qualified people, including doctors, under the age of thirty would be liable to be called for up to four years to serve wherever required by the state. However, the Act has not been implemented, in spite of occasional threats to use it to fill empty medical posts in rural areas. As a result of the refusal to consider compulsion, the only options open to the state have been financial incentives (positive and negative), career incentives, and the attempt to change the orientation of the doctor toward rural life.

Positive financial incentives have been tried in a number of ways since 1947, either to encourage private practice by paying a supplementary income or to encourage the acceptance of a rural posting by offering a rural allowance. More sophisticated proposals have involved additional educational allowances for a doctor's children. None of them can be demonstrated to have had the slightest impact. Essentially, as has been pointed out many times, doctors are drawn from the urban middle and upper classes, and expect to live in a similar way when they have qualified. This means they expect not just a sufficient income but access to social and physical infrastructures, such as electricity, sanitation, schooling, and so on. Inevitably, rural areas have a lower standard of such provision than towns. The problem will not be solved in the short run by raising the quality of rural amenities, since some of these are positional goods, which gain their value not from their intrinsic merit but because of their short supply. Schooling is the prime example; just improving rural schools is not enough, because urban schooling improves faster. The differential advantages of elite schooling count in getting ahead, which seems to weigh very heavily with young married doctors. Additional pay can provide access to urban schooling only if children are sent to the towns for their education; this does not create a willingness to accept rural conditions.

Negative financial incentives have been restricted to the taking of "bonds" in which medical students face the loss of quite substantial sums of money if they do not honor promises to work for the state government in a rural posting for two or three years after graduating. These have rarely had any impact. Often, more doctors graduate each year than there are jobs in state employment in rural areas. Escape clauses allow most new doctors to avoid any financial penalty. They cannot be forced to take up jobs that do not exist. They may take up the post formally but actually not work in the rural areas at all, or for only a very brief period.

Career incentives have also been tried, particularly by restricting access to postgraduate courses to those with rural experience, or preventing promotion for those without it. These constraints obviously apply only to those in government service and suggest something of the difficulties faced by administrators who attempt to control their medical personnel. No realistic assessment of the success of these barriers exists. Many doctors cynically suggest that those with "pull" can leap them with ease, and that only those without contacts suffer their full force, but evidence of a more substantial kind is lacking.

The vast majority of Indian doctors, then, leave medical colleges with a preference for clinical (rather than public health) work in urban settings or abroad (rather than in rural posts). Given the record of doctors elsewhere in the world, it would be very surprising if matters were any different. Indeed, the most surprising feature of the situation is that politicians and social scientists have held onto the view that some change in this orientation could be produced through exhortation or rural exposure. In turning to look at the conditions of work in urban clinics and hospitals, I want to stress two more features of medical work: the nature of hospital power structures; and limitations to the autonomy of private clinical practice.

Hospitals

Two of the very few sociological studies of the working of Indian hospitals (Kirkpatrick 1970; Minocha 1974) focus on the nature of the discrepancies between staff and patients in patterns of expectations, deriving much of their theoretical focus from American sociological discussions of doctor-patient relationships and the nature of "sick" roles. In general, while doctors seem to want to approximate the kinds of social relationships with patients which characterize medical roles in Western Europe or North America, patients attempt to bring very different patterns of expectations to bear. The most pervasive of the patients' expectations relate to the attempt to turn the relationship into a more personal one (see Gould 1965). Cooperation, flattery, and providing a financial inducement are all used to improve the quality of treatment received from doctors (Kirkpatrick 1970:161). The financial payments may be open, such as consulting the surgeon or physician privately before attending the hospital, or by making it clear that successful treatment will be followed by a substantial *inam*, or "voluntary" gift (Mathur 1975). Or the payments may be covert, in the form of various kinds of bribes to ensure access to the hospital, particularly where private practice of hospital doctors is illegal.

Junior doctors seem to find these social processes unpalatable, complaining about "illiterate, stupid, ignorant" patients and attempting to restrict their relationships to a formal, medical plane (Minocha 1974:192–194; Mathur, 1975:100–109). Senior doctors, by repute, are more willing to become involved in these relationships, usually, it would seem, because they cream most of the financial or other benefits to themselves (Mathur 1975:170–171; Venkataratnam 1979:180). Junior hospital doctors thus find themselves caught between unchangeable pressures from patients and senior doctors. Their patients rightly assume that their treatment will be affected by the kind of relationship they have with the medical staff, but the junior doctors they usually see and can influence are not the ones who count. The senior medical staff obviously adapt their working behavior to financial and other pressures from patients, but expect their junior staff to obey unquestioningly while gaining very little from what are seen as "unprofessional" activities (Venkataratnam 1979:253).

This situation can be described as one where professional values are adhered to by doctors, at least formally, but in practice the structural conditions necessary to implement them are absent (Jeffery 1977). While doctors have many of the formal trappings of professional organization (a medical council, university-level entry, a privileged position in state employment, etc.) the state does not, in fact, guarantee professional privileges. Further, in the private sector competition from "outsiders" (indigenous practitioners or unqualified competitors from within the Western mode) is fierce, leaving individual doctors subject to strong pressure to safeguard their incomes at the cost of their ethical codes. The absence of a strong independent profession means that state-employed doctors are in a weak bargaining position when negotiating public-sector employment conditions. There are, of course, private hospitals in the larger cities and successful private clinics. But these are the exception rather than the rule, and show little tendency to become the dominant mode of private practice.

Few mechanisms maintain medical autonomy, or doctors' ability to determine their own conditions of work, beyond the very narrow field of actual diagnosis. Decisions of hospital admission or different kinds of outpatient treatment seem to be very vulnerable to the personal characteristics of the patients. Such extramedical concerns enter into the heart of the medical encounter, in part because career advancement and security are not under the control of doctors alone. Doctors have failed to stake out and protect a professional sphere, and collegial control is insufficient to permit the development of collegial norms. It is difficult to find evidence to show the extent of interference in medical judgments, but few doubt wider political or financial interests are significant in all important occupational decisions. In this taken-for-granted understanding of the medical world it is difficult to show that a particular doctor was promoted because of the quality of his or her work or where degree candidates were examined impartially. A widespread cynicism is one result, a cynicism that also affects those working in other government positions.

Primary Health Centers

The concept of the primary health center was first elaborated in the report on health services in England, produced by a committee under the chairmanship of Lord Dawson of Penn in 1920 (Dawson Report 1920). It was not taken up in a substantial way in Britain until the 1960s, but the idea had already spread to other parts of the world, forming part of the ideas promoted by the League of Nations Health Organization, partly implemented in China (Lucas 1982). The concept was discussed at a Far Eastern Conference on Medical Relief in 1938, at which India was represented. The Bhore Committee took advice from Dr. John Grant, who had worked in China until the Japanese invasion and then moved to Calcutta until 1945. The Bhore Report endorsed the idea of a basic unit of health-service provision that would combine curative and preventive services, but it took ten years before the first steps were taken to implement the proposal. Under the Community Development Program, efforts were made to establish such centers for each Community Development Block, with its population of about 80,000 people. The Bhore proposals had called for a primary health center for a population of 20,000 by 1966, but by that date many blocks (now with populations nearer 100,000) had not been provided with the basic primary health center facilities.

To begin with, the primary health center building was often merely a dispensary renamed, with most of its activities indeed curative in focus. But as time passes, more and more staff members have been added, more PHCs have purpose-built facilities according to a national or statewide design, and the focus of their activities has shifted to include family planning as one of their central tasks. The standard PHC should have six beds for inpatients; more recently, a quarter of all the centers have been designated "upgraded" and are eventually to have thirty beds and attached specialist obstetricians and pediatricians. Originally each center was to have five or six subcenters attached, with a female health worker (auxiliary nurse-midwife or trained dai); current targets call for twelve or thirteen subcenters (1 for 8,000 people) as a step toward twenty or more (1 for 5,000 people, or 1 for 3,000 in tribal areas with sparse populations and poor communications). The increasing problems of supervising such a large number of subcenters have led to new proposals for the upgrading of some subcenters, or the establishment of sub-primary health centers. In this way, perhaps by the year 2000, the population served by a PHC will come down to about 20,000.

The most common criticism of the primary health center program has shifted somewhat since the first centers were established in 1952. Four main sets of problems have been voiced in the Central Council of Health or in other national forums:

1. Clinical and curative concerns have predominated over the intended emphasis on preventive work;

2. staff have been unwilling to work in primary health centers, resulting in understaffing and/or poor motivation;

3. the balance of expenditures has tended heavily toward salaries and wages, leaving very little for drugs, transport, and maintenance; and

4. there is little or no evidence of "people's participation" in the organization of health services by the centers and this is reflected in a general underutilization of facilities.

In addition, a fifth issue has been identified but is less often voiced in authoritative settings: the undesirable consequences of having integrated health services with family-planning or contraceptive provisions.

Of these problems, the first two were identified as early as the 1959 Central Council of Health meeting, when two basic points were made: staff were unwilling to work at PHCs; and there was a danger, as the health minister put it, that the centers would "degenerate into glorified dispensaries" because they neglected preventive work (GOI [CCH] 1960:30,99–102). At the 1967 Central Council of Health the major problem was expressed in almost identical terms: a shortage of staff, caused by a reluctance of doctors and nurses to serve in these posts because of a shortage of housing for them and poor schooling for their children, the absence of incentives for rural work and low pay scales in state government health services (GOI [CCH] 1968:22). The concern to improve conditions for primary health center staff has, indeed, dominated all official discussions of the problems of the centers.

As staff have been appointed and rates of vacancies declined, however, other problems have been highlighted. In 1968 the director-general of health services pointed again to the greater load of clinical work and the lack of attention to prevention (GOI [CCH] 1969:27). In 1969 insufficient drug and transport budgets were noted (GOI [CCH] 1970:110). However, only more recently has one point, made in 1959 by Director-General of Health Services Barkat Narain, been followed up: the argument that "the people's participation is essential which can only be secured by the new methodology of approach—call it extension technique, health education, or social education" (GOI [CCH] 1960:101). A further criticism is that the existing facilities are largely underused because of the way doctors work. They wait for patients to come to them, rather than attempting to take their services to the people.

I will follow these themes through by looking at three levels of primary health center work, dealing first with the Primary Health Center itself (or the "headquarters"); then with the work of field personnel—auxiliary nurse—midwives and male health workers; and finally with the newly created categories of trained dais and community health workers (or volunteers, also known as village health guides). Table 40 sets the context for this dicussion.

AT HEADQUARTERS

The staffing at a PHC has always focused on a doctor. Initially one doctor was to be attached, but by 1956 the number was raised to two; one a generalist and one specializing in family planning. In 1978 a third medical officer was added, specifically to deal with the training of community health workers and preferably a

TABLE 40
ESTABLISHMENT OF PRIMARY HEALTH CENTERS

	1956	1961	1966	1969	1974	1978
No. of blocks	1,564	3,137	4,724	5,265	5,123	5,005
No. of PHCs	67	2,565	4,631	4,909	5,283	5,400
(percent)	4	82	98	93	103	108
No. of subcenters		1,649		22,826	33,509	38,115
Doctors in posts				5,294		

SOURCES: GOI 1979:19, 65; GOI (CCH) 1970:51
NOTE: Data as at 31 March in each year. Comparable data are not available for each year. Some Community Development Blocks have more than one PHC; others have none.

graduate from one of the indigenous systems of medicine. All these posts have taken a long time to be filled. As late as 1972 only about half the centers had their full complement of doctors. On March 31, 1978, 61 PHCs had no doctor at all, 771 had only one doctor, and the remaining 4,568 had 2 or more. There were 115 centers still to be established, though some blocks had more than one (GOI 1979:66–67).

The centers that are less fully staffed are, not surprisingly, more remote and less well equipped. In a study that involved interviewing thirty-nine center medical officers in the early 1960s, low salaries, poor living conditions, inadequate facilities, and social isolation were reported as the most important obstacles to the recruitment of doctors for rural work (Takulia et al. 1967:49). A study in central Uttar Pradesh in 1971–72 classified PHCs into three categories by location (closeness to urban centers), facilities (electricity and water supply), and local amenities (schools, markets, etc.) (Misra et al. 1981). The nineteen most accessible centers in their survey had fifty-four supervisory staff members in post, whereas the eight most remote ones had only ten supervisors. However, not all those "in post" were "present and working." As Misra and others point out, those posted to remote primary centers may devote all their energies to achieving a transfer to a more desirable center, visiting the district or state headquarters for long periods to lobby and persuade senior staff to change their posting. Staff members may disappear on long leaves until they receive a better posting or they may be moved to other positions. These are two of the means by which posts may be filled-up, although the staff may be almost permanently absent. A possibly extreme example is provided by a study of a primary health center in Uttar Pradesh in 1977–1978, during the post-emergency collapse of the family planning program, when five staff members spent 75 percent of their time absent or on personal business (Sutherland 1978:42).

Despite the emphasis given to public health, preventive and promotive functions in job descriptions, most staff time is actually spent on curative work. One study carried out in 1968 in Punjab and Mysore (Alexander et al. 1972:1,852) weighted staff time by salaries and estimated that about 60 percent of staff time at the center headquarters went on illness services, 25 percent on family planning, and 12 percent on control of communicable diseases. The rest of the time was spent on maternal and child health, with no time spent on environmental health. In Takulia's study (1967:37–39), center doctors estimated a median of about 27 percent of their time spent on preventive activities, with half the doctors saying lack of interest was the main reason for spending little time on this work.

Even within this clinical focus, the quality of care seems to be poor. Quality is of course difficult to assess, and relatively few studies have produced more than anecdotal evidence. Most patients spend a very short time with the doctor; two studies at the end of the 1960s estimated the median time spent with the doctor at two minutes or less (Murthy and Parker 1973; Seth 1973). Average times are not likely to have risen since then. Sutherland (1978:37) reported that in prenatal consultations in a center in the Varanasi district (Uttar Pradesh), women were never weighed nor were hemoglobin levels determined; instruments were not sterilized and blood pressure was not always recorded. A number of other small-scale studies in the same center demonstrated inappropriate prescribing, little or no advice given by the doctor, and a minimal level of care (ibid.:47).

One reason for poor quality is probably the shortage of funds under the control of the center's staff for services to patients. Studies of the patterns of center expenditures are rare. One (Alexander et al. 1972:1,852) estimated that 10 percent of total annual expenditures went for drugs for headquarters and subcenters, and 74 percent on salaries and allowances for staff. Satpathy (1978) estimated that of the total Chiraigaon PHC budget of Rs. 332,000 in 1977, 85 percent went for salaries, leaving 9.4 percent for drugs, 1.4 percent for transport charges, and 4 percent for all other items. By contrast, Singh (1983:28) reports that some 40 percent of expenditure on medical care for the population insured under the Employees' Social Insurance Scheme goes on medicines, which are the fastest-growing category of expenditure between 1975–1976 and 1979–1980.

The drugs budget for the population served by PHCs has grown very slowly. It was pegged at Rs. 20,000 per center in 1965 (Reddy 1983:273), irrespective of its population or outpatient coverage. Since 1980 the budget has increased largely because of the sums allocated to an increasing number of subcenters and to community health workers. Thus, in 1983, a common annual drugs budget for a center was Rs. 12,000, with a further Rs. 3,000 for each subcenter and Rs. 600 for each community health worker. In a "standard" center there would thus be a total drug bill of Rs. 30,000 for ten subcenters, Rs. 60,000 for 100 community health workers as well as the Rs. 12,000 at headquarters, giving a total of Rs. 102,000, or about Rs. 1 per head of population nominally served per year. (Each person insured under the Employees Social Insurance scheme receives, on average, medicines worth about Rs. 13 per year [Singh 1984:28].) David and Narayana (1983:48–60) report that in Orissa delays in the release of funds, in the acceptance of tenders, and in the placing of orders, combined with an excessively long list of permitted drugs and poor ordering and stocking arrangements, meant that few primary health centers had a drug supply that matched the demands on them. Periodic press reports suggest that the medicines that are supplied are often substandard or out of date (Shepperdson 1986). Reddy (1983:275–276), using material from Karnataka and Andhra Pradesh, gives a similar picture. Studies of PHCs suggest that most prescriptions require the patient to purchase the drug from the market, because only a very small range of basic drugs are provided from center stores. The only exception to this general pattern—and a very significant one—is that the drugs required for tubectomies or vasectomies are provided from a special allocation and patients do not normally have to buy these themselves.

Because primary health center work has such a strong clinical orientation, it reaches a relatively small proportion of its nominal clientele. As in other parts of the world, patients do not travel far to consult a doctor except in emergencies or in chronic cases when patients may make very long trips (Ramachandran and Shastri 1983:185). Most patients attending a center come from within two or three miles (80 percent or more in three studies cited by Takulia from the mid-1960s [1967:28]). In a teaching block associated with Banaras Hindu University (Chiraigaon), in the mid-1970s, Marwah and others (1978) estimated that no more than 7.3 percent of pregnancies more than two miles from the health center were registered for prenatal care, compared with about 25 percent inside that distance. Staff find it difficult to travel far from the center headquarters to hold clinics in subcenters or in more remote parts of the block because they have inadequate vehicles and fuel allowances. Often doctors tour their blocks, if at all, on their own cycles or motorcycles. Once again, the main exception is that a special allocation for transport is made from incentive money for family-planning sterilizations. A health center with a large number of sterilizations to its credit receives an additional allocation for transport costs.

Even within the population which does use the primary health center, according to Banerji (1973:2,263) the "poor and the oppressed" are discriminated against. He suggests that these groups use the center less frequently than wealthier groups. Other sources suggest a different picture, in which use rates may not vary very much by socioeconomic background (e.g., Seal and Bose 1973:64; Ramachandran and Shastri 1983:181–183). However, the quality of care for the poor may be worse, with wealthier clients able to jump queues, receive longer attention from the doctor, and gain privileged access to scarce drugs held in the center.

FIELD STAFF

The male and female field staff of the PHC have rather different histories, because the women were originally in family-planning personnel, while the men were employed in the various "vertical" campaigns (including family planning) before the "multipurpose" reforms of the late 1970s. I shall therefore deal with these two categories separately.

Male Staff: Prior to the introduction of the multipurpose-worker scheme, male health workers were organized in a bewildering range of positions. The various national programs (malaria, smallpox, leprosy, tuberculosis, family planning) all had separate hierarchies. In addition, there were school health workers, sanitary inspectors and subordinate public-health staff. Each PHC had a different group of field staff, depending on local conditions, historical accident, or state policy and provision, and these staff would be paid from different budget heads and at different pay scales. Because of this complexity, a smooth conversion into a multipurpose system has been difficult to achieve. In most states substantial income differences remain and workers still tend to identify themselves with the single-purpose program where they began (Narayana and Acharya 1981:96).

Male health staff have not been the subject of much study, except for those in the family-planning cadres (e.g., Elder 1974; Misra et al. 1981). These accounts accord with that of Narayana and Acharya (1980:102–103) in suggesting little commitment to health and family planning work per se, but rather an economic orientation to work. In addition, these male paramedical workers are subject to conflicting lines of authority, with many of them naming four or more direct supervisors. However, they work very much on their own, with 75 percent saying that they meet a supervisor once a week or less often (ibid.:114–115). In this context, supervision tends to focus on an assessment of the written records kept by the worker. All his supervisors will request reports on their particular area of concern, and record keeping has become a major time user by these workers. Thus Alexander and others (1972:1,853) estimated that more than 40 percent of expenditures could be regarded as administrative (record keeping, travel, liaison with other agencies, etc.) and a further 17 percent to 20 percent as nonproductive or personal; unfortunately they do not classify this information by staff category or distinguish "headquarters" from "field" operations.

A major issue in supervision is that of transfers and promotions, a well-established feature of the Indian bureaucracy at all levels. Frequent transfers are explained as the only way to prevent a number of corrupt practices. For health workers, these might include illegal private practice as a healer; preference being shown to particular villages or villagers when spraying against malaria; conniving with supervisory staff to permit long leaves of absence, and selling health inputs such as drugs. But for these workers, familiarity with the villages where they work may be crucial. Knowing the geography, particular local problems of access, and obtaining the confidence of villagers could make the difference between the success or failure of a health program. Transfers every three or four years militate against this and, in trying to stay put, health workers are not helped by their objective performance but by the very kind of political influence the system is supposed to prevent.

The introduction of multipurpose working was partly justified as a way of reducing the time spent traveling between villages. Any single visit could be used for several purposes. Most workers seem to welcome the chance to reduce the population they are expected to serve. However, while the family-planning workers welcomed the chance to add health duties to their work, the other workers were less happy about their increased family-planning responsibilities (ibid.:132). Workers who "motivate" a "case" for sterilization are expected to spend a lot of time with that person. They go with them to the operating site to look after their needs and to ensure that they go through with the operation and to make sure that the worker gets credit for the "motivation." Since 1977 most sterilizations have been of women, and these are more often "motivated" by female workers, so this may not now be significant in the everyday working patterns of most male workers.

Male workers have a number of problems in their work which female workers face less often, most notably, access to houses. In general, people resist aspects of public-health work, such as the collection of blood slides for malaria surveillance and attempts to ensure complete coverage of immunizations. On occasion, minority groups have resisted the entry of workers from other sections of the population: Muslims, underrepresented in the health workforce, are most likely to restrict access. Some workers also face difficulties because they come from "untouchable" origins (ibid.:126–127). But more general criticism has questioned the capacity of workers to maintain their work at a sufficiently high level to produce results; Harrison's account of the problems of motivation and performance in malaria control has already been cited (1978). There is little reason to believe that these limitations of unipurpose preventive campaigns will now be overcome. The prevailing ethos of management is more akin to authoritarian supervision; a one-way flow of communication from the top down the hierarchy, targets fixed and punishment for those who do not meet them, little attempt to work beside subordinates to identify problems and help to solve them. This model is poorly adapted to create enthusiasm and job satisfaction, and the absence of promotion prospects for most staff compounds the difficulties. None of these problems has been addressed by the recent reforms, though the Area Development Programs described in chapter 11 have included management education as one of their elements.

Female Staff: The position of female-health staff is more straightforward. Women were not recruited for the single-disease campaigns, either because they were seen as suitable only for maternal and child health ("women's issues") or because of a realistic assessment of the supply of educated staff for the tasks these campaigns involved. Essentially there are two cadres of female staff—Auxiliary Nurse-Midwives and Lady Health Visitors—who were originally employed either as family-planning or maternal- and child-health staff. Since reorganization into a multipurpose scheme, they have all been reclassified as health workers.

One early study of the work of ANMs stressed several main points that have been frequently repeated. Reid (1969:1,55) argued that the range of duties expected was too vast. The worker could not possibly cover the geographical area assigned to her and the traveling time was disproportionately large (about 25 percent). The time spent on record keeping (about 20 percent) seriously interfered with the time available for work, and family-planning work was the most difficult aspect of their jobs. The estimates of Alexander and others (1972), cited above, are in line with these figures.

An additional problem for these female workers is their vulnerability in rural settings. They complain most bitterly about the housing provided for them—not just its availability but its security—and the dangers of traveling unchaperoned from village to village (IIM 1980). In many places they have the reputation of being loose women, and it is also reputed that they come under heavy sexual harassment from their superiors and from locals, unless they are protected by some male kinsmen or their husbands.

Finally, these workers are most seriously affected by the family-planning campaigns. Motivating family-planning cases (particularly for tubectomy—sterilization—but to a lesser extent for intrauterine-device [IUD] insertions) has always been a substantial element in their training and work, with varying importance at different times. It is overwhelmingly dominant during family-planning drives—around the time of camps (when special operating facilities are established), during 1976–1977, or during the one or two special family-planning months every year. Despite recent attempts to widen the job description to encourage female health employees to spend more time on maternal and child health, the only criterion by which staff performance is seriously measured is their ability to provide sterilization cases; this is reflected in the amount of time and effort they spend in family-planning work (IIM 1980:97–108). Under the Congress government of 1980 onward, a number of health elements appeared in the New 20-Point Program;

one of which was family planning. "Sterilization achievements" for each unit had to be collected and checked and passed up the bureaucratic system so that the month's figures could be on the prime minister's desk by the fifteenth of the following month. No other national health program has the same kind of central surveillance. Village women are well aware of the significance to health workers of motivating sterilizations. As a result they are cautious of becoming indebted to these staff and vulnerable to moral pressure to be sterilized (Jeffery et al. 1985).

VILLAGE-LEVEL PERSONNEL

Health departments had no "village-level" personnel before 1977. Prior to this, under the Community Development Program village-level workers were supposed to be concerned with some health matters, though it seems that they concentrated on agricultural development. But they were not really village-based in the way that term has come to be used. Village-level now usually means that the person is a long-term resident in the area, has no more than part-time employment, is subject to some form of control by village institutions, is trained outside the framework of formal training institutions, and is without a marketable qualification. By contrast, the village-level workers (and other health staff) are usually prevented from serving in their own village and are regularly transferred. The two categories of village-level health personnel (in the recent usage) who were the focus of the 1977 policy were called community health workers and dais. They were organized in different ways and for different purposes, so I will deal with them separately.

Community Health Workers: Unlike all other health personnel, the community health worker was supposed to be nominated by the village, and the primary health center medical officer would merely select trainees from among those nominated. The successful candidates would then undergo a three-month training course, held at the health center, when the trainees would receive a stipend of Rs. 200 a month. On successful completion of the course they would return to their own villages. There they would merely be paid Rs. 50 a month as a retainer, or honorarium, and would be provided with drugs and dressings to the value of Rs. 50 a month. They would be expected to spend two to three hours a day in health-related activities, but would not be under the formal bureaucratic control of the district medical officer. Dismissal could only follow a formal request from the village, and this was discouraged by making village institutions liable for paying the training stipend of any replacement. In general, the tasks to be carried out for which training was given would be first aid, preventive medicine, and community hygiene (NIHFW, 1978:1–3).

The scheme was introduced in 741 PHCs in 1977. Almost all blocks were to have been included in the program by the end of the Sixth Plan in March 1985. The program has changed through time: sometimes in response to findings based on research carried out on the first blocks covered, sometimes because of the change of political power when Congress governments were returned in Delhi and most of the states in 1980. But the basic principles remain unchanged. The program has been politically very sensitive, with doctors organized to oppose it on the grounds that it increased quackery and exposed villagers to second-class services. Perhaps for this reason, there have been several social-science research studies, so we have a fair amount of basic information about who the community health workers are, how they were selected, and about perceptions of their work by health staff and others. We have less information on what community health workers usually do or about the major factors that might have an effect on it.

Most health workers are relatively young (the modal age group is 20 to 29 in most studies, in line with official guidelines) and educated to secondary level. Very few are illiterate, and only 30 percent or so have only primary schooling (NIHFW 1978:Appendix V[c]). In the northern states of Bihar, Uttar Pradesh, and Punjab, a sizable minority (17 percent to 25 percent) of the first two batches had some college education (ibid.). Most community health workers are male, despite the evidence from voluntary projects that women are better suited to the work, particularly in services for the priority categories of mothers and children (Hardiman 1984). The percentage of women in the first two batches was 6 percent, with a regional variation from a high of 26 percent in West Bengal and surrounding eastern states, to no women at all in Rajasthan, one each in Haryana and Madhya Pradesh, and 4 (0.7 percent) in Uttar Pradesh (NIHFW 1978:Appendix V[b]). Recruitment guidelines for later batches stressed more strongly the desirability of choosing more women.

The selection procedure actually followed was radically different from the model outlined by the official documents and demonstrates very clearly the nature of village-level institutions and the political process in rural India. In principle, the village councilors (the panchayat) were to nominate several candidates from each village, and the medical officers were to assess their suitability in choosing among them. In practice, panchayats seemed to prefer to nominate only one candidate—the National Institute of Health and Welfare study (ibid.:41) noted that 47 percent of the 299 community health workers from the first two batches they studied said that there were no competitors for the post; Narayan and Acharya (1980:176) found that 62 percent of the 127 health workers in their study had had no competitors.

Doctors might be expected to prefer selecting the most appropriate candidate from a range of options, but it seems that the reverse is the case. Most doctors prefer a "least-risks" option, insisting that the panchayat come up with only one name; the political problems posed for the doctor by unsuccessful applicants make the task of selection one the doctor would like to avoid. The politicization of selection probably went farthest in west Bengal, where the Communist party government ensured that most candidates came from their own mass peasant organizations (Jobert 1985:15). Far from being an open procedure, involving villagers in discussion about the program and the relative merits of alternative candidates, in most places it became merely a question of one more minor political favor to be distributed.

Dais: By contrast, the very few studies of the new schemes for training traditional birth attendants and integrating their work into the maternal and child-health services have not been widely published or discussed. Dais involved in training in Uttar Pradesh were significantly older than community health volunteers (CHVs)—with a mean age of about forty—and almost all were illiterate. Nearly one-quarter were widowed, and nearly three-quarters were from scheduled (formerly Untouchable) castes (Kumar et al. 1982:14–18). The selection of dais for training does not seem to have aroused the same issues as with CHVs: most of the selection was carried out by female health workers, and the village leadership (after all, male and usually clean-caste) was hardly involved. The rewards for training are much lower for dais than for CHV training, though the stipend paid during training was a considerable financial incentive for poor women, because no honorarium was paid after the training was over. Trained dais are entitled to Rs. 2 for every prenatal case they refer, but such items are very low in budget priorities and often accumulate for many years unpaid.

Narayanan and Acharya (1980:134–164) report that training was generally carried out in inaccessible language and little more than stress on cleanliness and hygiene was actually understood by the dais they interviewed. Changes in the everyday practices of the dais seem to have been few and after training was completed they received little further support from the PHC staff. In Uttar Pradesh, trained dais are more likely to encourage pregnant women to be immunized against tetanus, to get some protection against anemia, and to report following more hygienic practices. But on some simple indicators (the percentage washing their hands with soap or boiling the instrument used to cut the umbilical cord) many of the trained dais reported practices little different from those of the untrained dais (Kumar et al., 1982:81).

PHC staff (especially the ANMs) tend to use the trained dai as an intermediary with the village, to allow them to find prenatal or potential family-planning cases, but very few dais receive the kits, or incentive payments, to which they are entitled (Jeffery et al. 1985; Gandhi and Sapru 1980). In a study based on interviews, 83 percent of trained dais said they liked to work with the ANM, whereas only 39 percent of untrained dais said so, and the trained dais referred about one case a month each to the ANM, whereas untrained dais made no referrals at all (Kumar et al. 1982:97–98). It would be unwise to generalize from this limited material, since the social characteristics of dais and of those selected for training, vary quite considerably throughout the country. The dai is far more significant in the north than in the east and the south, where many infant deliveries take place without a traditional birth attendant being involved; increasing numbers are taking place in clinics and health centers (Jeffery et al. 1985).

Health Services: The Lay Perspective

How do different patients, or potential clients, understand the range of medical options open to them? Posing the question in this way helps to avoid some of the difficulties raised by asking how people choose between medical systems. In a rather unproductive debate along these lines, Banerji (1981) and Djurfeldt and Lindberg (1975) argued that where Western medicine is available, cheap, and of good quality, it will invariably be preferred despite its inability to deal effectively with major diseases of poverty. Western medicines are seen as more powerful and faster-acting, hospitals are overcrowded, and the incomplete information on use rates suggests that Western facilities provide most consultations and consume most health expenditure. In this perspective, indigenous medicine continues only because of the inadequacies of Western medicine, its failure to penetrate throughout the country, or because of the bureaucratic rigidities of government services and the expense of private ones. By contrast, Nichter (1981) and Van der Veen (1981) point out the continuities between the categories of indigenous medicine and those of everyday thought —with prime examples being the use of humoral concepts (hot, cold, windy, etc.) in everyday discussions of the characteristics of climate, food, personality, and body type. Much Western treatment is interpreted through the use of these cultural categories, and many patients who are treated in Western facilities or by Western medicines will also take indigenous therapies to round out their treatment or to deal with likely side-effects of the excessive heat or power of Western remedies.

In addition, Nichter and Van der Veen point to the social context of indigenous therapy, which is usually more sensitive to local social norms than are western-style clinics and hospitals. Thus, Gould (1957) and Marriott (1956) noted that a personal relationship with the healer is important for most patients, but this is unlikely to occur and is unpopular with the staff in large urban institutions. Carstairs (1956), Khare (1963), and Marriott (1956) also point to contrasts in healing style, with indigenous healers more confident in prognosis, less dependent on detailed questioning for diagnosis, and more likely to refer to their personal qualities as a sign of the likely success of their treatment. Patients use patterns of expectations derived from these models as yardsticks to understand and evaluate Western medical practice, which tends to be very different.

The discussion of this question in the past fifteen years has shown, if nothing else, that nobody (either in India or elsewhere) "chooses" a system of medicine, not for one episode of illness, or for all forms of illness, or for one kind of patient or another. The question of choice is sometimes posed in order to demonstrate the superior attractiveness to the Indian populace of one system or another, or to argue that those who "choose" one system are more rational or educated than those who choose another. But research results using this approach have not produced clear-cut distinctions. Thus Madan's study in Ghaziabad concluded that no significant differences existed between those expressing a "preference" for Western medicine, with respect to their urban or rural origin, age, income, and education (1969:1,483–1,484). He also noted that for some people cost was the most important factor. If you belong to an occupational health-insurance scheme, you may use Western medicine just because it is free.

Leslie (1983) suggests that the lay person's search for therapy in India can be characterized as a pluralistic one. People guide their behavior using sets of ideas that may appear logically incompatible (such as ideas of "humoral balance" as well as the "germ theory" of disease). Using this knowledge which they often accept as incomplete, people have to act and they do so in a pragmatic way. They tend to assume that most events have more than one cause and that different types of treatments may be appropriate for each cause. Deciding whom to consult and what treatments to use will be guided by patients' past histories, their relationships with different available healers, costs, and other benefits involved in consultations as well as by a theory about what causes particular illnesses and what treatments are therefore most suited to treat them.

Thus very few people in India make an ideological commitment to a system of medicine. They may, as Djurfeldt and Lindberg (1975) suggest, make commitments to individual healers who are seen as especially useful for particular patients, but these commitments are unlikely to depend on that healer's choice of therapies nor will the commitment necessarily be inherited by whoever replaces that healer. Many healers do not make rigid distinctions among therapies, making use of medicines from more than one system in conjunction, and most patients do the same. Furthermore, patterns of "hierarchies of resort," or tendencies to consult certain kinds of healers first and then others, for some illnesses or for some patients are not consistent or commonly followed. Gould (1957) described a pattern of consulting indigenous medicine for "chronic, nonincapacitating dysfunctions," and Western medicine for "acute, incapacitating" ones. But he himself later argued that this was too simple a model (Gould 1965) and others have similarly found great difficulty in linking diseases (as defined by Western medicine) to healing choices. This is not surprising, since diseases are mediated by social processes and perceived in social terms as illnesses with social meanings already embedded in them. Slightly more surprising is the evidence of a lack of fit between diagnosis and treatment; illnesses may be seen as "caused" by supernatural means but taken to "somatic" healers, or vice versa (Kakar et al. 1972).

In general, then, someone consulting a practitioner does not necessarily accept the philosophical basis of the therapy he or she receives. This is true even for the most complete submission to the moral authority of the healer in hospital wards. Thus Minocha (1974:166–198) discusses the mismatch between patients' and staff's understanding of Western medicine. Patients often mistook diagnostic and curative procedures, queried the role of blood samples and the use of injections, and restricted the information they passed on to the doctor, especially about alternative remedies they had used or continued to take while in the hospital. Kirkpatrick (1976) describes patients who remain oriented to familial expectations rather than those of the hospital staff, and who explain their illness in terms of a diffuse variety of causes (based on karma) despite their willingness to undergo surgery.

Western medical facilities often ignore cultural guidelines in the way they treat patients. As a result, the healing process may be weakened and patients may fail to comply with doctor's orders. Conversely, indigenous healers are much more closely in tune with cultural guidelines and are better able to bring social and psychological forces into play to assist with healing—though we do not know if they are any better at getting patient compliance. But all patients tend to see the systems of medical belief and practice they consult as efficacious—they produce expected results. When several healers are consulted during the same illness episode, allocating success or failure decisively to one or other treatment becomes impossible. In this sense, India is little different from anywhere else.

The balance of choices of healers and treatments will probably continue to shift toward the Western style. Western medicine has more money, more symbolic and practical official support, and weak ideological barriers to its use. But medical pluralism will remain, in part at least, because government services are so often unpopular. Patients, or potential patients, object to the pressures placed on them to limit their family size through sterilization. Often they also find their treatment by health staff humiliating. In this respect, health-staff members are little different from other government employees for whom illiterate peasants are an unwanted burden. Indeed, an indicator of the value placed on Western medicine is how long people are prepared to wait in order to spend a very short time with a doctor who may then insult them while writing an inadequate prescription that may be dispensed by junior staff only after a further wait, taunts, or a bribe.

Conclusion

Since 1947, medical institutions have come under considerable pressure to respond to the major health problems of the mass of the population in rural areas. In some measure they have done so, notably in the establishment of single-disease control programs, and in their management through a structure of PHCs. However, they still do not respond creatively to disease problems. Field staff have followed bureaucratic guidelines during their work, but initiative has remained resolutely in the hands of the people at the top. In the case of malaria control, once the pressure was removed staff relaxed and malaria returned; in the case of smallpox, the program only met its targets after external agencies took a direct interest. Most junior staff follow a least-risk strategy, with staff members filling their forms and keeping their noses clean while collecting enough money and political credit to protect themselves against unwanted transfers.

None of the current models for ensuring competent and motivated health activities is applicable in India. The political party structure cannot provide a local watch on state employees to ensure that they carry out their jobs in a satisfactory manner. Professional structures using internalized norms to provide commitment do not exist. Senior staff may attempt to employ a coercive model, using supervision as a way of finding fault. This is poorly suited to health work. In any case it is not consistently employed. Supervisors cannot implement this model fully because junior staff can call upon political or financial resources to produce support from higher up in the system. The legitimacy of the senior staff is further undermined by the cynicism with which its motives and decisions are usually viewed. How far these conditions are likely to be changed by the new models that underly current proposals forms the subject of the final chapter.

CHAPTER ELEVEN

New Directions in Health Policy?

Around 1970, a watershed occurred in thinking about health-sector organization and the role of international aid, reaching India through international agencies and elite doctors oriented to new ideas from abroad. The new thinking affected international aid and Indian policies on medical personnel during the 1970s. In 1977 the Janata government claimed credit for implementing several of these "new" proposals, derived from plans made during the previous Congress government. These policies have been continued by the new Congress government, if with less enthusiasm. Foreign assistance has supported this shift. The main feature of community health that takes it beyond health planning (Rifkin 1985) are people's participation, integration, and the use of auxiliary health workers. In this concluding chapter I will assess the impact of the new ideas on international aid and on Indian health services, and the prospects for Indian health services in the 1990s.

Health Sector Organization

People's participation had been on the agenda in discussions of primary health centers since 1960 but only became central in a more sophisticated way after 1977. Participation can take a number of forms, depending on which areas of decision making are involved, what the sociopolitical orientations of the organizations are that offer participation, and what the sociopolitical structure and context of the communities are that are being offered participation. Integration has also been an item in discussions of health policy. During the early attempt (under the Community Development Program in the 1950s) to integrate health work with the general work of rural development, little health work was done, perhaps because neither villagers nor workers placed health high on their lists of priorities (Taylor et al 1965). Later discussions in the 1950s and the 1960s merely concerned implementing the integration of curative and preventive care, at the level of the doctors or the administrative structure, which Bhore had called for. In the 1970s integration of the different preventive health campaigns with separate cadres of paramedical workers was a central issue. In both cases, however, integration was restricted to health workers.

Now, the new voluntary sector projects again attempted integration with nonhealth development by addressing the "felt needs" of its members, or on the grounds that water supply or poverty are the main causes of ill health. The expanded use of auxiliary health workers is a final element. Village-level workers are generally drawn from the villages where they work, but projects have varied according to the minimum education they demand. Ideological differences occur between projects using untrained personnel to demystify medicine and those that accept auxiliaries only because of shortages of trained personnel.

Several voluntary projects, some church-related, have been pioneers in implementing the new ideas; others have seen their roles as action research. Yet others have crossed the boundary between the government and voluntary sectors. Despite these differences, I can make some generalizations about what distinguishes the voluntary sector from the government programs.

PARTICIPATION

In implementation or in decision making?: Voluntary sector projects have had varying commitments to participation in decision making. Narangwal, in keeping with its research orientation, hardly involved local people in planning. Gwatkin (Gwatkin et al. 1980:54–55) summarizes the organization as follows:

Community leaders were consulted regularly during the project's execution and community organisations provided support and assistance—

buildings for village health and feeding centres, for example—and financial contributions to the continued operation of project-initiated day-care
centres. Principal responsibility, however, rested with the project
leaders who determined what service would be provided, recruited and
supervised project personnel, and covered well over 90% of project costs
with funds raised from external sources.

At Jamkhed, by contrast, villages could only participate if they
were prepared to make fairly substantial inputs and, in return, their
priorities affected the program. Tube wells, farmers' associations,
and curative services were provided at least in part because of village demands. By 1978, 75 percent of costs were met from local
resources (Hardiman 1984:131). Most other projects have fallen between these examples or involved even less local participation than
in Narangwal. In three of the Maharashtra projects, services have
been delivered with no requirement of village input (Pyle
1979:15–16). Similarly, the larger projects discussed by Faruqee
and Johnson (1982:22–23) have had limited participation by payment for services or provision in kind of some basic material
resources.

In several projects village health committees were given no
resources or power and have failed to create any substantial local
participation. In Tilonia, the staff is made up of young professionals who offer technical services to villages for payment, but
they have also created several social institutions with considerable
local participation (Franda 1979:162–163). Size and the decisions
of charismatic "founders" seem to determine the extent of lay participation. The more conservative organizations (missions, or those
close to right-wing political parties like the Jan Sangh) generally
do not offer participation beyond the chance to be a patient. Participation in implementation seems to depend on participation in
decision making.

In government programs, participation receives no more than
cursory mention. In practice, participation in the selection of village health workers rarely gained any meaning. The further
proposals for local participation involved village health committees
to oversee the work of community health volunteers and to carry
out environmental improvements. While health committees are
part of the received orthodoxy, examples of their successful introduction into government schemes are lacking. Villagers see the
health committee either as part of normal political activity, so that

dominant factions ensure that they control their membership, or as a means of increasing the village's access to government services. Consequently, health committees cannot deliver village-level resources (labor, in kind, or cash) for health improvements. Government plans contain no proposals that might overcome these weaknesses and generate local involvement in environmental sanitation, collective rural insurance, or whatever.

Sociopolitical orientation: Most voluntary organizations offering participation have a social reformist orientation. Organizations with more revolutionary outlooks have rarely been involved in local, small-scale, health projects. An exception is the Left Front government in West Bengal under its Communist party (Marxist) leadership, which has introduced its cadres into the government health machinery through the Community Health Volunteer scheme, but no published reports indicate what this policy has achieved. The least reformist projects are those closest to the government or with a research orientation. Neither Narangwal nor Project Poshak had policy objectives beyond health, nutrition, and family planning. By contrast, the Indo-Dutch project in Andhra hoped to stimulate sufficient local change to allow the original organizers to withdraw, leaving a functioning institution behind them, but they did not succeed in this (Faruqee and Johnson 1982:68–69).

Other projects have tried to generate social change, either working through local institutions (panchayats) as in Maharashtra, or by effectively undermining them by establishing alternative ones. Both Tilonia and the Rural Unit for Health and Social Affairs (RUHSA) threaten local power holders because they offer alternative means of access to scarce, mainly nonhealth, public resources, such as loans and grants. But even the more narrowly health-based projects working with the panchayat may have much wider effects. In Jamkhed, for example, panchayats have been involved from the start. They took little interest at the outset, seeing health issues as nonthreatening, but successful village health workers have now developed political support and can provide alternative perspectives on political issues (Pyle 1979:16–17). Political protection for these projects then becomes vital if they are to continue, despite the absence of revolutionary rhetoric or intent.

In most of India, state governments are run by the Congress party or (in the south) by regional parties. None of these makes great claims that they are trying to change local social structures and, in practice, they are even less reformist. The Congress party is closely tied into local structures of power, economic and social, and tends to draw on the institutions of government (the police, the civil service) to support local party people. When Congress dominates, the political orientation is, at best, reformist, but more usually, it is conservative; if Congress politicians control health committees, participation is unlikely to progress very far.

Local social structures: Most voluntary projects work in socially and economically stratified areas. Those projects that have been reasonably documented are predominantly in states marked by considerable inequality. (None of them is in Kerala, for example.) The Palghar project in Maharashtra included fifteen tribal villages, where inequalities are usually less marked, but the impact of this on project success has not been discussed. In the absence of proposals to change local structures of inequality, the health needs of the poor are unlikely to receive any priority.

INTEGRATION

The application of integration of services has been as varied as participation. Almost all the voluntary projects have attempted some integration, mostly restricted to the health sphere. Exceptions are four of the projects covered by Faruqee and Johnson (1982:18), which dealt only with nutritional inputs and had few contacts even with local primary health care services. In Narangwal, variations in integration set the experimental framework: experimental groups were offered health, medical, nutrition, and family-planning services in different combinations. The focus has often been on services for mothers and children because they are regarded as the most vulnerable sections of the population.

By contrast, projects such as Jamkhed, RUHSA, and Tilonia, offer health services as part of a much broader package. Tilonia is not primarily a health project, though the health component is important. Jamkhed and RUHSA consider general social development as a vital contribution to health goals. As the Aroles, project directors in Jamkhed, put it in 1975 (quoted in Hardiman, 1984:131),

"Local resources such as building, manpower, and agriculture should be used to solve local health problems." The development of local resources is a health goal that can become a priority in itself. Such nonhealth developments may have the greatest chance of affecting health status, particularly of the poorest groups, and may also bring the most integrated projects into conflict with powerful local groups and individuals.

Integrating government services has gone no farther than integration within the health sector. Health assistants and health workers are now expected to turn their hands to whatever work, curative or preventive, is required of them, but the multipurpose program is still not fully implemented in all states. In some measure, integration is a way to bring more workers (especially men) into family planning work. Family planning is the only program of sufficient importance to enable the health services to require support or involvement from other government agencies—revenue, rural development, and police. Can this really be regarded as integration? During the emergency, and, to a lesser extent, since 1981 it has instead been seen by most people as the use of coercive agencies to meet sterilization targets.

At the level of day-to-day dovetailing of health with other social development programs so that they reinforce one another, integration is conspicuous by its absence. Even in the Integrated Child-Development Scheme (ICDS), where the resources are available and both health and education ministries have overt health goals in common, integration is at best partial and inadequate. Integration of plans in New Delhi or at the state capital is so diluted by the time it reaches the district or the block that integration where it really counts—where services are delivered—is almost indiscernible.

AUXILIARY PERSONNEL

Finally, auxiliary personnel are common to voluntary projects and the new government policies, but they vary considerably. In Narangwal, the ANMs and LHVs or their equivalents, who were running most of the experimental programs, were the lowest levels of auxiliary personnel. Village women were only recruited to run crèches. In Jamkhed, village health workers have usually been illiterate middle-aged women. However, as Hardiman

(1984:132) points out, the project founders had intended to use ANMs until they encountered problems in recruiting and placing such women in the project villages. Pyle (1979:20–21) reports that several Maharashtran projects discovered that village workers with less education performed better than educated ones. Almost all report better experience with women than with men, partly because many of these projects have focused on maternal and child health.

Using such women in part-time work with relatively little financial reward is a feature common to the innovative projects. The tasks the women have been expected to perform have varied, developing through experimentation, with new tasks added as workers become more skilled. In Jamkhed, weekly discussions are essentially in-service training to improve diagnostic and other skills. Entrusting increasing responsibilities to these workers generally does not result in any apparent loss of quality of care. Village workers are particularly good at improving the coverage of services compared with workers who are more highly trained and expensive but who lack local knowledge and social contacts with the population to be served. Extensive home visits are almost impossible without cheap, committed local workers, and projects without them (such as Project Poshak) have reported low coverage and high dropout rates (Faruqee and Johnson, 1982:28).

The government programs have failed to deal with the problems posed by using auxiliary health workers without adequate social and political support. At the lowest level, community health volunteers have usually been men, who often see the position as a step in a career ladder toward earning a full-time living through medicine. Women have, in general, been restricted to dai training programs. Further, government programs are hidebound by occupational boundaries; categories are rigidly divided, and cooperation, sharing knowledge, or raising the quality of services through improving morale are incompatible with hierarchical organization and the use by superiors of punishment to achieve conformity. Government staff are not committed to the improvement of health in a particular area because their tenure is limited. No health indicators are used to evaluate their work, only family-planning ones, and even if they are supportive of the program of using local health workers, they will be moved to a new posting almost as soon as they have discovered the contribution different individuals can make.

EFFECTIVENESS OF THE NEW APPROACHES

The results of the innovative voluntary programs, with their differing degrees and types of participation, integration, and use of auxiliary personnel, are interesting, though hardly clear-cut. Narangwal successfully made a considerable impact on local health indicators at relatively low cost despite being narrowly defined in health terms, having little local participation, with considerable integration of health services but little contact with wider development programs, and relying on well-motivated paramedicals, not village health workers. This may be because Punjab has high mortality and morbidity indicators given its relative wealth. Such an approach might be able to overcome a lag in providing health care behind wider social changes, but it might not be suitable in poorer parts of the country. By contrast, the Jamkhed project has also improved health indicators, using very different emphases. Faruqee and Johnson (1982:44) conclude that programs should be tailored to local conditions and that no one model is likely to be suitable everywhere.

The other general conclusion is that the success of these projects is owing largely to the commitment of their founders. Within the organization the enthusiasm of the directors, and their face-to-face contact with the fieldworkers fosters much higher levels of commitment and achievement by the employees than is common in larger organizations. Two major consequences follow: expanding the project beyond a relatively small area is very difficult; and integrating these new proposals within formal bureaucratic structures is likely to be unsuccessful.

The experience of governmental approaches to participation, integration, and the use of auxiliary workers support the argument that these innovations cannot be applied as if they are techniques divorced from a social, economic, and political context. The two lessons of local flexibility and committed leaders cannot be transferred to a government structure which allows initiative to be exercised only by those at the top and in which communications are transferred down the hierarchy but almost never up. Health services follow a health planning model; in India, community development still has to be effectively related to issues of health.

New Patterns in Aid

Does international aid offer any opportunity for over-coming these constraints? Aid following the old orthodoxy was in-tended to modernize by transferring Western institutions and technologies to India. "Best practices" were regarded as universal, and the benefits, for example, of big metropolitan hospitals were expected to trickle down to the mass of the surrounding popula-tion. The new orthodoxy advocates relating technology to economy and culture, calls for a new emphasis on primary care using para-medical workers, simplified techniques appropriate for use in un-derdeveloped countries, and facilities accessible to the mass of the population. It supports linking population programs to maternal and child-health programs, involving local communities in plan-ning and controlling health services, and using indigenous prac-titioners. This requires liberalizing aid terms to increase the grant element and reduce the practice of tying aid to purchases from abroad (World Bank 1975; ODM 1975).

These changes are not very radical. Although the new orthodoxy acknowledges that the sources of ill health might be found in so-cial, political, environmental, and economic arrangements, it nevertheless focuses only on changing the medical infrastructure. The impact of these changes on health may be marginal; but health-aid policies have changed substantially.

RECENT PROJECTS

The Integrated Child-Development Scheme: One feature of more re-cent aid programs has been assistance (largely from UNICEF) to the ICDS. This program was designed in the mid-1970s as a pilot at-tempt to bring together the health services (under ministries of health) and nutrition support (under ministries of social welfare and education). The Community Development Blocks included in the ICDS have an additional doctor attached to the primary health center, and some additional paramedical staff that work with so-cial education officers in monitoring the health and nutrition of children who attend feeding centers run by village nutrition or *an-ganwadi* (courtyard) workers. ICDS blocks are in every district in India, and they have higher funding than ordinary blocks.

However, problems of integration remain and the medical staff often has no real contact with its social-welfare counterpart. Coverage with ICDS blocks is scheduled to expand steadily over the next few years, but the scheme does not have a high profile in the health ministry.

Area Development Projects: Area development is a second feature of aid from 1977 to 1984. The first example was the first India Population Project (IPP-1) in six districts in Uttar Pradesh and three in Karnataka. In 1972 the World Bank agreed to provide loans in "social infrastructure" with substantial amounts for water supply and sanitation projects ($70 million being spent up to 1980) and in health and family planning. The population project received $21 million in loans from the World Bank, $11 million from the Swedish government in grants, and $12.5 million from the Indian government as counterpart funds. The new project was much bigger than most previous ones. Its main aim was to improve rural health delivery, nurse training, management systems, and the integration of family planning with maternal and child-health services. It was intended to be an example to the rest of the country but relatively little was published about the project. Still, it formed the basis of the Model Plan, a document that laid down guidelines for similar projects developed since 1977.

Five projects followed the general pattern established by the Model Plan, each one expected to last five years and dependent on counterpart funds coming from the government of India. One was partially funded by the Danish government grant of $35 million in selected districts of Tamil Nadu and Madhya Pradesh; a second was funded in part by the UNFPA in selected districts of Bihar and Rajasthan; a third, the second India Population Project in parts of Uttar Pradesh and Andhra Pradesh was funded in part by the World Bank for $46 million in loans (the Swedish government withdrew its offer of an additional $23 million in grants); a fourth was partly funded by the British government in Orissa for $25 million; and the fifth was a project partially funded by the United States Agency for International Development (USAID) in districts of five states (Gujarat, Haryana, Himachal Pradesh, Maharashtra, and Punjab) for $33 million.

The projects share a common core derived from the Model Plan, though they vary in detail. (For a comparison of three of these proposals see table 41). The Model Plan's main principle was to speed up the provision of services along the patterns laid down in the plans of the ministry of health and family welfare in New Delhi; this means concentrating expenditures on primary health, in general, and on subcenters (clinics manned by a female multi-purpose workers/auxiliary nurse-midwives) in particular.

The money spent under these projects primarily built new sub-centers, improved multipurpose worker training, provided facilities at primary health centers (e.g., with water supplies or new operation rooms and equipment), and supported family welfare education through films and other simple audiovisual aids. The staff included mainly indigenous midwives, community health workers, and multipurpose workers. The aid agencies, however did not pay honorariums or supply indigenous midwives and CHVs: these were provided from the government of India contribution. Equipment support was low compared to salary, training, and construction.

The common core of these proposals explains their similarities. However, local variations were acknowledged and donor agencies have different approaches. Thus the Danish proposal stressed more community involvement; the British proposal allowed for an extension to the rest of Orissa after a few years; and the American proposal emphasized management training. But all basically accepted that what is needed is more (and better) of what is currently being provided.

In many respects, these projects follow the new orthodoxy, and attempt to apply some of the lessons learned from the voluntary projects. Most funding is available in local currency and for primary care. The focus is on training and employing female health workers, and improving maternal and child health care. Nevertheless, the projects' limitations are obvious. The only community involvement lies in selecting candidates for employment and training as community health workers and indigenous midwives. Community input is virtually nonexistent in planning and executing the project, even in the Dutch program which has a "community chest" for funding elements of felt need that the program does not cover.

While integration of services is an important aspect of the proposals, it may be very lopsided. These are purely "health" programs, with no integration with other aspects of social development. They do not even have any clear relationship with the ICDS.

TABLE 41

Area Development Project Proposals

Category	Tamil Nadu (Danida) %	5 states (USAID) %	Orissa (UK) %
Administration	5	1	2
Construction	25	54	39
Maintenance and utilities	12	*	4
Supplies, equipment and drugs	12	7	16
Transport	*	3	6
Staff training, management, etc.	11	8	3
Additional staff salaries	14	23	27
Nutrition	4	*	1
Communication and media	4	2	1
Community fund, innovations, etc.	11	4	1
Total (Rs. million)	(144)	(518)	(295)
(Donor share)	(88%)	(62%)	(62%)

SOURCES: Strengthening Health Care and Family Welfare in two Districts of Tamil Nadu, mimeo, October 1980; Integrated Rural Health and Population Project—Project Paper, USAID, New Delhi, August 1980; Proposed Area Programme, Government of Orissa, mimeo 1979.

* Categories are not separately recorded.

KEY: USAID, (United States Agency for International Development); UK, United Kingdom.

But though the primary goal is the reduction of the high levels of maternal and infant morbidity and mortality, in the past the services to be financed have been used mainly for family-planning purposes. Few mechanisms can ensure that they will not be suborned in this way again. These aspects of the World Bank-sponsored IPP-2 were the main reasons that the Swedish government withdrew its proposed contribution. They might support the claim by Banerji (1981) that international agencies have encouraged a return to greater compulsion in family planning. This analysis is too simplistic because the donors have all publicly opposed compulsion, and they would face considerable political pressure from domestic constituencies to withdraw support if compulsion were reintroduced. But the agencies may be unable to make their views heard once the projects are completed. The Indian government has been fairly forceful in negotiating this assistance and the donor agencies have had to accept the terms on which they could offer it. The withdrawal of the Swedish contribution suggests the degree of Indian inflexibility.

Finally, the projects depend on the existing health services to deliver and manage the various programs. But two key elements in the success of voluntary-sector projects have been coverage through home visits and personal direction by a committed leadership. Neither of these can be provided by the current government structure. In some states (notably, Bihar) this management structure is so corrupt that it has proved almost impossible to introduce the new program. Elsewhere, state governments have tended to accept the new resources as yet further means of fueling a clientage structure—new jobs to be allocated, new contracts to be awarded, new benefits available to be offered to favored villages and constituencies.

In 1984 the area-development concept lost its preeminence in guiding international aid in India, partly because of some of these problems. Donor agencies have felt that without changing state health services, changes in particular districts can easily be nullified. More emphasis is now placed on training, population propaganda, social research, and improved service delivery. It is too early to assess the impact of this changed emphasis.

Conclusion

It would perhaps be easy to conclude that health policy in India is so closely dominated by national and international class interests that little scope remains for major change. However, that would be only part of the story.

In the first place, it ignores the very real achievements of Indian health policy. Health planners have ensured that resources are allocated to preventive medicine, rural areas, and paramedical workers. Substantial preventive campaigns have been waged against malaria and smallpox. Large numbers of PHCs and subcenters have been built and equipped, and staff have been appointed. In some areas—such as Kerala, or parts of Gujarat—staff have worked fairly conscientiously, albeit generally in those areas that are relatively well-equipped and favored in other ways too. Beneficiaries may have been disproportionately drawn from the higher classes and castes, but the poor have not been totally excluded. The numbers of paramedical staff (admittedly trained and employed on the cheap) have continued to rise, and those now in place could potentially supply most of the population with something approaching a reasonable health service. Some of these services have probably supported the declines in mortality, halting and uncertain though these have clearly been.

One reason for these, perhaps surprising—if qualified—achievements is that the various buttresses of class domination, health policies, health-sector assistance, and even the operations of pharmaceutical companies, are not the most crucial. It is often remarked that health concerns are not very high in people's common priorities, except at times of personal suffering. Radical health-sector proposals (such as nationalization of drug production) are of course energetically opposed by those whose interests are directly affected. Equally, the redistribution of local resources, which might overcome health inequalities or significantly reduce the diseases of poverty, will also be fiercely resisted. But very few health proposals come at all close to such radical ideas. The more notable features of Indian health policy are the shifts toward "appropriate" models. Factors internal to the government and political party structure have limited implementation of even these relatively modest proposals, but still they have been introduced.

Further, the Indian government's achievements appear considerable when measured against those of its neighbor, Pakistan, which shares India's historical legacy. In addition, per capita income levels in Pakistan have been comparable to those in India. Even though Pakistani health policy prior to 1971 allocated public-sector health resources to West Pakistan at the cost of East Pakistan (now Bangladesh), resource constraints have been at much the same levels. However, the Pakistani government has not articulated a coherent health policy or shifted resources toward those sectors identified as priorities—such as rural preventive health campaigns using paramedical personnel.

As in India, allocations to health services in the Plans have been underspent, but in Pakistan the health sector has spent a smaller proportion of its allocation than the other social services (Shepperdson 1981). In the Third Plan (1965–1970) only 59 percent of the health allocation was spent, without taking into account inflation. Hospitals and medical education have generally spent more than they were allocated, though this pattern was disrupted when malaria control programs went wrong more drastically in Pakistan than in India. Rural health programs have been allocated relatively little and have spent even less (ibid.:13–14). Shepperdson notes that "the allocation of development funds continues to be mainly inconsistent with general policy objectives such as the aim to expand rural services rapidly" (ibid.:18). Differentials in the availability of health services are much higher in Pakistan than in India. The ratios of health personnel per 1,000 population are much lower, and the imbalance toward doctors is much greater; in 1974 there were more doctors (10,000) than almost all other health personnel put together, with only dispensers (8,000) approaching that figure. Similarly, there were only 130 rural health centers (1:500,000 population) and 400 subcenters (1:150,000 population) (GOI, 1975:298).

Since the mid-1970s, allocations and expenditures for rural health programs have begun to rise, in real terms and proportionately. New proposals, based on rural health centers for populations of about 100,000, have been introduced. However, even in wealthy Punjab staffing levels in 1980 were very low, with only 30 percent of doctors in post, for example (Asian Development Bank (ADB) 1981:50). Finally, the massive differential in health provisions for government servants on the one hand, and rural peasants on the other, has not declined during the 1970s (Shepperdson 1981:8; Jeffery 1972).

India's position thus depends on the comparative framework employed: If Pakistani experience is used, India looks quite good; if the ideals of the planners and proponents of the "new perspectives" are used, India fares a great deal less well. These patterns are probably owing to features of social organization that are well-captured in Alavi's discussion of levels of the state and their degree of integration. Contrasts between "tight" states and "loose" ones are akin to Myrdal's distinction between hard and soft states. "Tight" states exhibit consistencies among the different levels of the state, and integration is close. In such states, whether conservative (Iran) or radical (China), the class interests dominating the state closely match the structural constraints in which they are set, and the political party system and bureaucracy respond to those interests. "Loose" states are those where integration is much less clear and contrasting pressures may operate to some effect.

In India the levels are less tightly related than in Pakistan. This can be attributed to several decisions made by the Indian political elite soon after independence—the creation of powerful planning mechanisms, the retention of state control over some crucial aspects of the economy, the elimination of *zamindari*—and to features of Indian social organization, such as the greater size and sophistication of the Indian capitalist class and the more secure base of the Indian civil service. This has made possible a political party structure more open in its organization than in most of the Third World, with a diversity of parties and competition for local political resources.

Thus, Indian decision making has been centralized, but it has not been consistent or able to ignore pressures for rural provisions, which socialist and Gandhian rhetoric helped to generate. Nor has it been unchanging. A break in Indian polity and economy occurred around 1964–1966 with the death of Nehru, the coming to power of Mrs. Gandhi, the crisis in planning, and the apparent downturn in industrial growth. This break can be seen (in retrospect) as a shift from "top-down" socialism, to a populist and potentially authoritarian regime. In health-policy terms, the Planning Commission lost much of its centrality, and its control over key aspects of policy (such as the numbers and quality of medical colleges) has become much more difficult to assert. I have termed the socialism "top-down" because, unlike Chinese communism, it involved no grassroots party structure that could either transmit demands up the political or bureaucratic structure or ensure that higher-level decisions were implemented. Indian socialism was largely a matter of the intellectual classes, with no popular roots. The absence of rural roots made it vulnerable to the changes that have largely overtaken politics since 1965: a populism often clearly at odds with the socialist inheritance. But the new populism has no strong village roots either, so its potential for improving health is also limited.

The thread that links the masses at the bottom to the planners at the top is a clientelist political structure. The state derives its coherence from the flow of resources (usually called "black" money) which moves between capitalists, landlords and their dependents, political parties (especially Congress), and members of the government machinery. This flow is essential to maintain the party structure, but it also ensures the protection of the propertied classes. The CHVs who obtain their jobs through patronage have to repay that patronage; the paramedical worker who wants a favorable transfer must please local elites and accumulate financial resources which will eventually end up recycled through the political machinery. The creation of rural resources (such as medical facilities) is part of the currency of local politics, not the implementation of clear-sighted solutions to underlying health problems.

The other factor which seems likely to grow in significance is the threat to health services posed by the family-planning program. Family planning has taken a steadily growing share of health-related expenditure; the Multi-Purpose Workers Scheme has drawn more and more staff into family-planning work, and an increasing share of foreign health aid is directly or indirectly supporting family planning. Family-planning targets are set for all health staff, and in some months family planning totally dominates their activities. This pressure undermines staff-client relationships, often destroying confidence, and staff are tempted into fraud or coercion to meet their targets and avoid punishment (India Today 31 July 1986). The 1986 policy decision for another big push to reduce fertility levels seems bound to exacerbate these problems.

No easy conclusions apply to the whole of the country. In states like Bihar, it is difficult to find any reason for hope. Here the state government is most tightly tied into class forces, and personnel at all levels have to work hard to retain their positions by any possible means. In Punjab and Haryana, relatively wealthy states are beginning to act more decisively against environmental disease. The pressure of rising expectations in these states is fueling greater demands on the clientelistic political structure as well as providing a market for private medical services. Similar pressures can be seen at work in West Bengal and Kerala, where the state governments are freer from class domination. Localized party structures, based on ideological party commitments and drawing support from the poor and landless as well as the landed, have been established in both states, though the effect on health-services organization and achievement is more marked in Kerala than in Bengal (Nag 1983). The only grounds for hope in the Indian experience is the possibility that such local social forces can be mobilized to control the resources which are finally arriving at village level. Such changes depend on prior social and economic changes, and can only progress on a knife-edge, if they are not to be repressed. But there are no signs that such changes are at all imminent in the "Hindi heartland" states of Uttar Pradesh, Madhya Pradesh, Rajasthan, and Bihar in the foreseeable future.

Glossary

ayah:	A female servant
Ayurveda:	"The science of life"—the system of high-culture medicine, looking to Sanskrit sources for its origins
Charaka:	The supposed author of one of the main *Ayurveda* texts
dai:	The Hindi term for a traditional birth attendant
hakim, hakeem:	A practitioner of *Yunan-i Tibb* (see below)
harijan:	"Son of Hari"—the name given by Mahatma Gandhi to untouchable casts
parda-nashin:	A woman living in strict parda
Siddha:	A Tamil variant of *Ayurvedic* medicine
Susruta:	The supposed author of one of the main *Ayurvedic* texts
takavi:	Advance of money to cultivators of sowing time in bad season, or for capital investment
vaid, vaidya:	A practitioner of *Ayurvedic* medicine; said in one text to be descendants of a Brahman father and a vaisya mother
vaisya:	One of the few broad categories of Hindu castes
Yunan-i Tibb:	"Greek medicine"—the system of high-culture medicine introduced to India by Muslim invaders and drawing its inspiration from Greek authors and Avicenna; often transliterated as *Unani* medicine

Bibliography

Aggarwal, A. 1978. "Malaria makes a come-back." *New Scientist.* 2 February, 274.

Ahmed, S. U. 1980. "Urban problems and government policies: A case study of the city of Dacca, 1810–30." In K. Ballhatchet and J. B. Harrison, eds. *The City in South Asia.*

Alavi, H. 1965. "Imperialism, Old and New." *Socialist Register* 241–275.

———. 1972. "The State in Post-Colonial Societies." *New Left Review* 74:59–81.

———. 1975. "India and the Colonial Mode of Production." *Socialist Register,* 160–197. *Economic and Political Weekly,* 10:33–35, 1,235–1,262.

———. 1981. "Structures of Colonial Formation." *Economic and Political Weekly* XVI: 475–486.

Alavi, H., and Shanin, T. 1982. "State and Class under peripheral capitalism." In *Introduction to the Sociology of "Developing Societies."* London: Macmillan.

Alexander, C. A. et al. 1972. "Cost Accounting of Health-Center Expenditures." *Indian Journal of Medical Research* 60: 1,849–1,863.

Alexander, C. A., and M. K. Shivaswamy. 1971. "Traditional healers in a region of Mysore." *Social Science and Medicine* 5, 6: 595–601.

Althusser, L. 1971. *Leninism and philosophy and other essays.* London: New Left Books.

Ambannavar, J. P. 1975. *Long-term Prospects of Population Growth and Labour Force in India.* Bombay: Ford Foundation.

Ambirajan, S. 1978. *Classical Political Economy and British Policy in India*. Cambridge: Cambridge University Press.

Anstey, V. 1936. *The Economic Development of India*. 3rd. ed. London: Longmans.

Antia, N. H. 1985. "An alternative strategy for health care? The Mandwa Project." *Economic and Political Weekly* XX, 51–52: 2,256–2,260.

Arnold, D. 1985a. "Medical Priorities and Practice in Nineteenth-Century British India." *South Asia Research* 5, 2: 167–186.

———. 1985b. "Review of McAlpin 1983." *Journal of Peasant Studies* 12, 4: 132–135.

Arora, V. L., Prakasam, C. P., and Karkal, M. 1980. "Infant Mortality and Its Correlates in Greater Bombay." *Health and Population* 2, 4: 289–299.

Asian Development Bank. 1981. "Appraisal of the Health and Population Project in Pakistan." Mimeographed. Manila: Asian Development Bank.

Balasubrahmanyan, V. 1986. "Towards a women's perspective on family planning." *Economic and Political Weekly* XXI, 2: 69–71.

Balfour, M. I., and Young, R. 1929. *The Work of Medical Women in India*. London: Oxford University Press.

Ballhatchet, K. 1980. *Race, Sex and Class under the Raj*. New Delhi: Vikas.

Ballhatchet, K., and Harrison, J. B., eds. 1980. *The City in South Asia*. London: Curzon Press.

Banerjee, G. N. 1981. *Hellenism in Ancient India*. New Delhi: Munshiram Manoharlal.

Banerji, D. 1971. *Family Planning in India*. New Delhi: People's Publishing House.

———. 1973. "Health behaviour of rural populations: impact of rural health services." *Economic and Political Weekly* VIII, 51: 2,261–2,268.

———. 1974. "Anatomy of the medical profession of India." Mimeographed. New Delhi: Centre of Social Medicine and Community Health, Jawaharlal Nehru University.

———. 1975. "Medical profession and social orientation of health services in India." Mimeographed. New Delhi: Centre of Social Medicine and Community Health, Jawaharlal Nehru University.

———. 1975a. "Social and cultural foundations of health services systems of India." *Inquiry* 12, 2: 70–85.

———. 1978. "Health as a lever for another development." *Development Dialogue* 1: 19–25.

———. 1981. "Treating the Symptoms." *Economic and Political Weekly* XVI, 25–26: 1095–1098.

———. 1983. "National Health Policy and its implementation." *Economic and Political Weekly* XVII, 4: 105–108.

———. 1985. *Health and Family Planning Services in India: an epidemiological, socio-cultural and political analysis and a perspective.* New Delhi: Lok Paksh.

Baran, P. A. 1958. *The Political Economy of Growth.* London: Penguin.

Bardhan, P. 1984. *The Political Economy of Indian Development.* Oxford: Blackwells.

Barnett, A. 1977. *An Introduction to the Health Planning and Budgeting System in India,* Discussion Paper 121. Brighton, Sussex: Institute of Development Studies.

Basham, A. L. 1976. "The practice of medicine in ancient and medieval India." In C. Leslie, ed. *Asian Medical Systems* 18–43.

Basu, B. D. 1936. *History of Education in India under the rule of the East India Company.* Calcutta: Modern Review.

Basu, R. N., et al. 1979. *The Eradication of Smallpox from India.* New Delhi: World Health Organization.

Bayly, C. A. 1979. "English language historiography on British expansion in India and Indian response." In P. C. Emmer and H. L. Wesseling eds. *Reappraisals in Overseas History.* Leiden: Leiden University Press.

Bhagwati, J. N., and Desai, R. 1970. *India: Planning for Industrialisation.* London and New York: Oxford University Press.

Bhang, A., and Patel, A. J. eds. (n.d.). *Health Care: Which Way to Go.* Pune: Medico Friends Circle.

Bhardwaj, 1981. "Homoeopathy in India." In G. R. Gupta, *The Social and Cultural Context of Medicine in India* 31–54.

Bhargava, G. 1983. "Sex-stereotyping and sex-congruency: Components in the role definition of medical specialities in India." *Social Science and Medicine* 17, 5: 1,017–1,026.

Bhatia, B. M. 1967. *Famines in India.* Bombay: Asia.

Bhatia, J. C., et al. 1975. "Traditional healers and modern medicine." *Social Science and Medicine* 9: 15–21.

Bhatt, R. V., et al. 1976. "Migration of Baroda medical graduates 1949–1972." *Medical Education.*

Block, F. 1980. "Beyond relative autonomy." *Socialist Register* 277–242.

Blomstrom, M., and Hettne, B. 1984. *Development Theory in Transition*. London: Zed.

Blunt, E. A. H. 1969. *Castes and Tribes of the North-West Provinces*. New Delhi (reprint of 1901 edition).

Blyn, G. 1961. "Agricultural Trends in India 1891–1947." Ph.D. Dissertation, University of Pennsylvania.

Boserup, E. 1970. *Woman's Role in Economic Development*. London: Allen and Unwin.

Bowers, J., ed. 1973. *Medicine in Chinese Society*. New York: Joseph Macey.

Bradfield, E. C. W. 1938. *An Indian Medical Review*. Delhi: Manager of Publications, Government of India.

Braibanti, R. 1961. *Tradition, Values and Socio-Economic Development*. Durham, N.C.: Durham University Press.

Brass, P. 1972. "The politics of Ayurvedic education." In L. H. and S. I. Rudolph, eds. *Education and Politics in India*. New Delhi: Oxford University Press, 342–371 and 452–459.

Briscoe, J. 1980. "Are Voluntary Agencies Helping to Improve Health in Bangladesh?" *International Journal of Health Services* 10, 1: 47–69.

Bryant, J. 1969. *Health and the Developing World*. Ithaca: Cornell University Press.

CARE. 1980. "Country Program Profile: India." Mimeographed.

Carstairs, M. 1956. "Medicine and faith in rural Rajasthan." In B. D. Paul, (ed.) *Health Culture and Community*. New York: Sage, 107–134.

Cassen, R. 1978. *India: Population, Economy, Society*. London: Macmillan.

Catholic Relief Services. 1979. "India Program: Annual Public Summary of Activities." Mimeographed.

Chandrachud, C. N. 1970. *Memories of an Indian Doctor*. Bombay: Popular Prakashan.

Chapin, G. and Wasserstrom, R. 1983. "Pesticide Use and Malaria Resurgence in Central America and India." *Social Science and Medicine*. 17, 5: 273–290.

Charlesworth, N. 1979. "Trends in the Agricultural Performance of an Indian Province: The Bombay Presidency 1900–1920." In K. N. Chaudhuri, and C. J. Dewey, eds. *Economy and Society*, 113–140.

————. 1982. *British Rule and the Indian Economy, 1800–1914*. London: Macmillan.

Chatterjee, M. 1985. "Health for All: Whither the Child?" *Social Action* 35, 3: 224–240.

Chattopadhyaya, D. P. 1977. *Science and Society in Ancient India*. Calcutta: Research India Publications.

Chaudhuri, K. N., and Dewey, C. J., eds. 1979. *Economy and Society*. New Delhi: Oxford University Press.

Chaudhuri, P. 1979. *The Indian Economy: Poverty and Development*. London: Crosby.

Chenery, H., et al., eds. 1972. *Redistribution with Growth*. London: Oxford University Press.

Chowdhury, Z. 1978. "The paramedics of Savar: An experiment in community health in Bangladesh." *Development Dialogue* 1: 41–50.

Chuttani, C. S., et al. 1973. "Study of private medical practitioners in rural areas of a few States in India." *Indian Journal of Medical Education* 12, 3 and 4: 248–252.

Clark, A. 1986. "Mortality, fertility and the status of women in India, 1881–1931." Paper given at the meeting of the Association for Asian Studies.

Cleaver, H. 1977. "Malaria, the politics of public health and the international crisis." *Review of Radical Political Economy* 9, 1: 81–103.

Cohen, J. M., and Uphoff, N. T. 1980. "Participation's place in rural developments: seeking clarity through specificity." *World Development*.

Cole-King, S. 1977. *Health sector aid from voluntary agencies: The British case study*. Discussion Paper 97. Brighton, Sussex: Institute of Development Studies.

Colombo Plan. 1969. *Annual Report*. Cmnd 9016. London: Her Majesty's Stationery Office.

Commerical Tariffs and Regulations. Resources and Trade. 1847–1848. C 974. London: Her Majesty's Stationery Office.

Coordinating Agency for Health Planning. 1975. *CAHP-TNAI Nursing Survey in India Report*. New Delhi: Coordinating Agency for Health Planning.

Crawford, D. G. 1914. *A History of the Indian Medical Service 1600–1913*. 2 vols. London: W. Thacker.

————. 1930. *The Roll of the Indian Medical Service*. London: W. Thacker.

Croizier, R. C. 1968. *Traditional Medicine and Modern China.* Cambridge, Mass.: Harvard University Press.

―――. 1970. "Medicine and cultural crisis." *Comparative Studies in Society and History* 12, 3: 275–291.

Cursetji, J. J. 1934. "Presidential Address." *Journal of the Indian Medical Association.* 3: 255–262.

Das Gupta, A. 1972. "Study of the historical demography of India." In D. Glass and R. Revelle, eds. *Population and Social Change.* London: Arnold. 419–435.

David, L. H., and Narayana, G. 1983. *Management of Health and Family Welfare Services.* Hyderabad: Administrative Staff College of India.

Davis, K. 1951. *The Population of India and Pakistan.* Princeton N.J.: Princeton University Press.

Dawe, A. 1970. "The two sociologies." *British Journal of Sociology* 21: 2. 207–218.

Dawson Report. 1920. *The Dawson Report on the Future Provision of Medical and Allied Services.* London: Her Majesty's Stationery Office.

de Kadt, E. 1981. "Ideology, social policy, health and health services: A field of complex interactions." *Social Science and Medicine* 15A, 741–52.

de Kadt, E., and Cole-King, S. 1976. *Dutch health aid via voluntary sector.* Discussion Paper 91. Brighton, Sussex: Institute of Development Studies.

Demerath, N. J. 1976. *Birth Control and Foreign Policy.* New York: Harper and Row.

Dewey, C. J. 1978. "Patwari and Chaukhidar: Subordinate officials and the reliability of India's agricultural statistics." In C. J. Dewey and T. Hopkins, eds. *The Imperial Impact.* London: Athlone. 280–314.

―――., eds. 1978. *The Imperial Impact.* London: Athlone.

Digby, W. 1901. *"Prosperous" British India: A Revelation from official records.* Calcutta: T. F. Unwin.

Directorate of Manpower. 1972. *Interim Report of the Working Group on Medical Manpower.* New Delhi: Ministry of Home Affairs.

Djukanovic, V., and Mach, E. P. eds. 1975. *Alternative Approaches to Meeting Basic Health Needs in Developing Countries.* Geneva: World Health Organization.

Donoso, G. 1979. "Weanling diarrhoea: An overview of its nutritional and public health importance." *Indian Journal of Nutrition and Dietetics* 16: 103–113.

Doyal, L., and Pennell, I. 1978. "Pox Britannica: Health, medicine and underdevelopment." *Race and Class* 18, 2: 155–172.

———. 1979. *The Political Economy of Health*. London: Pluto Press.

Dua, B. R. 1981. "India—a study in the pathology of a federal system." *Journal of Comparative and Commonwealth Politics* 19, 3: 257–275.

Dutt, A. K., Akhtar, R., and Dutta, H. M. 1980. "Malaria in India with reference to two west-central States" *Social Science and Medicine*. 14: 317–330.

Dutt, P. R. 1963. *Rural Health Services in India: Primary Health Centre*. New Delhi: Central Health Education Bureau.

Dyson, T. 1979. "A working paper on fertility and mortality estimates for the States of India." Mimeographed.

———, and Crook, N., eds. 1984. *India's Demography*. New Delhi: South Asian Publishers.

———, and Moore, M. P. 1983. "On kinship structure, female autonomy and demographic behaviour in India." *Population and Development Review* 9, 1, 35–60.

Elder, R. E. 1974. "Targets versus extension education: The family planning programme in Uttar Pradesh, India." *Population Studies*, 28, 2: 249–261.

Elling, R. 1979. *Cross-National Studies of Health Services*. New Brunswick: Transaction.

Farmer, B. H. 1986. "Perspectives on the 'Green Revolution' in South Asia." *Modern Asian Studies* 20, 1: 175–199.

Farrell, J. S. 1973. *The siege of Krishnapur*. London: Penguin.

Faruqee, R., and Johnson, E. 1982. *Health, Nutrition and Family Planning in India*. Staff Working Paper 507. Washington D.C.: World Bank.

Filliozat, J. 1964. *The Classical Doctrine of Indian Medicine*. Delhi: Munshiram Manoharlal.

Foster-Carter, A. 1978. "The mode of production controversy." *New Left Review* 107: 47–77.

Franda, M. 1979. *India's Rural Development*. Bloomington: Indiana University Press.

Frank, A. G. 1967. "The sociology of development and the underdevelopment of sociology." In his *Latin America: Underdevelopment or Revolution?* New York: Monthly Review Press, 21–94.

Frankel, F. 1978. *India's Political Economy 1947-77*. Princeton, N.J.: Princeton University Press.

Frankenberg, R. 1981. "Allopathic medicine, profession and capitalist ideology in India." *Social Science and Medicine* 15, 2: 115-125.

Frankenberg, R., and Leeson, J. 1972. "The Sociology of Health Dilemmas in the Post-Colonial World." In E. de Kadt and G. Williams, eds. *Sociology and Development*. London: Tavistock, 255-278.

Frykenberg, R. K. 1965. *Guntur District: 1788-1848*. Oxford: Oxford University Press.

Gaborieau M., and Thorner A., eds. 1981. *Asie du Sud*. Paris: Mouton.

Gadgil, D. R. 1959. *The Industrial Evolution of India in Recent Times*. 3rd. ed. Delhi: Oxford University Press.

Gandhi, H. S., and Sapru, R. 1980. "Dais as Partners in Maternal Health." Mimeographed. New Delhi: National Institute for Health and Family Welfare.

George, K. K., and Gulati, I. S. 1985. "Centre-State Resource Transfers 1951-84: An appraisal." *Economic and Political Weekly* XX, 7: 287-295.

Gill, S. S. 1985. "Return of malaria." *Economic and Political Weekly* XX, 11: 440-441.

Gillion, K. L. O. 1968. *Ahmedabad: A Study in Indian Urban History*. Berkeley: University of California Press.

Gish, O. 1971. *Doctor Migration and World Health*. London: Bell.
———. 1976. "Medical brain-drain revisited." *International Journal of Health Services* 6, 2: 231-237.

Goody, J. 1976. *Production and Reproduction*. Cambridge: Cambridge University Press.

Gopalan, C. 1983. "Development and deprivation." *Economic and Political Weekly* XVIII, 51: 2,163-2,168.
———. 1985. "The Mother and Child in India." *Economic and Political Weekly* XX: 159-166.

Gould, H. A. 1957. "The implications of technological change for folk and scientific medicine." *American Anthropologist* 59: 507-517.
———. 1965. "Modern medicine and folk cognition in rural India." *Human Organisation* 24: 201-208.

Government of India. 1946. *Report of the Health Survey and De-*

velopment Committee (Chair, Sir J. Bhore). 4 vols. New Delhi: Superintendent of Government Printing.

————. 1952. *First Five Year Plan. 1951–1956.* New Delhi: Planning Commission.

————. 1956. *Second Five Year Plan 1956–1961.* New Delhi: Planning Commission.

————. 1960. *Third Plan Draft Outline.* New Delhi: Planning Commission.

————. 1961. *Third Five Year Plan. 1961–1966.* New Delhi: Planning Commission.

————. 1961a. *Report of the Health Survey and Planning Committe.* (Chair, A. L. Mudaliar). New Delhi: Ministry of Health.

————. 1964. *Draft Fourth Plan.* New Delhi: Planning Commission.

————. 1966. *Annual Plan, 1966–1967.* New Delhi: Planning Commission.

————. 1967. *Annual Plan, 1967–1968.* New Delhi: Planning Commission.

————. 1968a. *Annual Plan, 1968–1969.* New Delhi: Planning Commission.

————. 1968b. *Fourth Five Year Plan, 1969–1974.* New Delhi: Planning Commission.

————. 1973a. *Draft Fifth Five Year Plan, 1974–1979.* New Delhi: Planning Commission.

————. 1973b. "Report of the Steering Group on Health, Family Planning, and Nutrition for the Fifth Five Year Plan." New Delhi: Planning Commission. Mimeographed.

————. 1975. *Pocket Book of Health Statistics 1975.* New Delhi: Central Bureau of Health Intelligence.

————. 1978a. *Pocket Book of Health Statistics 1978.* New Delhi: Central Bureau of Health Intelligence.

————. 1978b. *Draft Sixth Five Year Plan, 1978–1983.* New Delhi: Planning Commission.

————. 1981a. *Sixth Five Year Plan, 1980–1985.* New Delhi: Planning Commission.

————. 1981b. *Economic Survey 1980–1981.* New Delhi: Planning Commission.

————. 1983. *Survey on Infant and Child Mortality, 1979.* New Delhi: Office of the Registrar-General.

————. 1983a. *Economic Survey, 1982–1983.* New Delhi: Planning Commission.

————. 1983b. *Sixth Five Year Plan 1980–1985: Mid-Term Appraisal.* New Delhi: Planning Commission.

————. 1984. *Indian Labour Year Book 1983.* New Delhi: Labour Bureau.

————. 1985a. *Sample Registration System 1982.* New Delhi: Office of the Registrar-General.

————. 1985b. *Economic Survey. 1985–1986.* New Delhi: Planning Commission.

————. Central Provincial Health Board. 1948. *Minutes of the Meeting of the Central Provincial Health Board.* New Delhi.

————. (Central Council of Health) "Minutes of the Central Council of Health." Mimeographed. New Delhi. As follows:

1953. First Meeting, Hyderabad: 1953.

1954. Second Meeting, Rajkot: 1954.

1955. Third Meeting, Trivandrum: 1955.

1956. Fourth Meeting, New Delhi: 1956.

1957. Fifth Meeting, Ranchi: 1956.

1958. Sixth Meeting, Bangalore: 1958.

1959. Seventh Meeting, Shillong: 1959.

1960. Extraordinary Meeting, New Delhi: 1960.

1961. Eighth Meeting, Jaipur: 1960; and Special Meeting, New Delhi: 1961.

1962. Ninth Meeting: 1961.

1963. Tenth Meeting, Mahabaleshwar: 1962.

1964a. Eleventh Meeting, Madras: 1963.

1964b. Special Meeting, New Delhi: 1963.

1965a. Twelfth Meeting, Srinagar: 1964.

1965. Special Meeting, New Delhi: 1965.

1967. Thirteenth Meeting, Bangalore: 1966.

1968. Fourteenth Meeting, New Delhi: 1967.

1969. Fifteenth Meeting, Bombay: 1968.

1970. Sixteenth Meeting, Bhopal: 1969.

1973. Seventeenth Meeting, Jaipur: 1972.

1974. Eighteenth Meeting, Bhubaneswar: 1973.

1975. First Joint Meeting of the Central Council of Health and the Central Family Planning Council, New Delhi: 1974.

————. Central Council of Health. 1985. "Agenda notes for the eleventh joint conference of the Central Councils of Health and

Family Welfare." New Delhi: Ministry of Health and Family Welfare.

Government of Orissa: Health and Family Welfare Department. *Annual Administration Reports of the Health and Family Planning (or Welfare) Department 1972–1973 to 1978–1979.* Bhubaneswar: Government of Orissa.

Government of Pakistan. 1975. *Working Papers for the Development Perspective.* Islamabad: Planning Commission.

Greenhough, P. R. "Variolation and Vaccination in South Asia, 1700–1865." *Social Science and Medicine* 14, 3: 345–347.

Griffiths, P. 1952. *The British Impact on India.* London: Cass.

————. 1967. *The History of the Indian Tea Industry.* London: Weidenfeld and Nicholson.

Gujral, J. S. 1973. "Population Growth and Issues in Indian Economic History," Ph.D. Thesis. Washington, D.C.: Georgetown University.

Gumperz, E. M. 1966. "English Education and Social Change in Late Nineteenth Century Bombay 1858–1898." Ph.D. thesis, University of California, Berkeley.

Gupta, G. R., ed. 1981. *The Social and Cultural Context of Medicine in India.* New Delhi: Vikas.

Gupta, S. P., and Datta, K. L. 1984. "Poverty Calculation in the Sixth Plan." *Economic and Political Weekly* XIX: 632–638.

Gwatkin, D. R. 1974. "Health and Nutrition in India." Mimeographed. New Delhi: Ford Foundation.

Gwatkin, D. R., Wilcox, J. R., and Wray, J. D. 1980. *Can Health and Nutrition Interventions Make a Difference?* Washington: Overseas Development Council.

Habib, I. 1982. "Population." In T. Raychoudhuri and I. Habib, eds. *Cambridge Economic History of India.* vol. 1. Cambridge: Cambridge University Press.

Hanson, A. H. 1966. *The Process of Planning.* London: Oxford University Press.

Hardiman, M. G. W. 1984. "Lessons to Be Learnt from Small-Scale Community Health Projects." In T. Dyson and N. Crook, eds. *India's Demography.* 127–140.

Harris, L. 1980. "The State and the Economy." *Socialist Register* 243–262.

Harrison, G. A. 1978. *Mosquitoes, Malaria and Man.* New York: Dutton.

Harrison, J. B. 1980. "Allahabad: A Sanitary History." In K. Ball-hatchet and J. B. Harrison, eds. *The City in South Asia.*

Hartog, P. 1936. *Some Aspects of Indian Education Past and Present.* London: Oxford University Press.

Harvey, W. 1895. "Presidential Address." In *Proceedings of the First Indian Medical Congress.* Calcutta: Indian Medical Gazette.

Hasan, Z. 1980. "Problems of Nationalisation: Case of the Indian Drug Industry 1947–1976." *Indian Journal of Political Science* 41, 2: 232–254.

Hathi, J. L. 1975. *Report of the Committee on Drugs and Pharmaceutical Industry.* New Delhi: Ministry of Petroleum and Chemicals.

Hawthorn, G. P. 1982. "Caste and politics in India since 1947." In D. B. McGillivray ed. *Caste Ideology and Interaction.* Cambridge: Cambridge University Press.

Heston, A. 1983. "National Income." In D. Kumar ed., *Cambridge Economic History of India* vol. 2. Cambridge: Cambridge University Press, 376–462.

Hill, P. 1984. "The Poor Quality of Official Socio-Economic Statistics Relating to the Rural Tropical World." *Modern Asian Studies* 18, 3: 491–514.

Hillier, S. and Jewell, J. A. 1983. *Health Care and Traditional Medicine and Communist China.* London: Routledge and Kegan Paul.

Hooton, J. 1928. "Medical Relief in Villages." *Indian Medical Gazette* 265–269.

Hughes, C. C., and Hunter, J. M. 1970. "Disease and Development in Africa." *Social Science and Medicine* 3, 4: 443–488.

Hume, J. 1977. "Medicine in the Punjab, 1849–1911." Ph.D. thesis, Duke University.

————. 1979. "Rival Traditions: Western Medicine and 'Yunan-i Tibb' in the Punjab, 1849–1889." *Bulletin of the History of Medicine* 51: 214–231.

————. 1984. "Colonialism and Sanitary Medicine: The Development of Preventive Health Policy in the Punjab 1860–1900." Mimeographed.

Illich, I. 1976. *Medical Nemesis.* London: Boyars.

Indian Council for Social Science Research. 1975. *Report of the Committee on the Status of Women in India.* New Delhi.

Indian Statutory Commission. 1928. "Memorandum Submitted by the Government of Punjab." Lahore.

Institute of Applied Manpower Research. 1971. *Supply of Doctors during Fourth and Fifth Plans.* New Delhi: Institute of Applied Manpower Research.

————. 1974. "Stock of High Level Manpower: Allopathic Graduates, 1971, 1974 and 1979." Mimeographed. New Delhi: Institute of Applied Manpower Research.

Islam, M. M. 1978. *Bengal Agriculture 1920-1946.* Cambridge: Cambridge University Press.

Iyengar, N. S., and Suryanarayana, M. H. 1984. "On poverty indicators." *Economic and Political Weekly* XIX: 897-902.

Jaggi, O. P. 1979a. *Western Medicine in India: Medical Education and Research.* Delhi: Atma Ram.

————. 1979b. *Western Medicine in India: Public Health and Administration.* Delhi: Atma Ram.

————. 1980. *Western Medicine in India: Social Impact.* Delhi: Atma Ram.

Jain, A. K., and Adlakha, A. L. 1984. "Estimates of Fertility Decline in India during the 1970s." In Dyson, T. and Crook, N. eds. *India's Demography.* 37-54.

Jain, J. K. 1974. "The Challenge." In Diamond Jubilee Celebration Souvenir. New Delhi: Delhi Medical Association.

Jeffery, P. M., and Jeffery, R., Lyon, A. 1985. *Contaminating States: Midwifery, the State and Women's Status in Rural North India.* New Delhi: Indian Social Institute.

Jeffery, P. M., Jeffery, R., and Lyon, A. 1988. Labour Pains and Labour Power. London: Zed Press.

Jeffery, R. 1972. "The Health System of Pakistan." Mimeographed.

————. 1973. "Hospital Casualty Departments in Bristol and Lahore." M.Sc. thesis, Bristol University.

————. 1974. "Health plans and Health Policies: The Case of Pakistan." in J. Cook et al. eds. *Appropriate Technology and Economic Development.* Edinburgh: Centre for African Studies, 443-454.

————. 1976. "Migration of Doctors from India." *Economic and Political Weekly* XI, 13: 502-507.

————. 1977. "Estimates of Doctors in Delhi." *Economic and Political Weekly* XII, 5: 132-135.

―――. 1978a. "Allopathic Medicine in India: A Case of Deprofessionalisation?" *Social Science and Medicine* 11, 10: 561–573.

―――. 1978b. "The State and Primary Health Care in India." Paper presented to the International Sociological Association, Uppsala, Sweden.

―――. 1979. "Recognising India's Doctors: The Establishment of Medical Dependency, 1918–39." *Modern Asian Studies*, 13, 2: 301–326.

―――. 1980. "Indian Medicine and the State." *Bulletin of the British Association of Orientalists* 11: 58–70.

―――. 1981. "Medical Policy-Making in India in the 1970s: Out of Dependency?" in M. Gaborieau and A. Thorner, eds. 525–530.

―――. 1982. "Policies towards indigenous healers in Independent India." *Social Science and Medicine* 16: 1835–1842.

―――. 1986a. "New Patterns in Health Sector Aid to India?" *International Journal of Health Services,* 16, 1: 121–139.

―――. 1986b. "Health Planning in India, 1951–79: The contribution of the Planning Commission." *Health Policy and Planning,* 1, 2: 127–137.

―――. 1987. "Doctors and Congress: The Role of Medical Men and Medical Politics in Indian Nationalism." In M. Shepperdson and C. Simmons, eds. *The Indian National Congress and the Political Economy of India, 1885–1985.* London: Gower.

Jobert, B. 1985. "Populism and Health Policy: The Case of Community Health Volunteers in India." *Social Science and Medicine* 20, 1: 1–28.

Johnson, T. J. 1972. *Professions and Power.* London: Macmillan.

―――. 1973. "Imperialism and the Professions." In P. Halmos ed. *Professionalisation and Social Change.* Keele: Sociological Review Monograph, 20.

―――. 1978. "The Professions in the Class Structure." In R. Scase, ed. *Industrial Society: Class, Cleavage and Control.* London: George Allen and Unwin, 93–110.

Johnson, T. J., and Caygill, M. 1973. *Community in the Making.* London: Institute of Commonwealth Studies.

Jolly, J. 1977. *Indian Medicine.* 2nd. ed. Delhi: Munshiram Mancharlal.

Kakar, D. N., Srinivas Murthy, S. K., and Parker, R. L. 1972. "People's Perception of Illness and Their Use of Medical Care Services in Punjab." *Indian Journal of Medical Education* 11, 4: 286–298.

Kakar, S. 1982. *Shamans, Doctors and Mystics.* Delhi: Oxford University Press.

Karkal, M. 1985. "Maternal and Infant Mortality." *Economic and Political Weekly* XX, 43: 1835–1837.

Kerr, I. J. 1980. "Social Change in Lahore, 1849–75." *Journal of Indian History* LVII: 281–302.

Kessinger, T. J. 1974. *Vilyatpur 1848–1968.* Berkeley, Los Angeles, London: University of California Press.

Khaliq, Z. 1976. "The Indian Government and Multinationals." Ph.D. Dissertation, Pennsylvania State University.

Khan, M. E., and Prasad, C. B. 1985. *Health Financing in India: A Case Study of Gujarat and Maharashtra.* Baroda: Operations Research Group.

Khare, R. S. 1963. "Folk Medicine in a North Indian village." *Human Organisation* 22, 1: 36–40.

Kidron, M. 1965. *Foreign Investments in India.* London: Oxford University Press.

Kiernan, V. G. 1974. *Marxism and Imperialism.* London: Arnold.

King, M., ed. 1966. *Medical Care in Developing Countries.* Nairobi: Oxford University Press.

Kirkpatrick, J. 1976. "Primary and Secondary Institutions in the Delivery of Hospital Services in South Asia." *Journal of the Institute of Bangladesh Studies* 1, 1: 169–190.

Klein, I. 1972. "Malaria and Mortality in Bengal, 1840–1921." *Indian Economic and Social History Review* 11: 132–160.

———. 1973. "Death in India." *Journal of Asian Studies* 32, 4: 639–659.

———. 1974. "Population and Agriculture in Northern India 1872–1921." *Modern Asian Studies* 8, 2: 191–216.

———. 1984. "When the Rains Failed: Famine, Relief, and Mortality in British India." *Indian Economic and Social History Review* 21, 2:185–214.

Kocher, J. E. 1980. "Population Policy in India." *Population and Development Review* 6, 2: 299–310.

Krishnaji, N. 1984. "Family Size, Levels of Living and Differential Mortality in Rural India." *Economic and Political Weekly* XIX: 248–258.

Kumar, A., Chauhan, A. S., and Pandey, S. K. 1982. *Report of Evaluation of Traditional Birth Attendants (Dais) in the State of Uttar Pradesh*. Lucknow: Population Centre.

Kumar, D. 1965. *Land and Caste in South India*. Cambridge: Cambridge University Press.

———. ed. 1983. *Cambridge Economic History of India*. Vol. II, c1757–c1970. Cambridge: Cambridge University Press.

Kumar, R. R. 1968. *Western India in the Nineteenth Century*. London: Routledge and Kegan Paul.

Kurien, M., ed. 1975. *India: State and Society*. Madras: Orient Longman.

Kutumbiah, P. 1962. *Ancient Indian Medicine*. Madras: Orient Longman.

Kynch, J. 1985. "Indian Women: Famine and Medical Relief." Mimeographed.

Lall, S. 1977. "Medicines and Multinationals." *Monthly Review* 28, 10: 19–30.

Lalonde, M. 1975. *A New Perspective on the Health of Canadians*. Ottowa: Information Centre.

Lampton, D. 1974. "Health Policy During the Great Leap Forward." *China Quarterly* 60: 668–698.

———. 1977. *The Politics of Medicine in China*. Kent: William Dawson.

Leitner, G. 1882. *History of Indigenous Education in the Punjab since Annexation and in 1882*. Calcutta: Superintendent of Government Printing.

Leslie, C. 1968. "The professionalisation of Ayurvedic and Unani Medicine." *New York Academy of Sciences*, Series 2, 30, 4: 559–572.

———. 1973. "The professionalising Ideology of Medical Revivalism." In M. Singer, ed. *Entrepreneurship and Modernisation of Occupational Cultures in South Asia*. Durham, N.C.: Durham University Program in Comparative Studies in South Asia, 216–242.

———. 1974. "The Modernisation of Asian Medical Systems." In J. J. Poggie and R. N. Lynch, eds. *Rethinking Modernisation*. New York: Greenwood, 69–108.

———. 1975. "Pluralism and Integration in the Indian and Chinese Medical Systems." In A. Kleinman et al., eds. *Medicine in*

Chinese Cultures. Washington D.C.: Government Printing Office, 401–417.

————. ed. 1976. *Asian Medical Systems*. Berkeley, Los Angeles, London: University of California Press.

————. 1981. "What caused India's Community Health Volunteer Programme." Mimeographed.

————. 1983. "Social Research and Health Care Planning in South Asia." Mimeographed.

Lipton, M., and Firn, J. 1976. *The Erosion of a Relationship: India and Britain since 1960*. London: Oxford University Press.

Lucas, A. E. 1982. *Chinese Medical Modernization*. New York: Praeger.

McAlpin, M. B. 1983. *Subject to Famine*. Princeton, N.J.: Princeton University Press.

McGuire, G. 1929. "Hints on the Village Nurse Scheme." *Indian Medical Gazette* 95–99.

McKeown, T. S. 1965. *Medicine in Modern Society*. London: Allen and Unwin.

Madan, T. N. 1972. "Doctors in a North Indian City: Recruitment, Role Perception and Role Performance." In S. Saberwal, ed. *Beyond the Village*. Simla: Indian Institute of Advanced Studies, 77–110.

————. ed. 1980. *Doctors and Society: Three Asian Case Studies*. New Delhi: Vikas.

Maddison, A. 1971. *Class Structure and Economic Growth*. London: George Allen and Unwin.

Marriott, M. 1955. "Western Medicine in a Village of Northern India." In B. F. Paul, ed. *Health, Culture and Community*. New York: Russell Sage, 239–268.

Marwah, S. M., et al. 1978. *Health Profile of Chiraigaon Block*. Varanasi: Banaras Hindu University Press.

Marx, K. 1973. "The Future Results of British Rule in India." In his *Surveys from Exile*. London: Penguin, 319–325.

Mathur, I. 1975. *Interrelations in an Organisation*. Jaipur: Aalekh.

Mathur, P. N. "Demand and Supply of Doctors in India, 1951–1986." *Manpower Journal* 7, 1–2: 58–96.

Medawar, C., and Freese, B. 1982. *Drug Diplomacy*. London: Social Audit.

Medical Reports Selected by the Medical Board from the Records of Their Office. 1850. Madras: Government Press.

Mejia, A., et al. 1979. *Physician and Nurse Migration*. Geneva: World Health Organization.

Meller, H. 1979. "Urbanisation and the Introduction of Modern Town Planning Ideas in India 1900–1925." In K. N. Chaudhuri and C. J. Dewey, eds. *Economy and Society*, 330–350.

Melrose, D. 1982. *Bitter Pills*. Oxford: Oxfam.

Metcalf, B. 1985. "Nationalist Muslims in British India: The Case of Hakim Ajmal Khan." *Modern Asian Studies* 19, 1: 1–28.

Meyer, M. L. 1967. "A Comparative Analysis of the Indian Government's Relationships with World Health Organization, United Nations Educational, Scientific and Cultural Organization, and the Economic Commission for Asia and the Far East." Ph. D. thesis, University of Pennsylvania.

Minkler, M. 1977. "Consultants or colleagues: the Role of U.S. Population Advisers in India." *Population and Development Review* 3: 403–419.

Minocha, A. 1974. "Some Aspects of the Social System of an Indian Hospital." Ph.D. thesis, Delhi University.

Mishra, S. C. 1983. "On the Reliability of Pre-Independence Agricultural Statistics in Bombay and Punjab." *Indian Economic and Social History Review* 20: 171–190.

Mitra, A. 1978. *India's Population: Aspects of Quality and Control.* 2 vols. New Delhi: Abhinav Publications.

Montgomery, E. 1976. "Systems and Medical Practitioners of a Tamil Town." In C. Leslie ed., *Asian Medical Systems*, 272–284.

Moore, M. P. 1980. "Public Bureaucracy in the Post-Colonial State: Some Questions on 'Autonomy' and 'Dominance' in South Asia." *Development and Change* 11, 137–148.

Moore, R. J. 1966. *Liberalism and Indian Politics 1872–1922*. London: E. Arnold.

Moreland, W. H. 1920. *India at the Death of Akbar*. London: Macmillan.

Morley, D. 1972. *Paediatric Priorities in the Developing World.* London: Butterworths.

Morris, M. D. 1963. "Toward a Reinterpretation of Nineteenth-Century Indian Economic History." *Journal of Economic History* 23, 4: 606–618.

———. 1968. "Trends and Tendencies in Indian Economic History." *Indian Economic and Social History Review* 5, 4: 319–388.

―――. et al. 1969. *Indian Economy in the Nineteenth Century.* Delhi: Indian Economic and Social History Association.

―――. 1974. "The Population of All-India, 1800–1951." *Indian Economic and Social History Review* 11: 309–313.

Mukherji, B. 1965. *Levels of Economic Activity and Public Expenditure in India.* Poona.

Muller, M. 1982. *The Health of Nations.* London: Faber and Faber.

Murthy, A. K. Srinivas, and Parker, R. L. 1973. "New Methods for Assessing Health Care Delivery System." *Indian Journal of Medical Education* 12, 3 and 4: 269–277.

Myrdal, G. 1968. *Asian Drama.* 3 vols. London: Allen Lane.

Nag, M. 1984. "Fertility differential in Kerala and West Bengal." *Economic and Political Weekly* XIX: 33–41.

Naoroji, D. 1901. *Poverty and Un-British Rule in India.* London: Sonnenschein.

Narayana, G. and Acharya, J. 1981. *Problems of Field Workers: Study of Eight Primary Health Centres in Four States.* Hyderabad: Administrative Staff College of India.

National Institute of Health and Family Welfare. 1978. *An Evaluation of Community Health Workers Scheme.* New Delhi: Technical Report 4.

National Planning Committee. 1946. *Report of the Subcommittee on Public Health.* Bombay: National Planning Committee of the Congress Party.

Navarro, V. 1974. "The Underdevelopment of Health and the Health of Underdevelopment." *International Journal of Health Services* 4, 1: 5–27.

―――. 1975. "The Industrialisation of Fetishism or the Fetishism of Industrialisation: A Critique of Ivan Illich." *Social Science and Medicine* 9, 7: 351–363.

Neelamegham, A. 1963. *Development of Medical Societies and Medical Periodicals in India 1780–1920.* Calcutta: Oxford.

Neumann, A. K., et al. 1971. "Role of The Indigenous Medicine Practitioner in Two Areas of India—Report of a Study." *Social Science and Medicine* 5, 2: 137–149.

Newell, K., ed. 1975. *Health By the People.* Geneva: World Health Organization.

Nichter, M. 1981. "Toward a Culturally Responsive Rural Health-Care Delivery System in India." In G. R. Gupta ed. *The Social and Cultural Context of Medicine in India.* New Delhi: Vikas. 223–236.

Oakley, A. 1985. *The Captive Womb.* Oxford: Blackwell.

Overseas Development Administration. 1971. *Medical Aid.* London: Overseas Development Administration.

Overseas Development Ministry. 1975. *More Aid for the Poorest.* London: Overseas Development Ministry.

———. 1978. *Review of British Health Aid to Developing Countries 1974-76.* London: Overseas Development Ministry.

Panikar, P. G. K. 1980. "Resources Not the Constraints on health improvement: a case study of Kerala." In M. Gaborieau and A. Thorner, eds. *Asie du Sud.* 549–557.

Papers Showing the Progress of Education Since the Year 1866. 1870. HC 397. London: Her Majesty's Stationery Office.

Papers Respecting the Organisation of the Medical Services. 1881. C 2921. London: Her Majesty's Stationery Office.

Patel, A. J., ed. 1977. *In Search of Diagnosis.* Pune: Medico Friends Circle.

Paul, S. 1984. "Mid-Term Appraisal of the Sixth Plan." *Economic and Political Weekly* XIX: 760–765.

Payne, P., and Cutler, P. 1984. "Measuring Malnutrition." *Economic and Political Weekly* 19, 34: 1485–1487.

Pfleiderer, B. 1981. "Patterns of traditional therapeutic drama in Northern India." Mimeographed.

Piotrow, P. T. 1973. *World Population Crisis: The U.S. Response.* New York: Praeger.

Powles, J. 1973. "On the limitations of modern medicine." *Science Medicine and Man* 1, 1: 1–30.

Preston, S. H., and Bhat, P. N. Mari. 1984. "New evidence on fertility and mortality trends in India." *Population and Development Review* 10, 3: 481–503.

Pyle, D. F. 1979. "Voluntary agency-managed projects delivering an integrated package of health, nutrition and population services: the Maharashtra experience." Mimeographed. New Delhi: Ford Foundation.

Quinn, J., ed. 1972. *Medicine and Public Health in the People's Republic of China.* Washington D.C.: Fogarty International Center.

Raffel, M. W. 1984. *Comparative Health Systems.* University Park: Pennsylvania State University Press.

Ram, R., and Schultz, T. W. 1979. "Life-span, health, savings and productivity." *Economic Development and Cultural Change*, 27, 3: 399–421.

Ramachandran, N., and Shastri, S. S. 1983. "Movement for Medical Treatment: A Case Study of Rural India." *Social Science and Medicine* 17, 3: 177–187.

Ramalingaswami, P., and Neki, K. 1971. "Students' preference of specialities in an Indian medical college." *British Journal of Medical Education* 5, 3: 204–9.

Ramalingaswami, P., and Shyam, A. 1980. "Perceptions of primary Health Care by Medical Students." Mimeograph. New Delhi: Centre of Social Medicine and Community Health, J.N.U.

Ramalingaswami, V. 1980. *Health for All: an Alternative Strategy* Report of the Indian Council of Social Science Research and Indian Council of Medical Research Joint Study. Mimeographed.

Ramasubban, R. 1982. "Public Health and Medical Research in India: Their Origins under the Impact of British Colonial Policy." Stockholm: SAREC Report No. 4, Swedish Agency for Research Cooperation with Developing Countries.

Ramasubban R. 1984. "The Development of Health Policy in India." In T. Dyson and N. Crook, eds. *India's Demography*. 97–116.

Rangarao, B. V. 1975. "Indian Drug Industry." *Mainstream* 1, 8, and 15 March.

Rath, N. 1985. " 'Garibi Hatau': Can IRDP Do It?" *Economic and Political Weekly* XX: 238–246.

Ray, K. S., ed. 1929. *The Problems of the Medical Profession in India*. Calcutta: All-India Medical Association.

Rayappa, P. H., and Prabhakara, N. R. 1981. "Patterns of Population Growth in Southern States." *Economic and Political Weekly* 18, 48: 2,018–2,031.

Reddy, K. N. 1972. *The Growth of Public Expenditure in India 1872–1966*. Delhi: Sterling.

Reddy, M. 1983. "Drug shortage in Primary Health Centres." *Indian Journal of Social Work* 44, 3: 273–278.

Reid, M. 1969. *A Study of the Activities of Auxiliary Nurse-Midwives in Haryana, Punjab and Gujarat States, India*. New Delhi: World Health Organization.

Report of the Select Committee on Indian Territories. 1852. C 533. London: Her Majesty's Stationery Office.

Rifkin, S. 1985. *Health Planning and Community Participation.* London: Croom Helm.

Rockefeller Foundation. 1972. *Directory of Fellowships and Scholarships 1917-1970.* New York: Rockefeller Foundation.

Roemer, M. I. 1977. *Comparative National Policies on Health Care.* New York: Dekker.

Rosenthal, D. B. 1970. "Deurbanisation, Elite Displacement and Political Change in India." *Comparative Politics* 2, 2: 169-201.

Roxbrough, I. 1979. *Theories of Underdevelopment.* London: Macmillan.

Roy, B. C. 1964. *Towards a Prosperous India.* Calcutta: Pulia Bihari Sen.

Rudolph, L. I., and Rudolph, S. H. 1981. "Judicial Review Versus Parliamentary Sovereignty: The Struggle Over Stateness in India." *Journal of Commonwealth and Comparative Politics* 19, 3: 231-256.

Ruzicka, L. T. 1984. "Mortality in India: Past Trends and Future Prospects." In T. Dyson and N. Crook, eds. *India's Demography.* New Dehli: South Asian Publishers, 13-36.

Ruzicka, L. T., and Hansluwka, H. 1982. "Mortality trends in South and East Asia: Technology Confronts Poverty." *Population and Development Review* 8, 3: 567-588.

Sanitary Commission. 1865. *Report of the Commission Appointed to Enquire into the Sanitary State of the Army in India.* C 3184. London: Her Majesty's Stationery Office.

Satpathy, S. K. 1978. "Cost Accounting of P.H.C. Expenditure." M.D. thesis. Banaras Hindu University.

Saul, J. S. 1974. "The State in Post-Colonial Societies: Tanzania." *Socialist Register* 349-372.

Scrimshaw, N. S., et al. 1968. *Interactions of Nutrition and Infection.* Geneva: World Health Organization.

Scrip. 1985. *Yearbook.*

Seal, A. 1968. *The Emergence of Indian Nationalism.* Cambridge: Cambridge University Press.

Seal, S. C., and Bose, J. 1973. *A Study of Morbidity Patterns and Standard of Medical Care in the Rural Health Centres of West Bengal.* New Delhi: Indian Council of Medical Research.

Segall, M. 1972. "The Politics of Health in Tanzania." *Development and Change,* 4, 1: 39-50.

Sen, A. K. 1980. *Poverty and Famines.* London: Oxford University Press.

Seth, R. K. 1973. "O. R. in Health Care Delivery—Rural Health Training Centre, Najafgarh." *Indian Journal of Medical Education* 12, 3 and 4: 256–263.

Shenoy, B. R. 1974. *PL-480 Aid and India's Food Problem.* New Delhi: Affiliated East-West Press.

Shepperdson, M. 1981. "Health Policies and Planning in Pakistan." Mimeographed. Swansea: Centre for Development Studies.

Shepperdson, M. 1986. "Aspects of Health Policy." Paper given at the 9th European Conference on Modern South Asian Studies, Heidelberg.

Shiva, M. 1985. "Drug Policy and Drug Issues." *Social Action* 35, 3: 267–277.

Siddiqi, M. Z. 1959. *Studies in Arabic and Persian Medical Literature.* Calcutta: Calcutta University.

Sidel, V. 1972. *Serve the People.* New York: Monthly Review Press.

Simmons, G., et al. 1982. "Post Neo-natal Mortality in Rural India." *Demography* 19, 3: 371–389.

Singer, H. W. 1965. "External Aid: For Plans or Projects?" *Economic Journal* 75: 539–545.

Singh, H. M. 1983. "Research and Policy Measures Concerned with Improving Economic Efficiency in the Health Care Delivery System of India." *International Social Security Association Studies and Research* 19: 77–85.

Sinha, N. P. 1976. "Malaria Eradication: What Went Wrong?" *Economic and Political Weekly* XI: 946–947.

Srivastava, J. B. 1975. *Report of the Group on Medical Education and Support Manpower.* Mimeographed. New Delhi: Ministry of Health and Family Planning, Government of India.

Steinthal, B. J. 1984. "The Ayurvedic Revivalist Movement in Early Twentieth-Century British India." B.A. thesis, Harvard University.

Stoker, A. 1984. "Technology Transfer in the Indian and Indonesian Pharmaceutical Industries." Ph.D. thesis, University of Edinburgh.

Stoker, A., and Jeffery, R. 1987. "Pharmaceuticals and Health Policy in India." *Social Science and Medicine* (in press).

Stokes, E. 1959. *The English Utilitarians and India.* Oxford: Clarendon Press.

Streeten, P., and Lipton, M. eds. 1968. *The Crisis of Indian Planning*. London and New York: Oxford University Press.

Sundaram, K., and Tendulkar, S. D. 1983. "Poverty in the Mid-Term Appraisal." *Economic and Political Weekly* XVIII, 45: 1,928–1,935.

————. 1984. "More on poverty in the MTA." *Economic and Political Weekly* XIX: 1,003–1,006.

Sutherland, W. D. 1978. "A Systems Analysis of a Rural Primary Health Centre in India." M. Community Health Thesis, University of Liverpool.

Sykes, W. H. 1847. "Statistics of the Government Charitable Dispensaries of India, Chiefly in the Bengal and North-Western Provinces." *Quarterly Journal of the Statistical Society of London*: 1–37.

Takulia, H. S. et al. 1967. *The Health Centre Doctor in India*. Baltimore: Johns Hopkins Press.

Tampi, N. K. 1931. "Rural health work in Travancore State, South India." *Indian Medical Gazette* 690–694.

Tata. 1982. *A Pocket Book of Indian Statistics*. Bombay: Tata Economic Services.

Taylor, C. C., et al. 1965. *India's Roots of Democracy*. Bombay: Orient Longman.

Taylor, C. E., et al. 1976. *Doctors for the Villages*. London: Asia.

Thompson, E. P. 1979. *The Poverty of Theory*. London: New Left Books.

Thorner, A. 1983. "Semi-Feudalism or Capitalism: Contemporary Debates on Classes and Modes of Production in India." *Economic and Political Weekly* XVIII, 49, 50, and 51.

Thorner, A., and Thorner, D. 1962. *Land and Labour in India*. Bombay: Asia Publishing House.

Times of India. (various years). *Directory and Yearbook*. Bombay: Times of India.

Tinker, H. 1974. *A New System of Slavery*. London: Oxford University Press.

Tomlinson, B. R. 1986. "Issues in the Economic and Social history of Modern South Asia: 1880–1960." Paper given at the Review Workshop on Modern South Asian Studies, Cambridge.

Toye, J. F. J. 1979. *Public Expenditure and Indian Development Policy 1960–1970*. Cambridge: Cambridge University Press.

Ullmann, M. 1978. *Islamic Medicine*. Edinburgh: Edinburgh University Press.

United Nations. 1961. *Mysore Population Study.* Delhi: Oxford University Press.

United Nations Children's Fund. 1975. *Master Plan of Operations for a programme of services in India.* New Delhi: UNICEF.

United Nations Conference on Trade and Development. 1975. *The Reverse Transfer of Technology.* TD/B/AC.11/25/Rev.1 New York: United Nations.

United Nations Conference on Transnational Corporations. 1983. *Transnational Corporations in the Pharmaceuticals Industry of Developing Countries.* New York: United Nations.

United Nations Industrial Development Organization. 1978. *Assessment of the Pharmaceuticals Industry in Developing Countries* ID/WG.292/2. Vienna.

————. 1980. *Global Study of the Pharmaceutical Industry.* ID/WG.331/6. Vienna.

Urry, J. N. 1980. *The Anatomy of Capitalist Societies.* London: Macmillan.

Van der Veen, K. 1981. "Socio-Cultural Aspects of Care in Valsad District, Gujarat State." In Gupta; G. R. ed. 168–193.

Venkataratnam, R. 1979. *Medical Sociology in an Indian Setting.* Madras: Macmillan.

Vicziany, M. 1983. "Coercion in a soft-state: the family planning programme of India." *Pacific Affairs* 55, 3: 373–402 and 55, 4, 557–592.

Visaria, L. 1985. "Infant mortality in India: level, trends and determinants." *Economic and Political Weekly* XX, 32: 1,352–1,359; 33, 1399–1405, and 34, 1,447–1,450.

Visaria, P. 1969. "Mortality and fertility in India, 1951–61." *Milbank Memorial Fund Quarterly.* 47, 1: 91–116.

————. 1971. *The Sex Ratio of the Population of India.* 1961 Census Monograph No. 10. New Delhi: Office of the Registrar-General.

Visaria, P., and Visaria, L. 1981. "Indian population scene after the 1981 Census." *Economic and Political Weekly* 16, 44: 1,727–1,780.

————. 1983. "Population (1757–1947)." In D. Kumar, ed. *Cambridge Economic History of India.* 462–532.

Wade, R. 1984. "Irrigation reform in conditions of populist anarchy." *Journal of Developing Economies* 14, 3: 285–303.

Warren, B. 1980. *Imperialism: Pioneer of Capitalism.* London: Verso.

Washbrook, D. A. 1976. *The Emergence of Provincial Politics: The Madras Presidency, 1870–1920*. Cambridge: Cambridge University Press.

————. 1978. "Economic development and social stratification in rural Madras." In C. J. Dewey and T. Hopkins eds. *Imperial Impact*. 68–82.

————. 1986. "Problems and progress: South Asian economic and social history c.1720–1860." Paper given to the review workshop on modern South Asian studies, Cambridge.

Whitcombe, D. 1972. *Agrarian Conditions in Northern India*. Berkeley, Los Angeles, London: University of California Press.

White, A. 1977. *British Official Aid in the Health Sector*. Discussion Paper 107. Brighton, Sussex: Institute of Development Studies.

Wilkinson, A. 1958. *A History of Nursing in India and Pakistan*. Madras: Trained Nurses Association of India.

Wise, T. A. 1845. *Commentary on the Hindu System of Medicine*. London: Smith, Elder.

Wood, G. 1978. "Bureaucracy and the Post-Colonial State in South Asia." *Development and Change* 11: 149–56.

World Bank. 1975. *Health Sector: Policy Paper*. World Bank: Washington.

World Health Organization. 1977. *The Selection of Essential Drugs*. Technical Research Series 619. Geneva.

————. 1978. *Drug Policies and Management*. New Delhi.

Worsley, P. 1980. "One World or Three." *Socialist Register* 298–338.

Wyon, J. B., and Gordon, J. E. 1971. *The Khanna Study*. Cambridge, Mass.: Harvard University Press.

Young, A. "Some Implications of Medical Beliefs and Practices for Social Anthropology." *American Anthropologist* 78, 1: 5–24.

Zimmerman, F. 1978. "From classic texts to learned practice." *Social Science and Medicine*. 12, 2B: 97–103.

Zurbrigg, S. 1984. *Bakku's Story*. Madras: George Joseph.

Series Consulted

Command papers:
    Moral and Material Progress of India
    Annual Abstract of Statistics for East India

Annual reports of the Sanitary Commissioner with the Government of India.

Quinquennial Review of the Progress of Education in India, 3rd (1891/2) to 11th (1936/7)

Indian publications:

Administration Reports for the main Indian provinces, 19th and 20th centuries, notably Punjab, United Provinces, Bombay, Bengal and Madras (referred to as *Administration Report*, Province, and date.)

Annual reports of the Inspector-General Civil Hospitals and Dispensaries, for the main Indian provinces (referred to by the province name and date).

Index

COMPARATIVE STUDIES OF HEALTH SYSTEMS
AND MEDICAL CARE

Designer: U.C. Press Staff
Compositor: Freedmen's Organization
Text: Melliza
Display: Melliza
Printer: Malloy Lithographing, Inc.
Binder: John H. Dekker & Sons